Functional Histology

Functional Histology
A TEXT AND COLOUR ATLAS

FIRST EDITION BY

Paul R. Wheater
BA Hons (York), B Med Sci Hons (Nott), BM BS (Nott)
The Queen's Medical Centre, University of Nottingham

H. George Burkitt
BDSc Hons (Queensland), FRACDS, M Med Sci (Nott), MB BChir (Cantab)
School of Clinical Medicine, University of Cambridge

Victor G. Daniels
BSc Hons (Lon), MB BChir (Cam), PhD (Sheff), Dip Pharm Med (RCP)
Medical Director, Kirby-Warrick Pharmaceuticals

SECOND EDITION REVISED BY

Paul R. Wheater

and

H. George Burkitt

Drawings by
Philip J. Deakin
BSc Hons (Sheff), MB ChB (Sheff)
General practitioner, Sheffield

CHURCHILL LIVINGSTONE
EDINBURGH LONDON MELBOURNE AND NEW YORK 1987

CHURCHILL LIVINGSTONE
Medical Division of Longman Group UK Limited

Distributed in the United States of America by
Churchill Livingstone Inc., 1560 Broadway,
New York, N.Y. 10036, and by associated
companies, branches and representatives
throughout the world.

First edition 1979
Second edition 1987
  Reprinted 1987
  Reprinted 1988 (twice)

ISBN   0-443-02341-7

British Library Cataloguing in Publication Data
Wheater, Paul R.
  Functional histology : a text and colour
  atlas.—2nd ed.
  A. Histology
  1. Title II. Burkitt, H. George III. Daniels, Victor G.
  599.08′24   QM551

Library of Congress Cataloging in Publication Data
Wheater, Paul R.
  Functional histology.

  Includes index.
  1. Histology. I. Burkitt, H. George, II. Daniels, Victor G.
  III. Title
  [DNLM: 1. Histology—atlases. QS 517 W556f]
  QM551.W47 1986   611′.018   86-17627

Produced by Longman Group (FE) Ltd
Printed in Hong Kong

Preface to the Second Edition

The response from both students and their teachers to the first edition of this book has been most gratifying and confirms our enthusiasm for the study of histology as a visual contribution to understanding the elegant workings of the body. At first publication, we were aware of certain shortcomings which needed time and further preparation to overcome, and these, along with gratefully received suggestions from readers, have been incorporated in this new edition.

Altogether, the contents have been expanded by about 25 per cent including coverage of the vestibulo-auditory apparatus and major regional variations of the central nervous system, unwisely omitted previously. Many other light and electron micrographs have been added whilst others have been improved or enlarged. The text has been updated throughout in accordance with recent developments in the biomedical sciences.

The subject matter has been expanded and rearranged from 16 to 21 chapters and subdivided into three basic sections, namely 'The Cell', 'Basic Tissue Types' and 'Organ Systems' which correlate readily with the way in which the subject is learned. Despite these additions, we hope that the emphasis continues to rest upon important principles rather than on esoteric detail, so continuing to meet the needs of the majority of readers for whom histology represents but a small part of their biological studies.

Cambridge, 1987
Paul R. Wheater
H. George Burkitt

Preface to the First Edition

Histology has bored generations of students. This is almost certainly because it has been regarded as the study of structure in isolation from function; yet few would dispute that structure and function are intimately related. Thus, the aim of this book is to present histology in relation to the principles of physiology, biochemistry and molecular biology.

Within the limits imposed by any book format, we have attempted to create the environment of the lecture room and microscope laboratory by basing the discussion of histology upon appropriate micrographs and diagrams. Consequently, colour photography has been used since it reproduces the actual images seen in light microscopy and allows a variety of common staining methods to be employed in highlighting different aspects of tissue structure. In addition, some less common techniques such as immunohistochemistry have been introduced where such methods best illustrate a particular point.

Since electron microscopy is a relatively new technique, a myth has arisen amongst many students that light and electron microscopy are poles apart. We have tried to show that electron microscopy is merely an extension of light microscopy. In order to demonstrate this continuity, we have included resin-embedded thin sections photographed around the limit of resolution of the light microscope; this technique is being applied increasingly in routine histological and histopathological practice. Where such less conventional techniques have been adopted, their rationale has been outlined at the appropriate place rather than in a formal chapter devoted to techniques.

The content and pictorial design of the book have been chosen to make it easy to use both as a textbook and as a laboratory guide. Wherever possible, the subject matter has been condensed into units of illustration plus relevant text; each unit is designed to have a degree of autonomy whilst at the same time remaining integrated into the subject as a whole. Short sections of non-illustrated text have been used by way of introduction, to outline general principles and to consider the subject matter in broader perspective.

Human tissues were mainly selected in order to maintain consistency, but when suitable human specimens were not available, primate tissues were generally substituted. Since this book stresses the understanding of principles rather than extensive detail, some tissues have been omitted deliberately, for example the regional variations of the central nervous system and the vestibulo-auditory apparatus.

This book should adequately encompass the requirements of undergraduate courses in medicine, dentistry, veterinary science, pharmacy, mammalian biology and allied fields. Further, it offers a pictorial reference for use in histology and histopathology laboratories. Finally, we envisage that the book will also find application as a teaching manual in schools and colleges of further education,

Nottingham, 1979

Paul R. Wheater
H. George Burkitt
Victor G. Daniels

Acknowledgements

With few exceptions, each of the illustrations was specially prepared for the book. Whilst accepting full responsibility for the contents, the authors are indebted to many individuals who have made invaluable contributions in their specialised fields.

Most of the tissue preparation and photomicrography for the original edition was performed in the Departments of Pathology and Human Morphology of Queen's Medical Centre, University of Nottingham, and the authors are thus extremely grateful for the generous co-operation of Professors I.M.P. Dawson and R.E. Coupland. Special thanks are due to Janet Palmer of the Department of Pathology who gave tireless assistance in the preparation of many of the tissues for light microscopy which were used in this book and many more preparations for which space was not available. Similarly, our thanks are conveyed to Paul Beck of the Department of Human Morphology for producing a large number of valuable specimens. Many of the electron micrographs were made available by John Kugler and Annette Tomlinson, also of the Department of Human Morphology; to both we are deeply indebted and hope that in this edition we have done greater justice to their work, having ironed out various technical problems in reproduction of the material.

Other people freely made available their resources: Peter Crosby of the Department of Biology, University of York, provided most of the scanning electron micrographs, and his colleague Brian Norman provided several light microscopic sections; Dr Robert Lang, also of York University, produced the freeze-etched preparation used in Figure 1.8, whilst Dr I.A.R. More, Department of Pathology, Western Infirmary, Glasgow, provided the example of peroxisomes used in Figure 1.5; the superb otolith specimen used in Figure 21.27(c) was lent courtesy of Mr Roger Gray, FRCS, Addenbrooke's Hospital, Cambridge and Professor N. Dilly, St. George's Hospital, Tooting; Donald Canwell of the Physiological Laboratory, University of Cambridge contributed many sections from his personal collection, several of which enhance this new edition; Dr Graham Robinson and Stan Terras of the Department of Pathology, University of Nottingham, each provided several electron micrographs, and they and their colleague Linda Burns, provided all of the thin resin sections used for light microscopy; Drs David Tomlinson and Terry Bennett of the Department of Physiology, University of Nottingham contributed Figures 7.11 and 7.12 respectively; Dr Pat Cooke of the Department of Genetics, City Hospital, Nottingham lent the chromosome preparation used in Figure 2.2; Dr David Ansell of the Department of Pathology, City Hospital, Nottingham, Dr Hugh Rice and Dr Peter James of the Department of Pathology, Nottingham General Hospital and Dr Pauline Cooper of the Department of Pathology, Addenbrooke's Hospital, Cambridge made available various tissue specimens and slides. Peter Squires and Hugh Pulsford of Huntingdon Research Centre, Cambridgeshire were a great source in providing the primate tissues used when suitable human tissues were unavailable. To all of these kind and co-operative people we express our sincere thanks.

Bill Brackenbury of the Department of Pathology, University of Nottingham, very skilfully performed much of the macrophotography and Leonard Beard of the Department of Medical Illustration, Hinchingbrooke Hospital, Huntingdon, photographed the two difficult thin sections in black and white. All of the remaining colour photomicrography was performed by one of the authors (P.R.W.), many of the new additions being photographed on a Leitz Vario-Orthomat photomicroscope. The onerous task of typing the manuscript was carried out with skill and great patience by Christine Stevens and Jane Richards.

The authors express their warmest thanks to Dr Alan Stevens of the Department of Pathology, University of Nottingham, who performed the role of scientific editor with seemingly limitless dedication, insight and enthusiasm.

Contents

Part One: The Cell

1. Cell structure and function   2
2. Cell cycle and replication   28

Part Two: Basic Tissue Types

3 Blood   36
4. Connective tissue   52
5. Epithelial tissues   64
6. Muscle   79
7. Nervous tissues   95

Part Three: Organ Systems

8. Circulatory system   118
9. Skin   130
10. Skeletal tissues   142
11. Immune system   161
12. Respiratory system   178
13. Oral tissues   191
14. Gastrointestinal tract   203
15. Liver and pancreas   225
16. Urinary system   236
17. The endocrine glands   258
18. Male reproductive system   277
19. Female reproductive system   289
20. Central nervous system   308
21. Special sense organs   316
Notes on staining methods   342

Index   343

PART ONE

The cell

1. Cell structure and function
2. Cell cycle and replication

1. Cell structure and function

Introduction

The cell, the functional unit of all tissues, has the capacity to perform individually all the essential life functions. Within the various tissues of the body, the constituent cells exhibit a wide range of specialisations which are, nevertheless, merely amplifications of one or more of the fundamental cellular processes. Reflecting their particular functional specialisations, mammalian cells have an extraordinary range of morphological forms yet all cells conform to a basic model of cell structure.

Even with primitive light microscopy, it was evident that cells are divided into at least two components, the *nucleus* and the *cytoplasm*, and as microscopical techniques advanced it became increasingly obvious that both the cytoplasm and the nucleus contain a number of subcellular elements which are called *organelles*.

The resolving power of the light microscope is limited to about 0.25 μm (250 nm) and the study of the ultrastructure of the cell had to await the advent of electron microscopy (EM). The capacity of electron microscopes in current use permits the resolution of structures as small as 3.0 nm (30 ångström units); however, this falls far short of many cellular processes which occur at the molecular level and which require biochemical methods of study. Nevertheless, in recent years, light and electron microscopy have been successfully combined with biochemical and immunological techniques to define the location of many biological processes; these techniques are known as *histochemistry* and *immunohistochemistry* respectively.

Fig. 1.1 The cell *(illustration opposite)*

(EM × 15 000)

The basic structural features common to all cells are illustrated in this electron micrograph of a hormone-secreting cell from the pituitary gland. All the cells are bounded by an external limiting membrane called the *plasma membrane* or *plasmalemma* **PM** which serves as a dynamic interface between the internal environment of the cell and its various external environments. In this particular example, the cell interacts with two types of external environment: adjacent cells **C** and intercellular spaces **IS**.

The nucleus **N** is the largest organelle and its substance, often referred to as the *nucleoplasm*, is bounded by a membrane system called the *nuclear envelope* **NE**. The cytoplasm contains a variety of organelles most of which are also bounded by membranes. A diffuse system of membrane-bound tubules, saccules and flattened cisterns, collectively known as the *endoplasmic reticulum* **ER**, pervades the cytoplasm. A more distended system of membrane-bound saccules, the *Golgi apparatus* **G**, is usually found close to the nucleus. Scattered free in the cytoplasm are a number of relatively large, elongated organelles called *mitochondria*

M which have a smooth outer membrane and a convoluted inner membrane system. In addition to these major organelles, the cell contains a variety of other membrane-bound structures, an example of which are the numerous, electron-dense *secretory vacuoles* **V** seen in this micrograph. Thus the cell is divided into a number of membrane-bound compartments each of which has its own particular biochemical environment.

Membranes therefore serve to isolate incompatible processes as well as being the site of many specific biochemical reactions. The cytoplasmic organelles are suspended in a fluid medium called the *cytosol* in which much of the intermediary metabolism of the cell takes place. Within the cytosol, there is a network of minute tubules and filaments collectively known as the *cytoskeleton* which provides structural support for the cell and its internal organelles as well as providing a mechanism for cellular and intracellular movement; elements of the cytoskeleton are only visible with very high magnification.

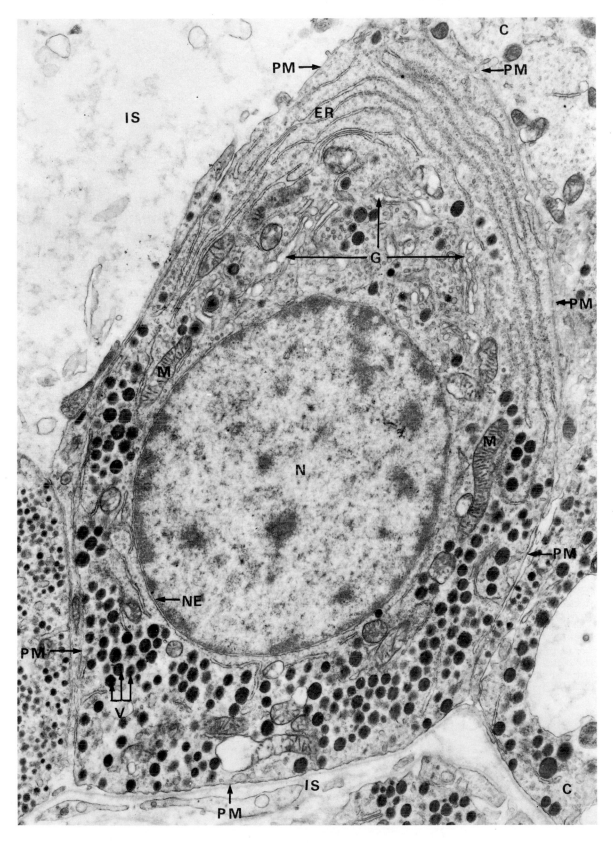

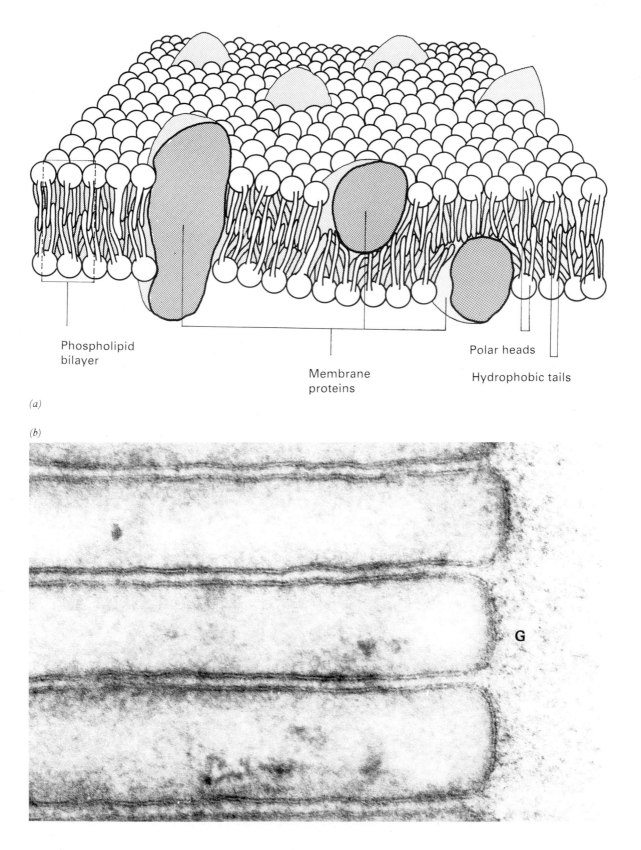

Phospholipid
bilayer

Membrane
proteins

Polar heads

Hydrophobic tails

(a)

(b)

G

Fig. 1.2 Membrane structure *(illustrations opposite)*

(a) Schematic diagram (b) EM × 300 000

Despite intensive investigation, the structure of cell membranes is sill not known with certainty; however, a theoretical model has been progressively developed which satisfactorily incorporates much of the currently available biochemical and histological evidence.

Towards the end of the last century, it was observed that lipids rapidly gain entry into cells, and it was postulated that the 'cell boundary' was composed of lipid. In the 1920s it was found that, by measuring the minimum area that could be occupied by a monolayer of lipids extracted from a defined number of red blood cells, there was enough lipid present in the monolayer to cover each cell twice. From this it was concluded that the cells were bounded by a double layer of lipid. Later, it was proposed that cell membranes are symmetrical structures consisting of a bilayer of phospholipid molecules sandwiched between two layers of protein. This model, however, failed to explain the selective permeability of most cell membranes to molecules which are not lipid-soluble such as glucose, sodium ions and potassium ions. These difficulties were theoretically overcome by postulating the existence of 'pores' composed of protein through which hydrophilic molecules could readily be transported by passive or active mechanisms.

Electron microscopic studies in the late 1950s revealed that all membranes have a three layered (trilaminate) structure and this led to the concept of the *'unit membrane'* in which it was proposed that all cell membranes have an identical structure.

The current concepts of membrane structure are shown diagramatically opposite. In this model, cell membranes consist basically of phospholipid molecules arranged as a bilayer. Phospholipid molecules are amphipathic, i.e. they consist of a polar, hydrophobic (water-hating) tail. The polar heads are mainly derived from glycerol conjugated to a nitrogenous compound such as choline, ethanolamine or serine via a phosphate bridge. The phosphate group is negatively charged whereas the nitrogenous group is positively charged. The non-polar tail of the phospholipid molecule consists of two long-chain fatty acids each covalently linked to the glycerol component of the polar head. In most mammalian cell membranes, one of the fatty acids is a straight-chain structural fatty acid whilst the other is an unsaturated fatty acid which is kinked at the position of the unsaturated bond. Because of their amphipathic nature, phospholipids in aqueous solution will spontaneously form a bilayer with the hydrophilic (polar) heads directed outwards and the hydrophobic tails forced together inwards. The weak intermolecular forces which hold the bilayer together allow individual phospholipid molecules to move relatively freely within each layer and sometimes between each layer. The fluidity and flexibility of the membrane is increased by the presence of unsaturated fatty acids which prevent close packing of the hydrophobic tails. Cholesterol molecules are present in the bilayer in an almost one-to-one ratio with phospholipids. Cholesterol molecules themselves are amphipathic and have a kinked conformation thus preventing too close packing of the phospholipid fatty acid tails whilst at the same time filling the gaps between the 'kinks' of the unsaturated fatty acid tails. Cholesterol molecules thus regulate the fluidity and stabilise the phospholipid bilayer.

Within the bilayer are scattered a variety of protein molecules some of them extending through the entire thickness of the membrane to be exposed to each surface; these transmembrane molecules may function as 'pores' through which hydrophilic molecules are transported either actively or passively. These proteins, and others which do not span the whole width of the membrane, are also freely mobile within the plane of the phospholipid bilayer. Whilst the lipid component of the membrane principally determines its mechanical properties, the dynamic functions of the membrane as an interface between biological compartments is a function of the membrane proteins. The model just described is known as the *fluid mosaic model* of membrane structure.

On the external surface of the plasma membranes of animal cells, many of the membrane proteins and some of the membrane lipids are conjugated with short chains of polysaccharide; these glycoproteins and glycolipids project from the surface of the bilayer forming an outer coating which may be analogous to the cell walls of plants, bacteria and fungi. This polysaccharide layer has been termed the *glycocalyx* and appears to vary in thickness in different cell types; whether an analogous layer exists on all membranes or only at the external surface is unknown. The function of the glycocalyx is obscure, but there is evidence that it may be involved in cell recognition phenomena, in the formation of intercellular adhesions, and in the adsorption of molecules to the cell surface. Alternatively, the glycocalyx may simply provide mechanical and chemical protection for the plasma membrane.

The electron micrograph in (b) provides a high magnification view of a plasma membrane; this example illustrates the minute surface projections (microvilli) of a lining cell from the small intestine. All membranes have a characteristic trilaminate appearance comprising two electron-dense layers separated by an electron-lucent layer. The outer dense layers are thought to correspond to the hydrophilic 'heads' of phospholipid molecules whilst the electron-lucent layer is thought to represent the intermediate hydrophobic layer mainly consisting of fatty acids. On the external surface of the plasma membrane an outer fibrillar coat, called the *'fuzzy coat'*, represents the glycocalyx **G**. This is an unusually prominent feature of small intestinal lining cells.

Transport across plasma membranes

Plasma membranes mediate the continuous exchange of molecules between the internal and external environments of the cell in four principal ways. These mechanisms enable the cell to control the quality of its internal environment with a high degree of specificity.

1. Passive diffusion: this type of transport is entirely dependent on the presence of a concentration gradient across the plasma membrane. Lipids and lipid-soluble metabolites such as ethanol pass freely through plasma membranes; plasma membranes also offer little barrier to the diffusion of gases such as oxygen and carbon dioxide. The plasma membrane is, in general, impermeable to hydrophilic molecules; nevertheless some small molecules including water and urea, and inorganic ions such as bicarbonate, are able to pass down osmotic or electrochemical gradients through the membrane via hydrophilic regions, the nature of which remains obscure.

2. Facilitated diffusion: this type of transport is also concentration-dependent and involves the transport of larger hydrophilic metabolites such as glucose and amino-acids. The process is strictly passive but requires the presence of so-called 'carriers' to which the metabolites bind specifically but reversibly in a manner analogous to the binding of substrate with enzyme.

3. Active transport: this mode of transport is not only independent of concentration gradients but also often operates against extreme concentration gradients. The classical example of this form of transport is the continuous transport of sodium out of the cell by the so-called 'sodium pump'; this process requires the expenditure of energy provided in the form of ATP. It is postulated that this form of transport occurs through 'dynamic pores' consisting of proteins or protein systems which span the plasma membrane. Both active and passive transport processes are enhanced by increasing the area of the plasma membrane by folds or projections of the cell surface as exemplified by the absorptive cells lining the small intestine (see Fig. 1.2).

4. Bulk transport: bulk transport involves engulfment of large molecules or small particles by cytoplasmic extensions, thus forming membrane-bound vacuoles within the cytoplasm. When this process involves the creation of small vacuoles it is known as *pinocytosis*, and when large vacuoles are formed it is called *phagocytosis*. The term *endocytosis*, encompassing both processes, is probably a more appropriate term for bulk transport into the cell. Endocytotic vesicles either discharge their contents directly into the cytoplasm or fuse with membrane-bound organelles called *lysosomes*; lysosomes contain more than 40 different enzymes which are capable of degrading carbohydrates, lipids, proteins, nucleic acids and other organic molecules. Lysosomal enzymes digest engulfed material which is then made available for metabolic processes. In many secretory processes, bulk transport also occurs in the opposite direction when it is termed *exocytosis*.

Histologically, the passive and active processes of transport can only be observed indirectly; for example, cells suspended in hypotonic solutions swell due to passive uptake of water whereas cells placed in hypertonic solutions tend to shrink due to outflow of water. Radio-isotope labelling techniques can be used to follow active transport processes. Bulk transport, however, is readily observable by microscopy.

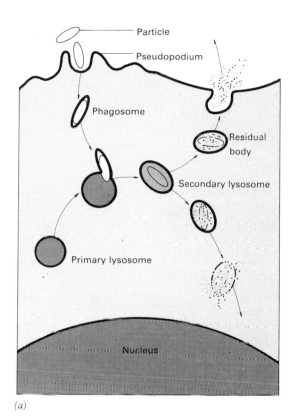

(a)

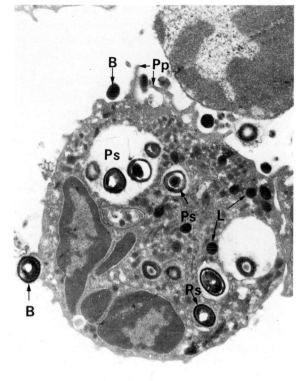

(b)

Fig. 1.3 Endocytosis

(a) Schematic diagram (b) EM × 11 750

This diagram summarises the main steps in endocytosis of particulate matter. The first stage of phagocytosis involves recognition of a particle; this then becomes surrounded by cytoplasmic extensions called *pseudopodia*. When the particle is completely surrounded, the plasma membrane fuses and the membrane surrounding the engulfed particle forms a vesicle, known as a *phagosome* or *endocytotic vesicle*, which detaches from the plasma membrane to float freely within the cytoplasm. The phagosome is then in some way recognised by one or more *primary lysosomes* which fuse with the phagosome to form a *secondary lysosome*. This exposes the engulfed material to a battery of lysosomal enzymes. When digestion is complete, the lysosomal membrane may rupture, discharging its contents into the cytoplasm. Undigested material may remain within membrane-bound vesicles called *residual bodies*, the contents of which may be discharged at the cell surface by exocytosis; alternatively

residual bodies may accumulate in the cytoplasm.

Lysosomes are also involved in the degradation of cellular organelles, many of which have only a finite lifespan and are therefore replaced continuously; this lysosomal function is termed *autophagy*. Most autophagocytic degradation products are re-utilised by the cell but some indigestible products accumulate and become indistinguishable from the residual bodies of endocytosis. With advancing age, residual bodies accumulate in the cells of some tissues and appear as brown so-called *lipofuscin granules*.

Micrograph (b) illustrates a highly phagocytic white blood cell, a neutrophil, in the process of engulfing and destroying bacteria **B**. Note the manner in which pseudopodia **Pp** embrace the bacteria before engulfment. Note also phagosomes **Ps** containing bacteria in various stages of degradation. Several primary lysosomes **L** are also visible.

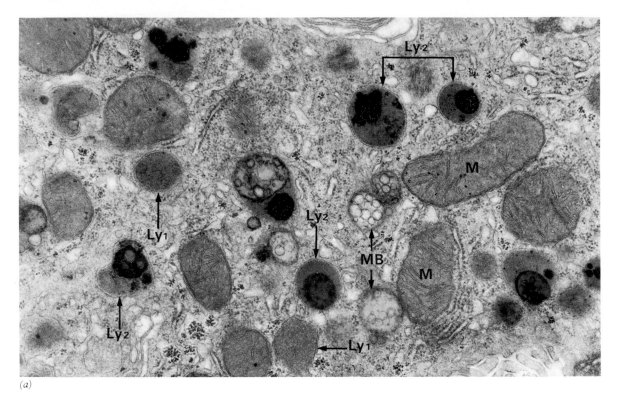

(a)

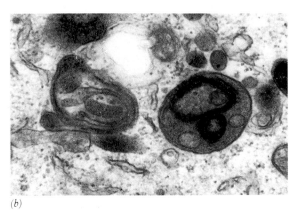

(b)

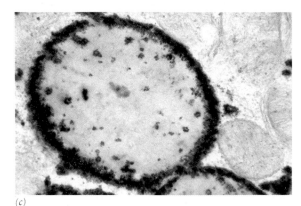

(c)

Fig. 1.4 Lysosomes

(a) EM × 27 000 (b) Residual bodies: EM × 50 000
(c) Histochemical method for acid phosphatase: EM × 30 000

These micrographs show the typical features of lysosomes and
residual bodies. Micrograph (a) shows part of the cytoplasm
of a liver cell. Primary lysosomes Ly_1 vary greatly in size
and appearance but they are recognised as membrane-bound
organelles containing a granular, amorphous material.
Secondary lysosomes Ly_2 are even more variable in
appearance but are recognisable by their diverse particulate
content some of which is extremely electron-dense. The
distinction between residual bodies and secondary lysosomes
is often difficult but one distinctive type of residual body,
the so-called *multivesicular body* **MB**, is seen in this
micrograph. Multivesicular bodies are membrane-bound
vesicles containing a number of smaller vesicles which are
thought to represent the debris of cell membrane
degradation. Note the size of lysosomes relative to
mitochondria **M.**

Micrograph (b) shows two residual bodies also from a
liver cell; both contain particulate material and small
fragments of membrane.

The lysosomal enzymes comprise more than 40 different
acid hydrolases which are optimally active at a pH of about
5.0. This may be a protective mechanism for the cell should
lysosomal enzymes escape into the cytosol where they would
be much less active at the higher pH.

Histochemical methods can be used to demonstrate sites
of enzyme activity within cells and thus act as markers for
organelles which contain these enzymes. Such a method has
been used in micrograph (c) to demonstrate the presence of
acid phosphatase, a typical lysosomal enzyme; the enzyme
activity is represented by a very dense deposit in the
lysosome.

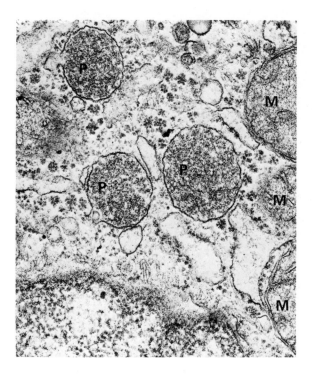

Fig. 1.5 Peroxisomes

(EM × 70 000)

Peroxisomes are small, spherical, membrane-bound organelles, also known as *microbodies*, which closely resemble lysosomes in electron microscopic appearance. They are, however, distinguished from lysosomes by their content of an entirely different set of enzymes which can be demonstrated by histochemical techniques. Peroxisomes contain at least three oxidases, namely, D-amino acid oxidase, urate oxidase and catalase. The first two enzymes catalyse various catabolic oxidative reactions which utilise molecular oxygen and produce hydrogen peroxide as a by-product; catalase then utilises the hydrogen peroxide in the oxidation of a variety of potentially toxic metabolites including phenols, alcohol and fatty acids.

Large peroxisomes are a feature of liver and kidney and, in some species, contain a central crystalloid structure.

In this micrograph, note the fine granular contents of several peroxisomes **P** the size of which can be compared with that of adjacent mitochondria **M**.

Protein synthesis

Proteins are not only a major structural component of cells but, in the form of enzymes, mediate every metabolic process within the cell. Thus the nature and quantity of proteins present within any individual cell determines the activity of that cell. Both the structural proteins and enzymes of the cell are subject to wear and tear and are replaced continuously. Many cells also synthesise proteins for export; such proteins include glandular secretions and extracellular structural components of tissues. Protein synthesis is, therefore, an essential and continuous activity of all cells and the major function of some cells.

The principal organelles involved in protein synthesis are the *nucleus* and *ribosomes*. The nucleus of every cell contains within its complement of DNA a template for each protein that can be made by that individual as a whole. However, most cells only synthesise a certain defined range of proteins which are characteristic of the particular cell type and therefore only part of the DNA template is utilised. The process of protein synthesis involves *transcription* of the DNA code for a particular protein by synthesis of the specific, complementary messenger RNA (mRNA) molecule. The mRNA molecule then enters the cytoplasm to associate with ribosomes upon which protein synthesis occurs; the amino acid sequence of the resulting protein is determined by *translation* of the mRNA code.

Ribosomes are minute cytoplasmic organelles, each composed of two subunits of unequal size. Each subunit consists of a strand of RNA (ribosomal RNA) with associated ribosomal proteins; the ribosomal RNA strand and associated proteins are folded to form a condensed, globular structure. Ribosomes are highly active structures with specific receptor proteins which align mRNA strands so that transfer RNA (tRNA) molecules carrying the appropriate amino acids may be brought into position prior to the addition of their amino acids to the growing polypeptide chain. Other ribosomal proteins are involved in catalysing peptide bond formation between amino acids. Individual ribosomes are too small to be clearly resolved by electron microscopy although they are visible as small electron-dense masses at high magnification; nevertheless, the detail of ribosome structure and function are well established at the molecular level. Ribosomes are seen lying free in the cytoplasm either alone or attached to messenger RNA molecules in small aggregations called *polyribosomes* or *polysomes*. Ribosomes and polyribosomes also may be attached to the surface of the extensive intracytoplasmic membrane system known as the endoplasmic reticulum (see Fig. 1.9).

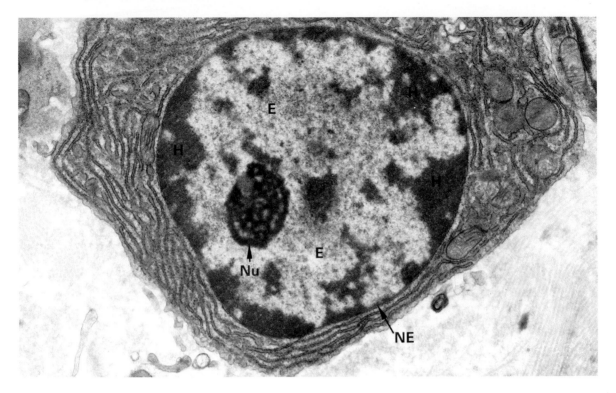

Fig. 1.6 Nucleus

(EM × 15 400)

This micrograph illustrates the typical nucleus of a highly active, protein-secreting cell. The nuclear envelope **NE**, separating the nuclear contents from the cytoplasm, is barely visible at this magnification.

The nucleus not only contains DNA, which comprises less than 20% of its mass, but also contains a large quantity of protein called *nucleoprotein*, and some RNA. Most of the nucleoprotein is closely associated with DNA; these DNA-binding proteins are of two major types, *histones* and *non-histones*. Histones, which comprise the bulk of DNA-associated protein, are relatively low molecular weight proteins with a high content of positively charged amino acids which bind them readily to the negatively charged DNA strands. Histones may be involved in the folding of DNA strands and the regulation of DNA activity. The non-histone DNA-associated proteins are a heterogeneous group which may also be involved in the regulation of gene activity. The remaining nucleoproteins include enzymes responsible for DNA and RNA synthesis. All nucleoproteins are synthesised in the cytoplasm and imported into the nucleus. The nuclear RNA represents newly synthesised messenger, transfer and ribosomal RNA which has not yet passed into the cytoplasm.

Except during cell division, the chromosomes, each comprising a discrete length of the DNA complement, exist as tangled strands which extend throughout the nucleus and cannot be visualised individually by direct electron microscopy. Nuclei appear as heterogeneous structures with electron-dense and electron-lucent areas. The dense areas, called *heterochromatin*, represent that portion of the DNA complement and its associated nucleoprotein which is not active in RNA synthesis. Heterochromatin **H** tends to be clumped around the periphery of the nucleus but also forms irregular clumps throughout the nucleus. In females, the quiescent X-chromosome (equivalent to the Y-chromosome of the male) forms a small discrete mass known as a *Barr body*; Barr bodies are seen at the edge of the nucleus in a small proportion of female cells when cut in a favourable plane of section. The electron-lucent nuclear material, called *euchromatin* **E**, represents that part of the DNA which is active in RNA synthesis. Collectively, heterochromatin and euchromatin are known as *chromatin*, a name derived from the strongly coloured appearance of nuclei when stained for light microscopy.

Many nuclei, especially those of cells highly active in protein synthesis, contain one or more extremely dense structures called nucleoli **Nu** which are the sites of ribosomal RNA synthesis and ribosome assembly. The many different ribosomal proteins are imported from the cytoplasm and conjugated with ribosomal RNA to form the different ribosomal subunits which then pass into the cytoplasm before being assembled into fully active ribosomes. Nucleoli are heterogeneous structures, the paler areas being the sites of DNA coding for ribosomal RNA and the dark areas being the sites of partially assembled ribosomes.

Each cell type has a characteristic nuclear morphology and, in general, the degree of activity of any cell may be judged by the ultrastructural appearance of its nucleus. Relatively inactive cells have small nuclei in which the chromatin is predominantly in the condensed form (heterchromatin) and in which the nucleolus is small or absent, whereas in highly active cells, the nuclear material is dispersed (euchromatin) and nucleoli are a prominent feature.

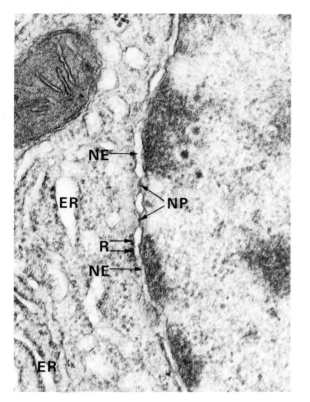

Fig. 1.7 Nuclear envelope

(EM × 67 500)

The nuclear envelope **NE** which encloses the nucleus consists of two layers of membrane which represent a specialised part of the endoplasmic reticulum. The intermembranous space is continuous with that of the endoplasmic reticulum **ER** and like the endoplasmic reticulum, the outer surface of the nuclear envelope is studded with ribosomes **R**. On the inner aspect of the nuclear envelope there is an electron-dense layer, the *nuclear lamina*, consisting of polypeptides bound to membrane proteins and linked with underlying chromatin.

The nuclear envelope contains numerous *nuclear pores* **NP** at the margins of which the inner and outer membranes become continuous. Each pore contains an electron-dense structure known as a *pore complex* which consists of a ring of proteins with a central channel, the whole complex being stabilised by the nuclear lamina. Experimental evidence suggests that nuclear pores permit and regulate the exchange of metabolites, macromolecules and ribosomal subunits between nucleus and cytoplasm.

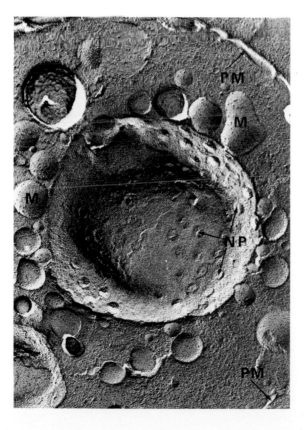

Fig. 1.8 Nuclear pores

(Freeze-etched preparation × 34 000)

This micrograph shows an example of a technique called *freeze-etching*. Briefly, this method involves the rapid cooling of cells to subzero temperatures; the frozen cells are then fractured. This exposes internal surfaces of the cell in a somewhat random manner although the fracture lines tend to follow natural planes of weakness. Further surface detail is obtained by 'etching' or subliming excess water molecules from the specimen at low temperature. A thin carbon impression is then made of the surface and this mirror image is viewed by conventional electron microscopy. Freeze-etching provides a valuable tool for studying internal cell surfaces at high resolution.

In this preparation, the plane of cleavage has included part of the nuclear envelope and nuclear pores **NP** are clearly demonstrated. Note also the outline of the plasma membrane **PM** and mitochondria **M**.

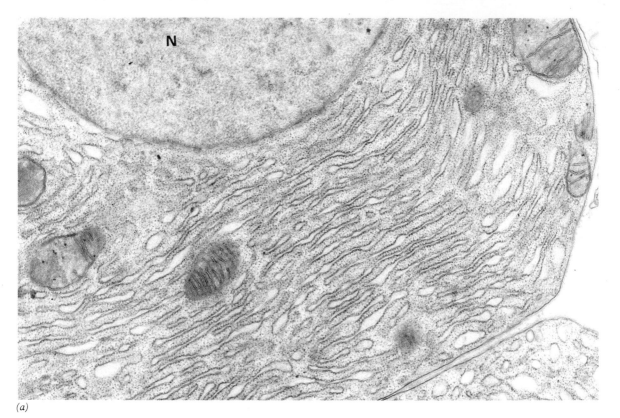

(a)

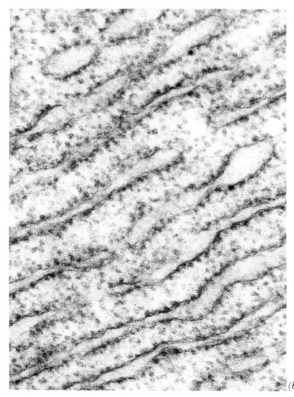

(b)

Fig. 1.9 Rough endoplasmic reticulum
(EM (a) × 25 000 (b) × 100 000)

As previously described, the endoplasmic reticulum consists of an anastomosing network of tubules, vesicles and flattened cisternae which ramifies throughout the cytoplasm. Much of the surface of the endoplasmic reticulum is studded with ribosomes giving the reticulum a rough or granular appearance; such endoplasmic reticulum is therefore called *rough* or *granular endoplasmic reticulum* (rER or gER).

These micrographs illustrate rough endoplasmic reticulum in a cell which is specialised for the synthesis and secretion of protein; in such cells rough endoplasmic reticulum tends to be profuse and to form closely packed parallel laminae of flattened cisternae. Proteins are synthesised on the ribosomes of the external surface of rough endoplasmic reticulum and some are then passed into the reticular lumen for distribution to other intracellular sites or for secretion later.

Micrograph (a) illustrates rough endoplasmic reticulum in a cell which is specialised for the synthesis and secretion of proteins. The cytoplasm is closely packed with parallel laminae of cisternae, and the chromatin in the nucleus **N** is dispersed (euchromatin) consistent with this great biosynthetic activity.

Micrograph (b) shows rough endoplasmic reticulum at high magnification. Numerous ribosomes stud the surface of the membrane system and numerous other ribosomes lie free in the intervening cytosol.

Lipid biosynthesis

Lipids are synthesised by all cells in order to repair and replace damaged or worn membranes. Many cells also synthesise lipid as a means of storing excess energy; in such cells lipid is stored as cytoplasmic droplets. The synthesis of all classes of lipid is based on the precursor molecules fatty acids, triglycerides and cholesterol. These precursors are available to the cell from dietary sources or as a result of mobilisation of lipid stored in other cells. Fatty acids, triglycerides and cholesterol, however, can be synthesised by most cells using simple sources of carbon such as acetyl-CoA and other intermediates of glucose catabolism. Fatty acids and triglycerides are mostly synthesised within the cytosol, whereas cholesterol and phospholipids are synthesised in areas of endoplasmic reticulum devoid of ribosomes called *smooth endoplasmic reticulum* (sER). Cells which are highly active in lipid biosynthesis, such as liver cells, tend to have well developed networks of smooth ER.

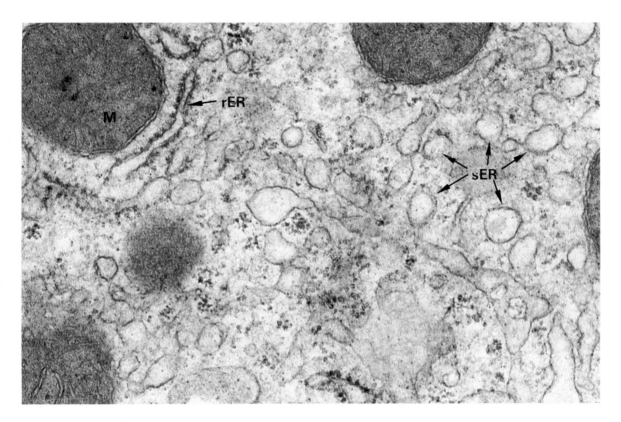

Fig. 1.10 Smooth endoplasmic reticulum

(EM × 100 000)

Smooth endoplasmic reticulum (sER) consists of an irregular network of membranous tubules and vesicles devoid of ribosomes in contrast to the flattened ribosome-studded cisternae of rough endoplasmic reticulum. It forms part of the intracellular membrane system being continuous with the rough endoplasmic reticulum and Golgi apparatus (see Fig. 1.11). The principal functions of smooth endoplasmic reticulum are lipid biosynthesis and intracellular transport; in liver cells, smooth endoplasmic reticulum also plays a major role in the detoxification of various noxious metabolic by-products and drugs. One particular enzyme, cytochrome P450, is present in large amounts in the smooth endoplasmic reticulum of liver; this enzyme hydroxylates water-insoluble

hydrocarbons which become dissolved in the lipid bilayer of the membranous vesicles.

In general, most cells do not have a prominent system of smooth endoplasmic reticulum but rather, scattered elements can be seen amongst the other organelles. The notable exceptions are those cells specialised for lipid biosynthesis such as the steroid hormone-secreting cells of the adrenal glands and the gonads, and the liver. In this micrograph from the liver, most of the membranous elements form part of the smooth endoplasmic reticulum **sER**; however, a small fragment of rough endoplasmic reticulum **rER** is present near a mitochondrion **M**.

Secretion

The export from cells of materials, which may be excretory waste products or secretory products, involves the four principal mechanisms outlined earlier for the transport of materials into cells. Excretion or secretion of small molecular weight compounds or lipid-soluble materials rarely involves bulk transport, whereas secretion of proteins and protein complexes almost exclusively involves bulk transport. Prior to release from the cell, proteins and other secretory products are packaged within membrane-bound vesicles which then fuse with the surface plasma membrane thus releasing their contents by the process of exocytosis. The Golgi apparatus (also called *Golgi body* or *Golgi complex*) is the organelle primarily responsible for the packaging process.

During the secretory process, large amounts of intracellular membrane become incorporated into the plasma membrane and the Golgi system recycles excess plasma membrane, returning it to an internal 'pool' of membrane. Recent studies have shown that the Golgi apparatus elaborates new membrane necessary for cell growth and formation of membrane-bound organelles such as lysosomes, as well as replacing membrane lost or damaged during normal metabolic activities.

Fig. 1.11 Golgi apparatus *(illustrations opposite)*

(a) Schematic diagram (b) EM × 50 000

The diagram illustrates the main structural features of the Golgi apparatus and summarises the probable mechanism by which secretory products are packaged within membrane-bound vesicles. The Golgi apparatus consists of a stacked system of saucer-shaped cisternae, with the concave surface facing the nucleus. Proteins, synthesised on ribosomes of the rough ER, are transported within the endoplasmic reticulum to the region of the Golgi apparatus. Membrane-bound vesicles containing protein, known as *transitional vesicles*, bud off from the endoplasmic reticulum and then coalesce with the convex surface of the Golgi apparatus, an area of the Golgi apparatus known as the *forming face*. By a mechanism still unresolved, secretory product is passed towards the concave surface, the *maturing face,* where new vesicles containing secretory product are formed. Some proteinaceous secretion products consist of protein-carbohydrate complexes; it is known that the carbohydrate component is added during passage through the Golgi apparatus. After release from the maturing face, the contents of *secretory vesicles* become condensed to form mature secretory vesicles, often termed *secretory granules,* which are then liberated at the cell surface by exocytosis.

The Golgi apparatus is a dynamically changing structure, the appearance of which varies enormously according to the functional state of the cell; for this reason the 'classical' appearance of the Golgi apparatus is, in practice, rarely seen, Moreover, a cell may contain from one to more than 100 Golgi stacks.

The micrograph illustrates a particularly well developed Golgi apparatus; transitional vesicles **T** and elements of the rough endoplasmic reticulum **rER** are seen adjacent to the forming face. A variety of larger vesicles **V** can be seen in the concavity of the maturing face, some of which appear to be budding from the Golgi cisternae **C**. A large number of intermediate vesicles can be seen close to the periphery of the cisternal stack.

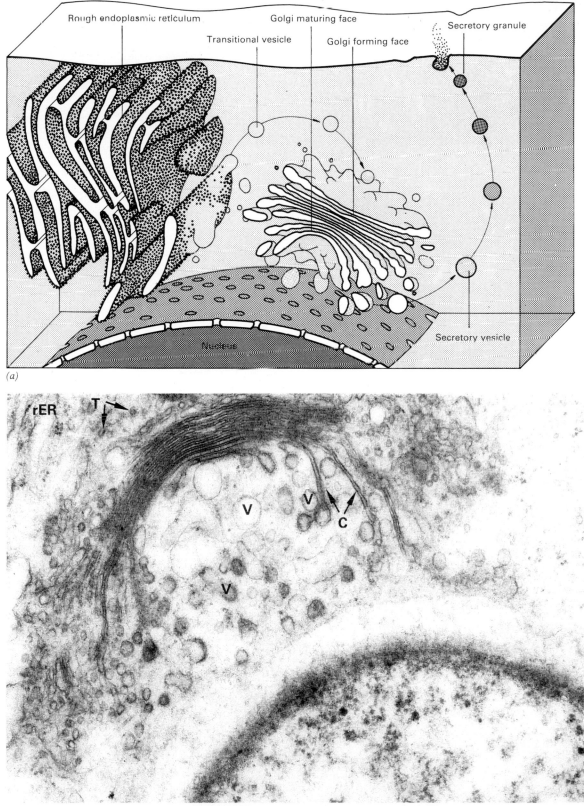

(a)

(b)

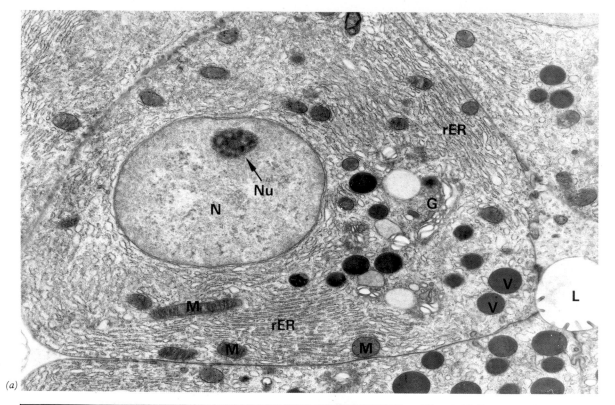

(a)

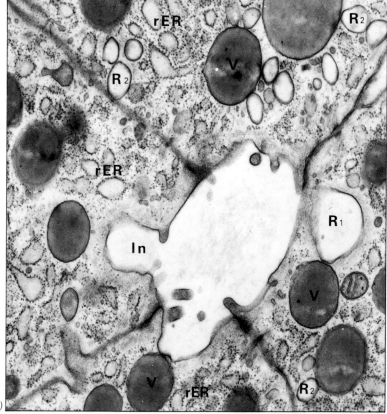

(b)

Fig. 1.12 Exocytosis

(EM (a) × 14 000 (b) × 30 000)

Micrograph (a) illustrates a typical protein-secreting cell; this example is from the pancreatic gland which produces a secretion rich in digestive enzymes. In the nucleus **N,** the chromatin is dispersed, and there is a prominent nucleolus **Nu,** both features indicative of intense RNA synthesis. The cytoplasm is packed with rough endoplasmic reticulum **rER** and there is a prominent Golgi apparatus **G.** Mitochondria **M** are scattered amongst the rough endoplasmic reticulum. Secretory vesicles **V** become increasingly electron-dense as they are concentrated towards the glandular lumen **L.**

Micrograph (b) shows the apical regions of four secretory cells converging on a tiny central excretory duct. Large, membrane-bound secretory vesicles **V** are seen approaching the lumen, one of which appears to be fusing with the surface plasma membrane. A deep invagination **In** in one of the plasma membranes probably represents a secretory vesicle which has just discharged its contents. A large vesicle R_1, and numerous smaller, apparently empty vesicles R_2 may represent vesicle membrane in the process of being recycled.

Energy production and storage

All cellular functions are dependent on a continuous supply of energy. Energy is derived from the sequential breakdown of organic molecules during the process of *cellular respiration*; the energy released from the breakage of chemical bonds during this process is ultimately stored in the form of ATP molecules. In actively respiring cells, ATP forms a pool of readily available energy for all the metabolic functions of the cell. The main substrates for cellular respiration are simple sugars and lipids, particularly glucose and fatty acids. Cellular respiration of glucose begins in the cytosol where it is partially degraded to form pyruvic acid by the process known as glycolysis, which yields a small amount of ATP. Pyruvic acid then diffuses into specialised organelles called *mitochondria* where, in the presence of oxygen, it is degraded to carbon dioxide and water in a process which yields a large quantity of ATP. In contrast, fatty acids pass directly into mitochondria where they are also degraded to carbon dioxide and water; this process also yields a large amount of ATP. Glycolysis may occur in the absence of oxygen and is therefore termed anaerobic respiration, whereas mitochondrial respiration is dependent on a continuous supply of oxygen and is therefore termed aerobic respiration. Mitochondria are the principal organelles involved in cellular respiration in mammals and are found in large numbers in metabolically active cells such as in the liver and skeletal muscle.

Under favourable nutritional conditions, most cells generate and store excess glucose and fatty acids in the relatively insoluble and non-toxic forms glycogen and triglyceride respectively. Cells vary greatly in their content of stored carbohydrate and lipid; extreme examples are nerve cells which contain almost no intracellular glycogen or triglyceride, and fat cells, the cytoplasm of which is almost entirely filled with stored lipid.

Fig. 1.13 Mitochondrion

Mitochondria vary enormously in size and shape but are most often elongated, cigar-shaped organelles. They are motile organelles and tend to localise at intracellular sites of maximum energy requirement. The number of mitochondria in cells is highly variable; liver cells each contain as many as 2000 mitochondria whereas inactive cells contain very few.

Each mitochondrion consists of two layers of membrane; the outer membrane is relatively permeable and contains enzymes that convert certain lipid substrates into forms that can be metabolised within the mitochondrion. The inner membrane is thrown into folds called *cristae* projecting into the inner cavity which is filled with an amorphous substance called *matrix*. The matrix contains a number of dense *matrix granules*, the nature and function of which are unclear. The inner mitochondrial membrane is closely applied to the outer membrane leaving a narrow intermembranous space which extends into each crista.

Aerobic respiration takes place within the matrix and inner mitochondrial membranes and this process is enhanced by the large surface area provided by the cristae. The matrix contains most of the enzymes involved in oxidation of fatty acids and the enzymes of the tricarboxylic acid cycle (Krebs cycle). The inner membrane contains the cytochromes, the carrier molecules of the electron transport chain, and the enzymes involved in ATP production.

Mitochondria, as organelles, have several most unusual features. The mitochondrial matrix contains a strand of DNA arranged as a circle in a manner analogous to the chromosomes of bacteria. The matrix also contains ribosomes which have a similar structure to bacterial ribosomes. There is evidence that mitochondria synthesise at least some of their own constituent proteins, others being synthesised by the cell in which they reside. In addition, mitochondria undergo self-replication by a process which is similar to bacterial cell division. On the basis of these features, it has been proposed that mitochondria are semi-autonomous organelles which arose during evolution as bacterial intracellular parasites of larger, more advanced cells.

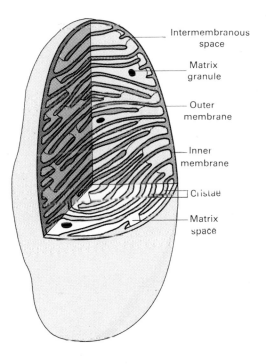

Intermembranous space

Matrix granule

Outer membrane

Inner membrane

Cristae

Matrix space

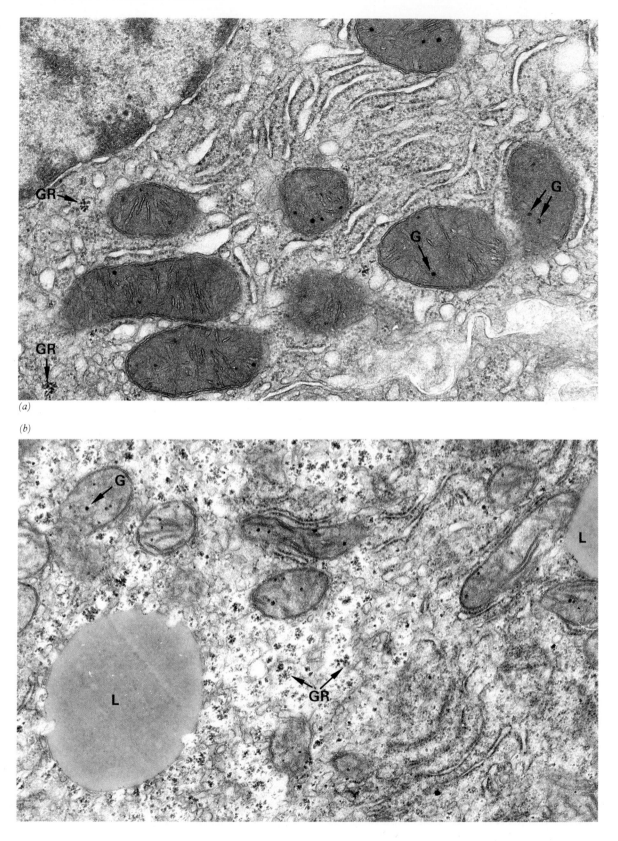

(a)

(b)

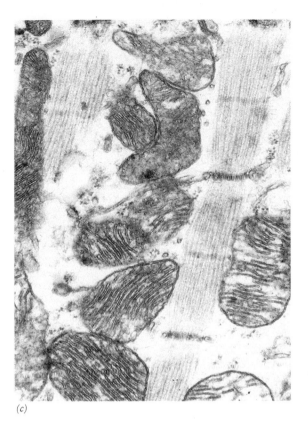

(c)

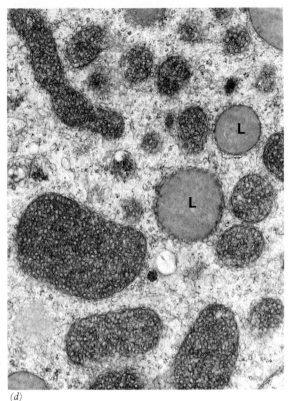

(d)

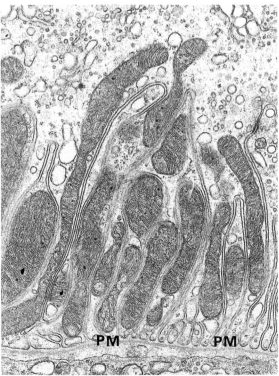

(e)

Fig. 1.14 Mitochondria, lipid droplets and glycogen *(illustrations (a) and (b) opposite)*

(EM (a) × 42 400 (b) × 36 400 (c) × 42 600 (d) × 32 400 (e) × 16 500)

All mitochondria conform to the same general structure but vary greatly in size, shape and arrangement of cristae; these variations often reflect the metabolic status of the cell type in which mitochondria are found. Mitochondria move freely within the cytosol and tend to aggregate in intracellular sites with high energy demands where their shape often conforms to the available space.

Micrographs (a) and (b), both of liver cell cytoplasm, show the typical appearance of mitochondria when cut in different planes of section; note the relatively dense matrix containing a few matrix granules **G**. Glycogen and lipid droplets are also seen in micrographs (a) and (b); glycogen appears either as single minute dense granules (called α *particles*) or as aggregations termed *glycogen rosettes* **GR**, (also called β *particles*). Lipid droplets **L** are of variable size and electron density and are not bounded by a membrane.

Mitochondria from heart muscle and steroid-secreting cells can be seen in micrographs (c) and (d) respectively; in each, the cristae are densely packed, reflecting the metabolic activity of the cell, and have a characteristic shape. The cristae of heart muscle mitochondria are laminar whereas those of steroid-secreting cells are tubular.

Micrograph (e) shows the base of an absorptive cell from a kidney tubule where there is intense active transport of ions. The basal plasma membrane **PM** is deeply infolded so as to increase the surface area, and elongated mitochondria are packed into the intervening spaces.

The cytoskeleton and cell movement

In order to maintain structural stability, there is within every cell a supporting framework of minute filaments and tubules known as the *cytoskeleton*. Nevertheless, the cell membrane and intracellular organelles are not rigid or static structures but are in a constant state of movement to accommodate processes such as endocytosis and phagocytosis. Some cells, e.g. white blood cells, propel themselves about by amoeboid movement, other cells have actively motile membrane specialisations such as cilia and flagella, whilst other cells, e.g. muscle cells, are highly specialised for contractility. In addition, cell division is a process which involves extensive reorganisation of cellular constituents. The cytoskeleton thus incorporates features which accommodate all these dynamic functions.

The cytoskeleton of each cell contains structural elements of three main types, *microfilaments*, *microtubules* and *intermediate filaments* as well as many accessory proteins responsible for linking these structures to one another, to the plasma membrane and to the membranes of the intracellular organelles.

1. Microfilaments. Microfilaments are extremely fine strands of a molecule known as *actin* which is made up of globular protein subunits. Each actin filament consists of two strings of bead-like subunits twisted together like a rope. The globular subunits are stabilised by calcium ions and associated with ATP molecules which provide energy for contractile processes. Actin filaments are best demonstrated histologically in skeletal muscle cells where they are arranged in bundles with a different type of filamentous protein called *myosin*. Contraction occurs when the actin and myosin filaments slide relative to one another due to the rearrangement of intermolecular bonds fuelled by the release of energy from associated ATP molecules; this process is described in more detail in Chapter 6.

Cells not considered to be overtly contractile also contain the globular subunits of various subtypes of actin which appear to assemble readily into microfilaments and then dissociate thereby providing a dynamically changing structural framework for the cell. Membrane specialisations such as microvilli (see Fig. 5.22) also contain a skeleton of actin filaments which not only provide structural support but also cause the microvilli to shorten and elongate.

2. Microtubules. Microtubules have a much greater diameter than microfilaments but, like them, are made up of globular subunits which can readily be assembled and disassembled to provide for alterations in cell shape and position of organelles. The microtubule subunits consist of molecules of a globular protein known as *tubulin* which are arranged so as to form a hollow tubule; when seen in cross-section, 13 tubulin molecules make up a circle. In cilia, nine pairs of microtubules are disposed in a cylindrical structure, and movement occurs by rearrangement of chemical bonds between adjacent pairs (see Fig. 5.21). In most cells, however, movement appears to be effected by the addition or subtraction of tubulin subunits from the microtubules causing them to become either lengthened or shortened. The function of the spindle during cell division is a classic example of this process on a large scale (see Fig. 2.3).

3. Intermediate filaments. Intermediate filaments are, as their name implies, intermediate in size between microfilaments and microtubules. However, in contrast, intermediate filaments have a stable fibrous structure made up of a variety of different irregular molecular strands which appear to be fairly specific to particular cell types. For example, in epithelial cells, the intermediate filaments are composed of the protein keratin and are known as *tonofibrils*; the filaments form a tough supporting meshwork within the cytoplasm and are anchored to the plasma membrane at strong intracellular junctions with the adjacent epithelial cells.

The organising centre for the cytoskeleton appears to be located near the nucleus in an area called the *centrosome* (cell centre) which contains a pair of *centrioles*. Each centriole consists of nine triplets of microtubules arranged in a cylindrical manner, the pair of centrioles being disposed at right angles to one another. Centrioles are illustrated in Figure 2.6. The centrosome appears to act as a nucleation centre for microtubules which radiate from here towards the cell periphery. Centrioles appear to be necessary for microtubular function. For example, prior to cell division the pair of centrioles is duplicated, the pairs migrating towards opposite ends of the cell. Here they act as organising centres for the microtubules of the spindle which controls distribution of chromosomes to the daughter cells. Likewise a pair of centrioles, known as a *basal body*, is found at the base of the microtubules of cilia.

The distribution of microfilaments and intermediate filaments tends to be complementary to that of the microtubules and there is experimental evidence that, at least in some situations, microtubules may form a temporary framework around which more permanent cytoskeletal structures can be built up. The elements of the cytoskeleton are attached to one another and to the plasma membrane and the membranes of cytoplasmic organelles by a variety of linking proteins. In addition, some of the metabolic enzyme systems of the cytosol appear to be bound to various elements of the cytoskeleton. Moreover, the cytoskeleton appears to provide a mechanism whereby some molecules can be transported within the cell; such molecules are bound to microfilaments and microtubules and as these elongate and shorten, the molecules are moved from one site to another. The cytoskeletal elements may then disassemble leaving the transported molecules in new positions.

In summary, the cytoskeleton consists of three main structural elements. The microfilaments and the microtubules are relatively labile and dynamically changing structures (except where they perform highly specialised functions such as in muscle and cilia respectively), whereas the intermediate filaments serve a more static supporting function. The organising centre for the cytoskeleton is located near the cell nucleus in the centrosome which contains a pair of centrioles which act as nucleation centres for microtubules. The functions of the cytoskeleton are fourfold. Firstly, it provides the structural support for the plasma membrane, cellular organelles and some cytosol enzyme systems. Secondly, it provides the means for movement of intracellular organelles, the plasma membrane and other cytosol constituents necessary for the routine function of all cells. Thirdly, the cytoskeleton provides the locomotor mechanism for amoeboid movements and specialised motile structures such as cilia and flagella. Finally, the cytoskeleton is responsible for the property of contractility in the cells of specialised tissues such as muscle.

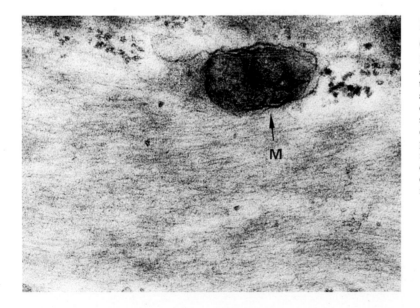

Fig. 1.15 Microfilaments
(EM × 76 500)

In general, individual microfilaments are difficult to demonstrate because of their small diameter and diffuse arrangement amongst other cytoplasmic components. In this example from a smooth muscle cell, a cell type in which cytoplasmic filaments are a predominant feature, parallel arrays of microfilaments are readily seen. The diameter of microfilaments may be compared with the diameter of a mitochondrion **M**.

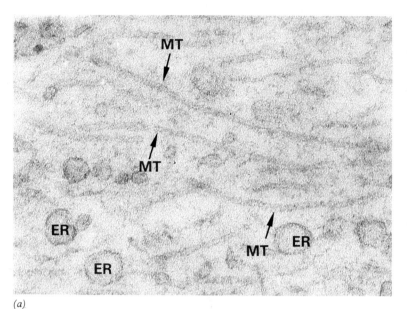

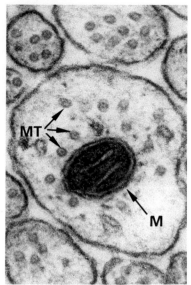

(a)   *(b)*

Fig. 1.16 Microtubules

(EM (a) LS × 171 500 (b) TS × 171 500)

These micrographs illustrate microtubules within nerve cells; each nerve cell has an extremely elongated cytoplasmic extension called an axon (see Ch. 7) in which microtubules are unusually prominent. The axonal microtubules probably provide structural support and direct intra-axonal transport. In longitudinal section, microtubules **MT** appear as straight, unbranched structures and in transverse section appear hollow. The small diameter of microtubules is evident when compared with a small mitochondrion **M** and elements of smooth endoplasmic reticulum **ER**. Microtubules may direct intracellular transport by acting as 'guide rails' for the movement of organelles such as mitochondria or secretory vesicles; alternatively microtubules may merely act as a system of internal tubes for conveying molecules within the cytoplasm.

Light microscopical appearances of cellular organelles and histochemical techniques

Knowledge of the ultrastructure of cells has mainly been obtained from electron microscopic studies, nevertheless light microscopy still has a useful role in the demonstration of intracellular components. A major advantage of light microscopy is that a wide range of empirical and specific staining methods are available to demonstrate cellular organelles and biochemical constituents. The empirical methods, the traditional staining techniques of histology, were developed from dyes used in the textile industry last century.

The specific staining methods, known as *histochemical techniques*, employ reagents known to react with defined cellular constituents, e.g. lipids, glycogen and DNA, thereby staining those constituents in a characteristic manner. The activity of enzymes can similarly be demonstrated by staining for their specific substrates or end products; such methods are examples of *enzyme histochemistry*. Antibodies can be raised against specific cellular components and then be conjugated with dyes or with enzymes. The antibodies are then applied to the tissue under study where they combine with their 'antigen' thus localising the dye or attached enzyme at the intracellular site of the 'antigen'; the dye can be viewed directly and the presence of enzyme can be demonstrated by an appropriate histochemical method. Such immunological methods (*immunohistochemistry*) have a high degree of specificity and are suitable for accurate localisation of cellular constituents. Histochemical, enzyme and immunological techniques have more recently been adapted for use in electron microscopy (for example, see Fig. 1.4c).

A problem common to both light and electron microscopy is the need to prevent autolytic degeneration and to preserve cellular ultrastructure; fixatives such as formaldehyde are therefore employed for this purpose. *Fixation* causes cross linking of macromolecules which arrests biological activity, at the same time rendering the cells more amenable to staining.

Most tissues are too thick to be examined directly in the microscope and must therefore be cut into very thin slices (*sections*). To facilitate the cutting of thin sections, the tissue is usually *embedded* in a hard medium such as paraffin wax or a plastic resin; fixed tissues generally require dehydration with organic solvents before embedding. Each stage in the fixation, dehydration, embedding, sectioning and final staining sequence may induce distortions or artefacts in the cellular architecture. When biological activity of cell constituents, e.g. enzymes must be preserved, thin sections can be obtained from unfixed frozen tissue; such *frozen sections* have their own peculiar artefactual distortions. It follows therefore that the image seen in the microscope is an artificially derived representation of the living architecture. The next section illustrates examples of histochemical methods employed in the study of cellular ultrastructure.

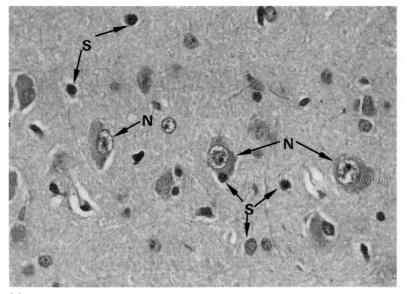

(a)

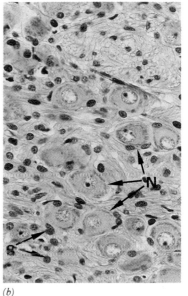

(b)

Fig. 1.17 Nuclei

(a) H & E × 480 (b) Azan × 320

Nuclei from different tissues vary greatly in morphology depending on function and level of activity with regard to protein synthesis. The nucleic acids DNA and RNA are negatively charged thus having an affinity for basic dyes i.e. *basophilic*. The intensity of nuclear staining with such dyes reflects the concentration of DNA and RNA in different parts of the nucleus. The nuclei of cells active in protein synthesis are generally large and relatively lightly stained since their chromatin is widely dispersed; nucleoli are usually prominent, reflecting ribosomal RNA synthesis. In contrast, inactive cells have condensed chromatin and therefore have small, densely stained nuclei and no visible nucleoli.

The cytoplasm of highly active cells often contains much rough endoplasmic reticulum of which the ribosomal RNA is also stained by basic dyes. The intensity of cytoplasmic staining is usually much less than that of the nucleus reflecting the lower concentration of nucleic acids.

The specimen shown in micrograph (a) is of brain tissue which has been stained with *haematoxylin and eosin* (H & E), the 'standard' histological staining method. Haematoxylin is blue in colour and eosin is pink. Haematoxylin, a basic dye, is principally employed to demonstrate nuclear form whereas eosin, an acidic dye, has affinity for positively-charged structures such as mitochondria and many other cytoplasmic constituents (excluding ribosomes which are basophilic as previously described); *acidophilic* structures are therefore *eosinophilic* when stained by the H & E method. The highly active nerve cells **N** seen in micrograph (a) have huge nuclei with relatively pale-stained, dispersed nuclear chromatin and prominent nucleoli. In contrast, the surrounding relatively inactive support cells **S** have small nuclei with densely-stained, condensed chromatin and no visible nucleoli. Note the cytoplasmic basophilia of the nerve cells due to their high content of ribosomes.

The specimen in micrograph (b) also shows nervous tissue but in this case is stained by the Azan method which contains a red basophilic dye and a blue-green acidophilic dye. Note how the nuclear form of the neurones **N** and support cells **S** corresponds to that in micrograph (a) despite the difference in colour.

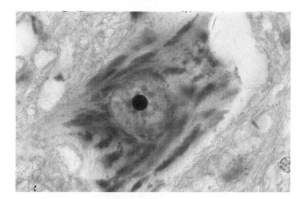

Fig. 1.18 Nuclei

(Cresyl violet × 800)

This micrograph shows a single nerve cell at very high magnification stained by another basophilic dye, cresyl violet. In this cell, the dispersed chromatin and prominent nucleolus are particularly well demonstrated and even the nuclear envelope can be distinguished. The basophilic clumps in the extensive cytoplasm represent areas of prolific rough endoplasmic reticulum.

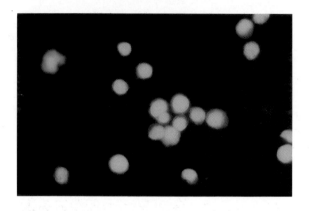

Fig. 1.19 Nucleic acids

(Acridine orange × 320)

In this micrograph, a fluorescent method has been used for localising DNA and RNA. The specimen has been stained with a dye which combines with DNA and RNA; when viewed in a fluorescent microscope, the DNA is seen as yellow-green fluorescence and the RNA as orange-red fluorescence thereby highlighting the nuclei and cytoplasm respectively. The micrograph shows plasma cells and lymphocytes in a smear of bone marrow aspirate; the plasma cells, which are very active in protein synthesis, have much cytoplasmic RNA whereas the quiescent lymphocytes have almost none.

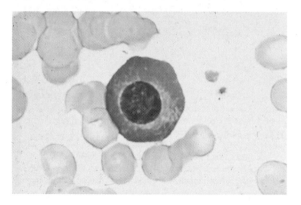

Fig. 1.20 Golgi apparatus

(Giemsa × 300)

This micrograph illustrates a plasma cell from a bone marrow smear; these cells are responsible for antibody production. The cytoplasm is packed with rough endoplasmic reticulum responsible for protein (antibody) synthesis and is thus strongly basophilic. There is a very well developed Golgi apparatus which packages the antibody prior to secretion; the Golgi, which mainly consists of lipid (membrane), remains unstained and appears as a pale area adjacent to the nucleus.

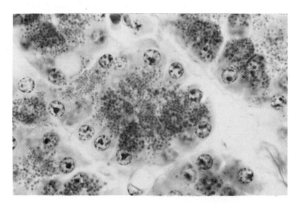

Fig. 1.21 Secretory granules

(Iron haematoxylin × 400)

This staining method is used to demonstrate the secretory granules of the pancreatic gland which secretes digestive enzymes. The secretory cells are grouped around a minute central duct and the secretory granules, which are stained black, are concentrated towards the luminal aspect of the cell. Correlate this appearance with the ultrastructural appearance shown in Figure 1.12.

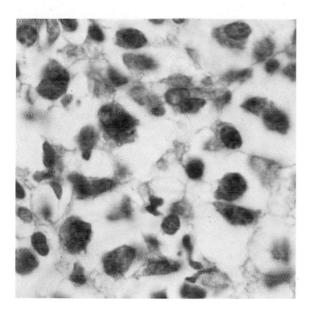

Fig. 1.22 Secretory products

(Immunoperoxidase × 480)

In this specimen, the intracellular location of IgA antibody within plasma cells has been defined using an immunological staining technique. The reagent consists of an antibody raised against the human IgA to be demonstrated, this raised antibody being conjugated to the enzyme, *horseradish peroxidase*. The brown deposits seen in the cytoplasm of some of the cells represents the reaction product of a standard enzyme histochemical method for horseradish peroxidase. Horseradish peroxidase is a commercially available enzyme which is frequently used in immunohistochemistry. A similar technique has been used to demonstrate glucagon secreting cells in Figure 17.21.

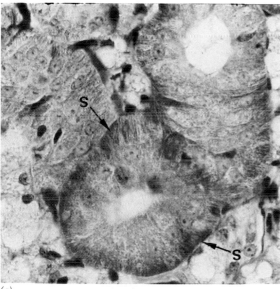

(a)

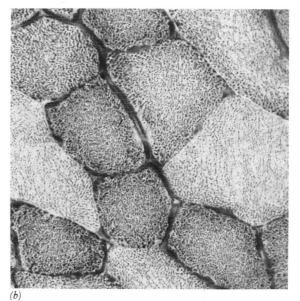

(b)

Fig. 1.23 Mitochondria

(a) Iron haematoxylin × 480 (b) Succinate dehydrogenase × 480

Mitochondria are in general not seen by light microscopy. However, they are acidophilic and with the standard H & E stain they are responsible for much of the eosinophilia (pink staining) of cytoplasm. In some cells, the mitochondria are profuse and may be concentrated in one region of the cell and can be demonstrated directly and indirectly by various staining methods.

Micrograph (a) shows a salivary gland duct made up of cells which are extremely active in secretion and reabsorption of a variety of inorganic ions. This takes place at the base of the cells (i.e. the surface away from the lumen) and is powered by ATP produced by extremely elongated mitochondria associated with numerous basal infoldings of the plasma membrane similar to that shown in

Figure 1.14 (e). The cells have been stained by a modified haematoxylin method which not only stains basophilic structures (i.e. DDA and RNA) but also acidophilic structures such as mitochondria which can be seen as striations **S** in the basal aspect of the cells.

In specimen (b), which shows skeletal muscle cells in transverse section, an enzyme histochemical method for succinate dehydrogenase has been employed. Succinate dehydrogenase is an enzyme of the citric acid cycle which is exclusive to mitochondria and therefore provides a marker for mitochondria. In skeletal muscle there are three different muscle types differing in mitochondrial concentration and such a staining method can be used to demonstrate their relative proportions (see also Fig. 6.12).

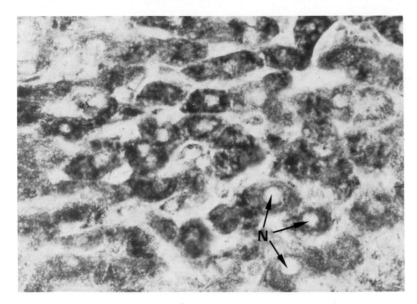

Fig. 1.24 Glycogen
(PAS/Alcian blue × 600)

This micrograph of liver cells has been stained by a histochemical method to demonstrate the presence of glycogen which is stained magenta. The cytoplasm of each liver cell is packed with glycogen thus leaving a negative (unstained) image of the nuclei **N**. The alcian blue component stains vascular lining cells blue.

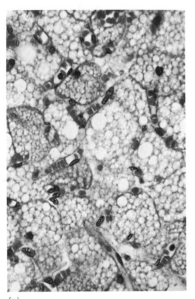

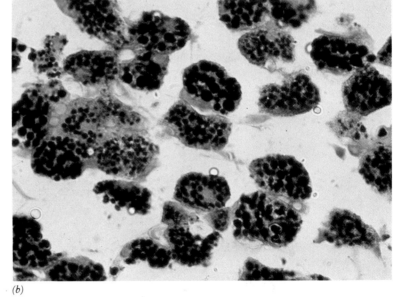

(a)   *(b)*

Fig. 1.25 Lipid
(a) H & E × 320 (b) Osmium × 320

Routine processing methods for microscopy generally extract lipid from tissues and therefore lipid droplets within cells appear as unstained vacuoles as in micrograph (a). Lipids are therefore best demonstrated in frozen sections stained by specific lipid methods such as osmium as in micrograph (b) with which lipid is stained black. Both micrographs show brown adipose tissue at similar magnifications.

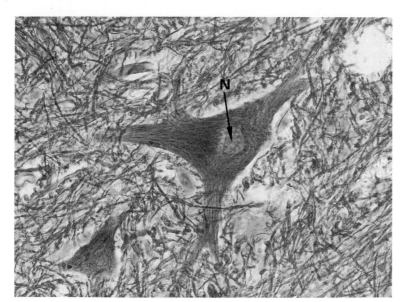

Fig. 1.26 Microtubules

(Silver impregnation method × 600)

Individual elements of the cytoskeleton are not easily visualised by light microscopy. However, in cells with prominent aggregations of cytoskeletal elements e.g. nerve cells or cells undergoing division, these can be demonstrated by impregnation with silver and gold.

In this micrograph, the silver impregnated cytoskeleton can be seen radiating from the vicinity of the nucleus **N** into various cytoplasmic extensions.

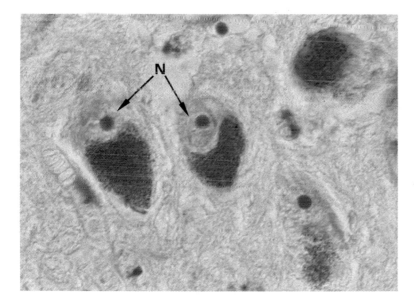

Fig. 1.27 Cellular pigment: melanin

(Modified azan × 600)

In general, mammalian tissues have minimal intrinsic colour when viewed in the microscope, thus the need for staining. A few tissues however, contain intracellular pigments, the most typical being melanin which is mainly responsible for skin colour (see Fig. 9.5). This pigment is also present in the nerve cells of one of the brain nuclei, the substantia nigra, shown in this micrograph. This specimen has been lightly stained to pick out the nuclei **N** which are stained pale blue with prominent red nucleoli.

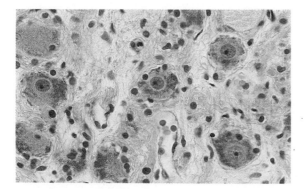

Fig. 1.28 Cellular pigment: lipofuscin

(H & E × 320)

Lipofuscin is an intracellular pigment which probably represents an insoluble degradation product of organelle turnover. It accumulates with increasing age particularly in sympathetic ganglion cells (as seen in this micrograph) other neurones and cardiac muscle cells, and is thus sometimes referred to as 'age pigment'.

2. Cell cycle and replication

Introduction

The development of a single, fertilised egg cell to form a complex, multicellular organism involves cellular replication, growth and progressive specialisation for a variety of functions. The mechanism of cellular replication in all but the male and female germ cells is known as *mitosis*. Mitosis or *mitotic division* of a single cell results in the production of two daughter cells, each genetically identical to the parent cell. After the period in which mitosis takes place, the daughter cells enter a period of growth and metabolic activity prior to further mitotic division. The time interval between mitotic divisions, that is the life cycle of an individual cell, is called the *cell cycle*. As development of the fertilised ovum progresses to produce a multicellular embryo, groups of cells and their progeny become increasingly specialised to form tissues each with different specific functions. The process whereby cells become specialised is called *differentiation*. In the fully developed organism, the differentiated cells of some tissues, such as the neurones of the nervous system, lose the ability to undergo mitosis, whereas certain cells of other tissues, such as the epithelial cells lining the gastrointestinal tract, undergo continuous cycles of mitotic division throughout the lifespan of the organism. Between these extremes are other cells such as liver cells which do not normally undergo mitosis but retain the capacity to undergo mitosis should the need arise.

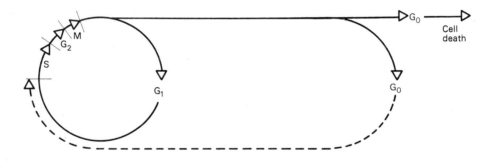

Fig. 2.1 The cell cycle

Historically, only two phases of the cell cycle were recognised: the *mitotic phase (M phase)* and the remainder of the cell cycle during which cell division does not take place. This second phase, called *interphase*, usually occupies most of the life cycle of the cell. With the development of radio-isotopes it was found that there is a discrete period during interphase when nuclear DNA is replicated; this phase, described as the *synthesis* or *S phase* of the cell cycle, is completed some time before the onset of mitosis. Thus interphase may be divided into three separate phases. Between the end of the M phase and the beginning of the S phase, the *first gap* or G_1 *phase* occurs; this is usually much longer than the other phases of the cell cycle. During the G_1 phase, cells grow and perform their specialised functions with respect to the tissue as a whole. The interval between the end of the S phase and the beginning of the M phase, the *second gap* or G_2 *phase*, is of relatively short duration and is the period in which cells prepare for mitotic division.

Some cell types progress continuously through the cell cycle as in the case of tissue growth or cell turnover whereas other cell types, e.g. nerve cells, lose the capacity for mitotic division and leave the cell cycle after the M phase and enter a protracted functional state designated as the G_0 *phase*.

Some other cell types enter the G_0 phase but retain the capacity to re-enter the cell cycle when suitably stimulated. Some liver cells appear to enter a protracted G_2 phase in which they are fully functional cells despite the presence of more than the usual complement of DNA.

The M phase is usually relatively short and is the period in which DNA, duplicated during the S phase, is equally distributed between the two daughter cells by cell division.

In general, the S, G_2 and M phases of the cell cycle are relatively constant in duration, each taking up to several hours to complete whereas the G_1 phase is highly variable, in some cases lasting for several days or even longer. The G_0 phase may last for the entire lifespan of the organism.

The cell cycle, and hence the rate of cell division, is controlled by both extrinsic and intrinsic factors. Hormones are among the extrinsic factors which regulate the cell cycles of many cells and thus co-ordinate tissue growth and function. At present, little is known about the intrinsic factors which control the cell cycle. An understanding of all the factors which control the cell cycle is likely to be a prerequisite for elucidation of the primary defect which occurs in conditions of uncontrolled cell division such as cancer.

Mitosis

Somatic cell division occurs in the M phase of the cell cycle, the process being completed in a matter of hours. The cell division occurs in two phases. Firstly, the chromosomes duplicated in the S phase are distributed equally and identically between the two potential daughter cells; this process is known as *mitosis*. Secondly, the dividing cell is cleaved into genetically identical daughter cells by cytoplasmic division or *cytokinesis*. Although mitosis is always equal and symmetrical, cytokinesis may, in some situations, result in the formation of two daughter cells with grossly unequal amounts of cytoplasm or cytoplasmic organelles. In other circumstances, mitosis may occur in the absence of cytokinesis as in the formation of binucleate and multinucleate cells.

Fig. 2.2 Mitotic chromosomes

(Giemsa × 1200)

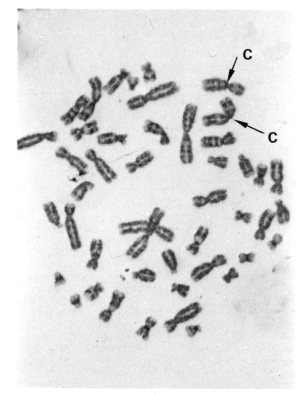

In general, the nuclei of all cells contain the same fixed complement of DNA, a quantity called the *genome*. The genome is identical in every cell (except the germ cells and a few odd exceptions) of the same individual. The DNA of the genome is intimately associated with proteins, called nucleoproteins, and is arranged as a number of discrete, folded strands called *chromosomes*. The cells of each species have a characteristic, fixed number of chromosomes (46 in man) known as *the diploid number*. Chromosomes function in pairs, called *homologous pairs*, the members of each pair having a similar length of DNA and a similar structure.

During interphase, chromosomes exist as an unravelled mass within the nucleus; this arrangement may facilitate gene expression, a process which takes place mainly within the G_1 and G_0 phases of the cell cycle. Histologically, individual chromosomes are not usually visible within the nucleus of cells in interphase. During the S phase, each chromosome is duplicated and the two identical chromosomes become tightly coiled and condensed such that they are readily visible with the light microscope. This arrangement of chromosomes is merely a mechanism for packaging the duplicated genome which may then be distributed identically and equally between the two daughter cells during mitosis.

This micrograph illustrates the chromosomes of a human cell cultured *in vitro* and arrested at the onset of mitosis; the chromosomes have been treated with the enzyme trypsin, thus revealing a cross-banding pattern along the length of each chromosome. Such mitotic chromosomes each consist of a duplicated chromosome, each member of the duplicate being referred to as a *chromatid*. The two chromatids are joined at a point called the *centromere* **C**.

Each member of a homologous pair of mitotic chromosomes is similar in length, centromere location and banding pattern. The significance of trypsin-induced chromosomal banding is not understood but the phenomenon provides a useful technique for the identification of chromosomes, especially in the investigation of chromosomal abnormalities.

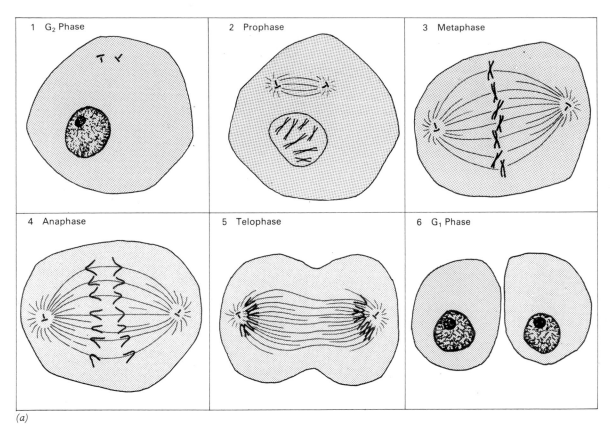

(a)

Fig. 2.3 Mitosis

(a) Schematic diagram (b) Mitotic series: Giemsa × 800 (opposite)

Mitosis is a continuous process which is traditionally divided into four phases: *prophase, metaphase, anaphase* and *telophase*, each stage being readily recognisable with the light microscope. Cell division requires the presence of a structure called the *mitotic apparatus* which comprises a spindle of longitudinally-arranged microtubules extending between paired structures called *centrioles* (see Fig. 2.6) at the two poles of the dividing cell. The mitotic apparatus is visible within the cytoplasm only during the M phase of the cell cycle since it disaggregates shortly after completion of mitosis.

Prophase: the beginning of this stage of mitosis is defined as the moment when chromosomes first become visible within the nucleus. As prophase continues, the chromosomes become increasingly condensed and shortened and the nucleoli disappear. Dissolution of the nuclear envelope marks the end of prophase.

During prophase, the microfilaments and microtubules of the cytoskeleton disaggregate into their protein subunits. Prior to mitosis, the pair of centrioles in the centrosome has duplicated and in prophase these migrate towards opposite poles of the cell whilst simultaneously a spindle of microtubules is formed between them. As the centriole pairs move apart, the microtubules progressively elongate by the addition of tubulin subunits.

Metaphase: the nuclear envelope having disintegrated, the mitotic spindle moves into the nuclear area and the duplicated chromosomes become attached to some of the tubules of the mitotic spindle. The area of attachment of each chromatid to the spindle is known as the *kinetochore*. The chromosomes then become arranged in the plane of the spindle equator, this being known as the *equatorial* or *metaphase plate*.

Anaphase: this stage of mitosis is marked by the separation of the centromere which binds the chromatids of each duplicated chromosome. The mitotic spindle becomes lengthened by addition of tubulin subunits to its pole-to-pole tubules; the centrioles are then pushed apart and the chromatids of each duplicated chromosome are drawn by the pole-to-kinetochore tubules to opposite ends of the spindle, thus achieving an exact division of the duplicated genetic material. By the end of anaphase, two groups of identical chromosomes (the former chromatids) are clustered at opposite poles of the cell.

Telophase: during the final phase of mitosis, the chromosomes begin to uncoil and to regain their interphase conformation. The nuclear envelope reforms and nucleoli again become apparent. The process of cytokinesis also takes place during telophase; the plane of cytoplasmic division is usually defined by the position of the spindle equator, thus producing two cells of equal size. The plasma membrane around the spindle equator becomes indented to form a circumferential furrow around the cell, the *cleavage furrow*, which progressively constricts the cell until it is cleaved into two daughter cells. In mammalian cells, a ring of microfilaments is present just beneath the surface of the cleavage furrow and it has been suggested that cytokinesis occurs as a result of contraction of this filamentous ring.

In the early G_1 phase, the mitotic spindle disaggregates and in many cell types the single pair of centrioles begins to duplicate in preparation for the next mitotic division. The series of micrographs, shown opposite, illustrates the mitotic process in actively dividing primitive blood cells from a smear preparation of human bone marrow.

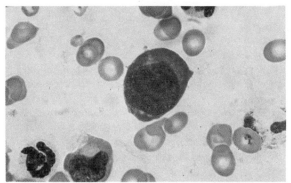

1. G₁ phase

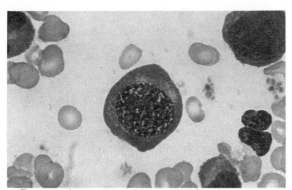

2. Early prophase

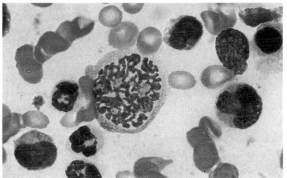

3. Late prophase

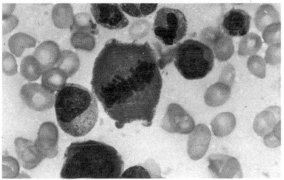

4. Metaphase

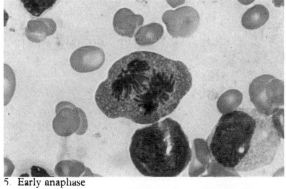

5. Early anaphase

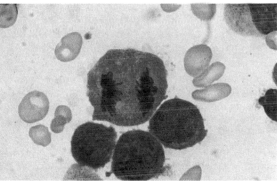

6. Late anaphase

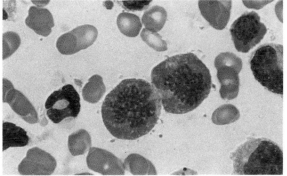

7. Early telophase and cytokinesis

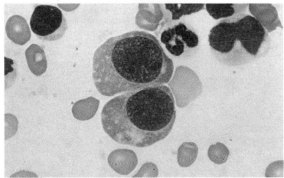

8. Late telophase and cytokinesis

(b)

Meiosis

In all somatic cells, cell division (mitosis) results in the formation of two daughter cells, each one genetically identical to the mother cell. Somatic cells contain a full complement of chromosomes (the diploid number) which function as homologous pairs as described earlier. The process of sexual reproduction involves the fusion of specialised male and female cells called *gametes* to form a *zygote* which has the diploid number of chromosomes. Each gamete thus contains only half the diploid number of chromosomes; this half complement of chromosomes is known as the *haploid number*.

The production of haploid cells involves a unique form of cell division called *meiosis* which occurs only in the germ cells of the gonads during the formation of gametes; meiotic cell division is thus also called *gametogenesis*. Meiosis involves two cell division processes of which only the first is preceded by duplication of chromosomes.

1. The **first meiotic division** results in the formation of two daughter cells; this process differs from mitosis in two important respects:

(a) Whereas in mitosis each duplicated chromosome divides at the centromere liberating two chromatids which migrate to opposite ends of the mitotic spindle, in the first meiotic division there is no such separation of the chromatids but rather one duplicated chromosome of each homologous pair migrates to each end of the spindle. Thus at the end of the first meiotic division, each daughter cell contains a half complement of duplicated chromosomes, one chromosome being derived from each homologous pair of the mother cell.

(b) During the first meiotic division, and preceding the process described in (a) above, there is an exchange of alleles between the chromatids of homologous pairs of duplicated chromosomes. This exchange, called *chiasmata formation*, results in chromatids with a different genetic constitution from those of the mother cell.

2. The **second meiotic division** merely involves splitting of each chromosome at the centromere to liberate chromatids which migrate to opposite poles of the spindle.

Thus, meiotic cell division of a single diploid germ cell gives rise to four haploid gametes. In the male, each of the four gametes undergoes morphological development into a mature spermatozoon whereas in the female, unequal distribution of the cytoplasm during meiosis results in one gamete gaining almost all the cytoplasm from the mother cell, whilst the other three acquire almost no cytoplasm; the large gamete matures to form an *ovum* and the other three, the so-called *polar bodies*, degenerate.

During both the first and second meiotic divisions, the cell passes through stages which have many similar features to prophase, metaphase, anaphase and telophase of mitosis. Unlike mitosis, however, the process of meiotic cell division can be suspended for a considerable length of time. For example, in the development of the human female gamete, the germ cells enter prophase of the first meiotic division during the fifth month of fetal life of the girl and then remain suspended until some time after she reaches sexual maturity; the first meiotic division is thus suspended for between 12 and 45 years!

The primitive germ cells of the male, the *spermatogonia*, are present only in small numbers in the male gonads before sexual maturity. After sexual maturity, spermatogonia multiply continuously by mitosis to provide a supply of cells which then undergo meiosis to form male gametes. In contrast, the germ cells of the female, called *oogonia*, multiply by mitosis only during early fetal development thereby producing a fixed complement of cells with the potential to undergo gametogenesis.

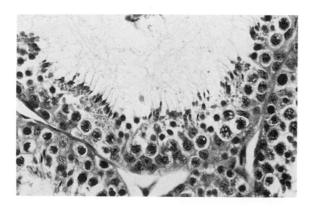

Fig. 2.4 Spermatogenesis

(H & E × 320)

This micrograph illustrates parts of a testicular tubule in which spermatozoa (male gametes) are being produced. The primitive male germ cells, the spermatogonia (which contain the same diploid chromosome complement as the body's somatic cells) lie in the basal layer; they undergo mitosis to provide a constant supply of germ cells which then divide by meiosis into male gametes (with a haploid complement of chromosomes).

In histological sections (as in this micrograph), as opposed to smear preparations, the different stages of mitosis and meiosis are always much more difficult to identify.

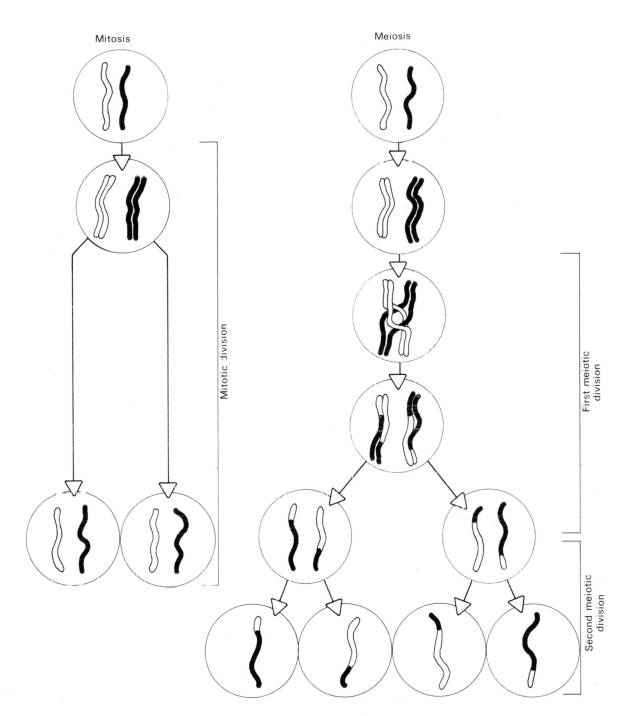

Mitosis

Meiosis

Mitotic division

First meiotic division

Second meiotic division

Fig. 2.5 Comparison of mitosis and meiosis

This diagram compares the behaviour of each homologous pair of chromosomes during mitosis and meiosis; note that only one homologous pair is represented here.

The key differences between the two forms of cell division are:

1. Chiasmata formation occurs in meiosis only

2. Meiosis involves two sequential cell divisions, the first meiotic cell division resulting in reduction of the chromosome complement to the diploid state and the second meiotic division resulting in the production of four haploid daughter cells, or gametes.

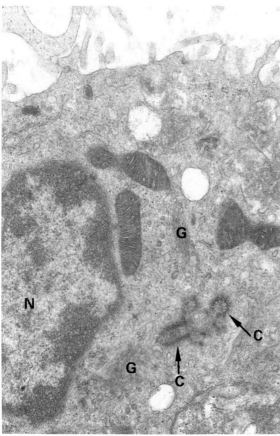

(a)

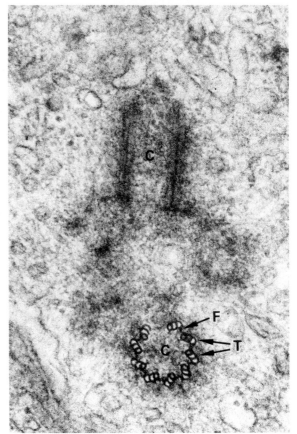

(b)

Fig. 2.6 Centrosome

(EM (a) × 9200 (b) × 48 000)

The *centrosome* is a zone of cytoplasm usually centrally located in the cell adjacent to the nucleus **N** and often surrounded by the Golgi apparatus **G**. The centrosome, the *cell centre*, contains a pair of centrioles **C** together known as a *diplosome*. Centrioles are structures involved in formation of the mitotic apparatus along which chromosomes migrate during mitosis. Each centriole is a hollow cylinder, closed at one end, and consisting of nine triplets of parallel microtubules; in transverse section, each triplet **T** is seen to consist of an inner microtubule which is circular in cross-section and two further microtubules which are C-shaped in cross-section. Each of the inner microtubules is connected to the outermost microtubule of the adjacent triplet by a fine filament **F**, thus forming a continuous cylinder. The two centrioles of each diplosome are arranged with their long axes at right angles to each other as can be seen in these micrographs; the significance of this arrangement is obscure.

During interphase, and even occasionally during late telophase, diplosomes reduplicate in readiness for the next mitotic division. In prophase, the two pairs of centrioles migrate towards opposite poles of the cell and the microtubule spindle develops between them. The pole-to-pole spindle microtubules become progressively elongated by addition of tubulin subunits from the cytoplasm, thus pushing the centrioles apart. The centrioles act as nucleation centres for the formation of microtubules. During metaphase, each chromatid becomes attached by its kinetochore to a spindle microtubule. During anaphase, the pole-to-pole microtubules of the spindle elongate, thus lengthening the spindle and the chromatids are drawn to opposite poles of the cell by the pole-to-kinetochore tubules which may also shorten by subtraction of tubulin subunits.

In the non-dividing cell, the centrosome acts as the organising centre for the microtubules of the cytoskeleton as described in Chapter 1. Structures apparently identical to centrioles form the basal bodies of cilia and flagella (see Figs. 5.21 and 18.7 and 18.8 respectively).

PART TWO

Basic tissue types

3. Blood
4. Connective tissue
5. Epithelial tissues
6. Muscle
7. Nervous tissues

3. Blood

Introduction

Blood is a tissue which consists of a variety of cells suspended in a fluid medium called *plasma*. Blood functions principally as a vehicle for the transport of gases, nutrients, metabolic waste products, cells and hormones throughout the body. Thus any sample of blood is composed not only of cells and molecules involved in transport processes but also cells and molecules in the process of being transported.

Plasma is essentially an aqueous solution of inorganic salts which is constantly exchanged with the extracellular fluid medium of all body tissues. Plasma also contains proteins, the *plasma proteins*, of three main types: *albumins, globulins* and *fibrinogen*. Collectively, the plasma proteins exert a colloidal osmotic pressure within the circulatory system which helps to regulate the exchange of aqueous solution between plasma and extracellular fluid. The albumins, which constitute the bulk of plasma proteins, bind relatively insoluble metabolites such as fatty acids and thus serve as transport proteins. The globulins are a diverse group of proteins which include the antibodies of the immune system (see Ch. 11) and certain proteins responsible for the transport of lipids and some heavy metal ions. Fibrinogen is a soluble protein which polymerises to form the insoluble protein *fibrin* during blood clotting. In general, the molecular components of plasma cannot be demonstrated by light and electron microscopy.

The cells of blood are of three major functional classes: *red blood cells (erythrocytes), white blood cells (leucocytes)* and *platelets (thrombocytes)*. Erythrocytes are primarily involved in oxygen and carbon dioxide transport, the leucocytes constitute an important part of the defence and immune systems of the body, and platelets are a vital component of the blood clotting mechanism. All these cell types are formed in the bone marrow by a process called *haemopoiesis*. Erythrocytes and platelets function entirely within blood vessels whereas leucocytes act mainly outside blood vessels in the tissues. Thus the leucocytes found in circulating blood are merely in transit between their various sites of activity.

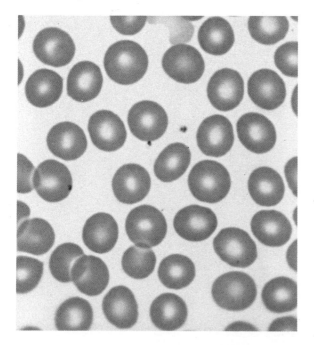

Fig. 3.1 Erythrocytes

(Giemsa × 1200)

The erythrocyte is highly adapted for its principal function, that is, the transport of oxygen and carbon dioxide. The erythrocyte develops from precursors in the bone marrow. During differentiation, vast quantities of the iron-containing respiratory pigment *haemoglobin* are synthesised. Before release into the general circulation, the nucleus is extruded and, by maturity, all cytoplasmic organelles degenerate. The fully differentiated erythrocyte thus consists merely of an outer plasma membrane enclosing haemoglobin and the limited number of enzymes which are necessary for maintenance of the integrity of the plasma membrane and the gaseous transport function.

This micrograph demonstrates the characteristic appearance of erythrocytes in a stained smear of peripheral blood. The cells are stained pink due to their high content of haemoglobin. The pale staining of the central region of the erythrocyte is a result of its unusual biconcave disc shape.

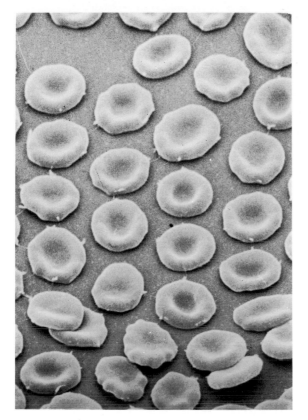

Fig. 3.2 Erythrocytes

(Scanning EM × 2400)

Scanning electron microscopy reveals the biconcave disc shape of erythrocytes. The unusual shape provides a large surface area relative to cell volume which greatly enhances gaseous exchange. The fluidity of the plasma membrane, combined with its biconcave shape allows the erythrocyte to deform readily, thus erythrocytes (average diameter 6–8 μm) are able to pass through the smallest capillaries (3–4 μm in diameter).

The biconcave shape of the erythrocyte is determined in part by its delicate cytoskeleton and in part by its water content; the volume of water in the cell is partially determined by the concentration of inorganic ions within the cell.

As with all other mammalian cells, sodium ions must be pumped out of erythrocytes continuously. The energy required for this process is derived, in the form of ATP, from anaerobic metabolism of glucose. The absence of mitochondria precludes aerobic energy production; hence erythrocytes are totally dependent on glucose as an energy source.

The lifespan of an erythrocyte, 120 days on average, may be determined by its ability to maintain the biconcave shape. In the absence of appropriate organelles, erythrocytes are unable to synthesise new proteins to replace deteriorating enzymes and membrane proteins. This leads to diminished ability to pump sodium ions from the cell and results in uptake of water, thereby producing spheroidal erythrocytes. Such cells are removed from the circulation and destroyed by the spleen and liver.

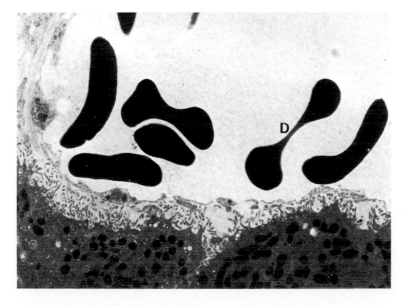

Fig. 3.3 Erythrocytes

(EM × 5700)

This micrograph illustrates the characteristic features of erythrocytes seen by transmission electron microscopy. With this technique, the observed shape of the erythrocyte depends on the plane of section through the cell. The classical dumb-bell shape **D** is only seen when the erythrocyte is cut through its thin central zone; more frequently, irregularly shaped erythrocytes are seen due to the deformation which normally occurs in the bloodstream. The high electron density of erythrocytes is due to the iron atoms of haemoglobin. Note the total absence of cytoplasmic organelles.

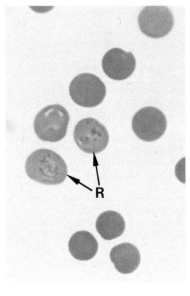

Fig. 3.4 Reticulocytes

(Cresyl blue/Eosin × 1200)

Reticulocytes are the immature form in which erythrocytes are released into the circulation from the bone marrow; they mature into erythrocytes within about one day of release. The rate of release of reticulocytes into the circulation generally equals the rate of removal of spent erythrocytes by the spleen and liver. Since the lifespan of circulating erythrocytes is about 120 days, reticulocytes constitute slightly less than 1% of the circulating red blood cells.

Reticulocytes cannot be readily distinguished in routinely stained blood smears, but when fresh blood is incubated with the basic dye, brilliant cresyl blue, a blue-stained reticular precipitate is formed in the reticulocytes but not in mature erythrocytes. This is due to the interaction of the dye with ribosomal RNA still remaining in the immature cells. This technique, called *supravital staining*, is illustrated in this micrograph. Note that reticulocytes **R** are usually slightly larger than the surrounding mature erythrocytes.

When severe erythrocyte depletion occurs, such as after haemorrhage and in certain disease states, the rate of erythrocyte production in the bone marrow increases and the proportion of reticulocytes in circulating blood rises. Thus the reticulocyte count provides a convenient measure of the rate of red blood cell formation in the bone marrow.

White cell series

There are five cell types in the white blood cell series and these are subdivided into two main classes, *granulocytes* and *agranulocytes*, according to the granularity of their cytoplasm and general nuclear characteristics:

1. Granulocytes: the granulocytes are characterised by prominent cytoplasmic granules and a single, multilobed nucleus which may give the erroneous impression that granulocytes are multinucleate cells. The highly variable shape of granulocyte nuclei has given rise to the common name of *polymorphonuclear leucocytes* or *polymorphs*.

There are three different types of granulocytes, *neutrophils, eosinophils* and *basophils* named according to the staining characteristics of their *specific granules*.

The specific granules of neutrophils have little affinity for either acidic or basic dyes whereas those of eosinophils are stained strongly by acidic dyes such as eosin, and those of basophils are stained intensely by basic dyes such as haematoxylin or methylene blue.

2. Agranulocytes: the agranulocytes, which comprise the *lymphocytes* and *monocytes*, are so named since they do not contain cytoplasmic granules readily visible with light microscopy. In contrast to the granulocytes, the nuclei of the agranulocytes are not lobed although they may be deeply indented; this nuclear feature led to the application of the misleading term *mononuclear leucocytes* in reference to the agranulocytes.

Leucocytes constitute an important part of the body's defences against foreign invaders. Neutrophils and monocytes are highly phagocytic and engulf microorganisms, cell debris and particulate matter in a non-specific manner; this activity may be enhanced and directed by immune responses to specific foreign agents (see Ch. 11). On the basis of their relative sizes, monocytes and neutrophils are often referred to as *macrophages* and *microphages* respectively.

Lymphocytes play the key role in all immune responses and, in contrast to the other leucocytes, their activity is always directed against specific foreign agents.

In general, all the leucocytes perform their functions in the tissues and merely use the blood as a vehicle for passage between sites of formation, storage and activity. It follows, therefore, that increased demand for particular leucocytes in various sites is reflected in increased numbers in the circulation. All leucocytes exhibit amoeboid movement which provides the means for migration in and out of the circulatory system and through the tissues.

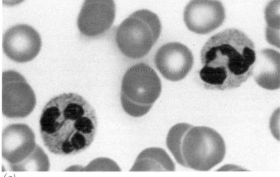

(a)

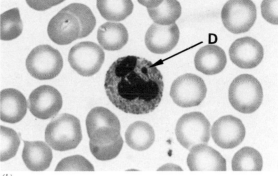

(b)

Fig. 3.5 Neutrophils

(Giemsa (a) × 1200 (b) × 1200)

Neutrophils are the most common type of leucocyte in blood and constitute from 40–75% of circulating leucocytes. The most prominent feature of the neutrophil is the highly lobulated nucleus. In the mature neutrophil there are usually five lobes connected by fine strands of nuclear material, but in the less mature neutrophil the nucleus is generally not as lobulated. In micrograph (a) two neutrophils in different stages of maturity are illustrated.

In neutrophils of females, the condensed, quiescent X-chromosome or Barr body (see Fig. 1.6) exists in the form of a small drumstick-shaped appendage of one of the nuclear lobes. This appendage, known as the *drumstick chromosome* **D**, is visible in about 3% of neutrophils in females as shown in micrograph (b).

The cytoplasm of neutrophils is lightly stippled with purplish granules called *azurophilic granules* which are merely large lysosomes often referred to as primary granules. The more numerous but much smaller specific granules are poorly stained and are thus not visible in this type of preparation.

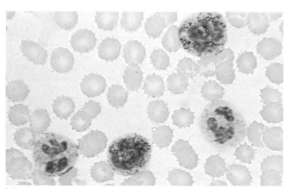

(a)

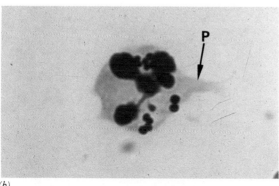

(b)

Fig. 3.6 Neutrophils

(a) Histochemical method for alkaline phosphatase × 800
(b) Giemsa × 1200

The specific granules of neutrophils contain a group of proteins with antibacterial action called *phagocytins* and the enzyme *alkaline phosphatase*, the function of which is not understood. Nevertheless, alkaline phosphatase activity is a useful marker for the specific granules of neutrophils and can be demonstrated by histochemical methods. In micrograph (a), enzyme activity is indicated by a brown, granular deposition in the neutrophil cytoplasm. Immature neutrophils, recognisable by their less lobulated nuclei, exhibit less enzyme activity since they contain fewer specific granules.

In contrast to the specific granules, the azurophilic primary granules, the lysosomes, contain a variety of hydrolytic enzymes plus potent antibacterial enzymes such as lysozyme, myeloperoxidase and D-amino-oxidase which destroy bacterial cell walls. The principal function of neutrophils is to engulf invading microorganisms, particularly bacteria; neutrophils are the main white cell type involved in acute inflammatory responses.

Micrograph (b) illustrates a neutrophil which has engulfed some coccoid bacteria; note the pseudopodia **P**. This specimen was obtained experimentally by incubating fresh blood with bacteria; under normal circumstances, neutrophils die after engulfing bacteria and do not re-enter the circulation.

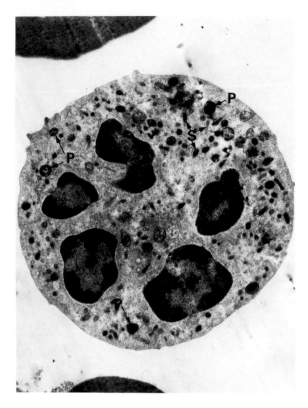

Fig. 3.7 Neutrophil

(EM × 11 400)

With electron microscopy, neutrophils have three distinguishing features. Firstly, the nucleus has up to five lobes which in section may appear as separate nuclei. Secondly, the cytoplasm contains numerous membrane-bound granules. The primary granules **P** are large, spheroidal and electron-dense, similar to the lysosomes of other cell types. The specific granules **S** are much more numerous, small and often rod-like, and of variable density and shape. Thirdly, all other cytoplasmic organelles are scarce although the cytoplasm is particularly rich in dispersed glycogen.

Neutrophils are the principal cells involved in the acute inflammatory response to tissue damage; they are highly mobile and migrate from small blood vessels to sites of tissue damage where they engulf and destroy cell debris and microorganisms by phagocytosis. Since the mature neutrophil has few appropriate organelles for protein synthesis, it has very limited capacity to regenerate expended lysosomal and specific enzymes which are rapidly depleted by phagocytic activity; the neutrophil is thus incapable of continuous function and degenerates after a single burst of activity. Defunct neutrophils are the main cellular constituent of *pus* and are therefore sometimes referred to as *pus cells*. The paucity of mitochondria and the abundance of glycogen in neutrophils reflects the predominance of the anaerobic mode of metabolism; this permits neutrophils to function in the poorly oxygenated environment of damaged tissues.

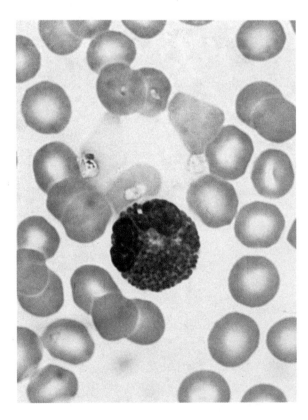

Fig. 3.8 Eosinophil

(Giemsa × 1600)

Eosinophils are much less common than neutrophils and account for 1–6% of leucocytes in circulating blood. Characteristically, eosinophils have a bilobed nucleus and the cytoplasm is packed with large, eosinophilic (dark-pink stained) specific granules of uniform size.

It has long been observed that the number of eosinophils in circulating blood increases in certain parasitic infestations such as hookworm, and in some hypersensitivity states such as hay fever, but the role of eosinophils in these processes is poorly understood.

During the last decade, the eosinophil has been found to have a variety of functions in inflammatory and immune responses, often in conjunction with other leucocytes. Eosinophils are highly phagocytic for antigen-antibody complexes (see Ch. 11) although they also exhibit some of the general phagocytic activity of neutrophils. Eosinophils are attracted to sites of inflammation by substances released from basophils (see Fig. 3.10) and their connective tissue analogues, the mast cells (see Fig. 4.15), and deactivate vasoactive substances such as histamine produced by these cells during the inflammatory response. More recent evidence suggests that eosinophils have a direct destructive effect on some parasites provided that specific antibodies are present (see also Ch. 11).

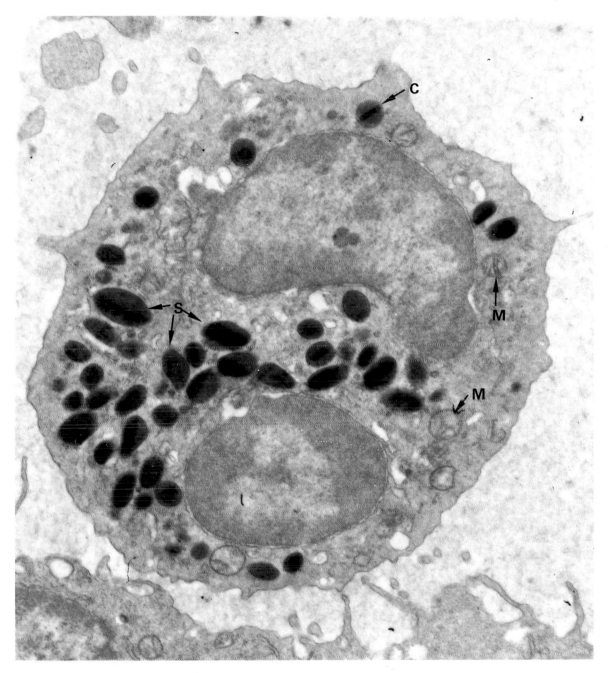

Fig. 3.9 Eosinophil

(EM × 21 200)

The most characteristic ultrastructural feature of eosinophils are the large, ovoid, specific granules **S**, each containing a dense crystalloid **C** in the long axis of the granule; in man, as in this micrograph, the crystalloids are irregular in form but in many other mammals they have a regular, discoid shape. The specific granules are membrane-bound and the matrix contains a variety of hydrolytic enzymes including *histaminase*. The crystalloids are thought to be composed of basic proteins but these are of unknown function. Other cytoplasmic organelles such as mitochondria **M** are relatively sparse and rough endoplasmic reticulum is absent. Note the characteristic bilobed nucleus.

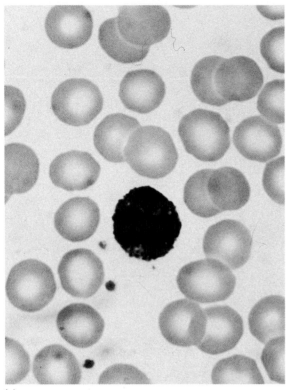

(a)

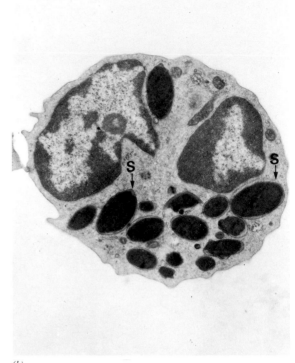

(b)

Fig. 3.10 Basophils

(a) Giemsa × 1600 (b) EM × 10 500

Basophils are the least common leucocyte and constitute less than 1% of leucocytes in circulating blood. Like eosinophils, basophils also have a bilobed nucleus but, in general, this is obscured by numerous large, densely basophilic (deep blue) specific granules. These granules are highly soluble in water and tend to be dissolved away during common blood smear preparation, thus adding to the difficulty of finding these rare cells.

With electron microscopy, the characteristic bilobed nucleus of the basophil is easily recognisable. The large specific granules **S** are membrane-bound and are filled with a closely packed, electron-dense material which contains *heparin, histamine*, other vaso-active amines, and *slow reacting substance of anaphylaxis (SRS-A)*. Heparin is a powerful anticoagulant while histamine and the other vaso-active amines cause dilatation of small blood vessels and increased capillary permeability thus promoting fluid exudation into the tissues; SRS-A stimulates smooth muscle contraction and thus constriction of internal viscera. The stimulus for exocytosis of the contents of the specific granules is the interaction of antigen with antibodies of the IgE group which are attached to the basophil cell membrane. This type of interaction typically occurs in hypersensitivity to external allergens, e.g. in hay fever and allergic asthma, and forms the basis of the Type I (immediate hypersensitivity, anaphylactoid) immune response.

Basophils bear a close resemblance to the fixed mast cells of connective tissue (see Fig. 4.15) in the structure and content of their specific granules, but there are important ultrastructural differences. Whilst basophils and mast cells are not thought to be two manifestations of the same cell type, they are considered to be functionally analogous since similar stimuli induce degranulation of both cell types producing similar physiological consequences.

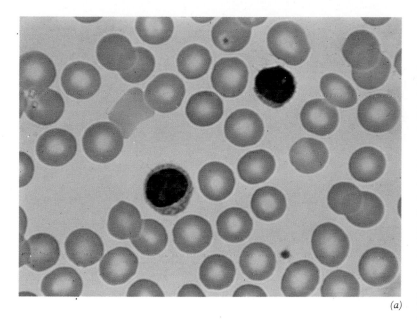

(a)

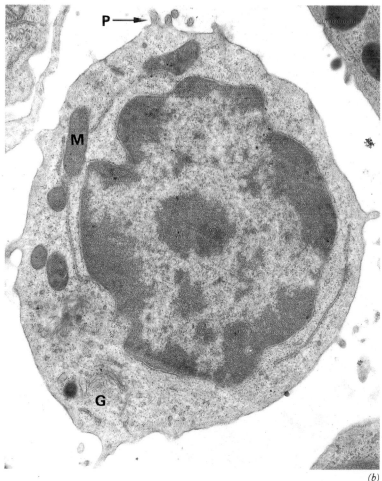

(b)

Fig. 3.11 Lymphocytes

(a) Giemsa × 800 (b) EM × 20 000

Lymphocytes are the smallest cells in the white cell series, being only slightly larger than erythrocytes. Lymphocytes are the second most common leucocyte in circulating blood and make up 20–45% of the differential white cell count.

Lymphocytes are characterised by a round, densely stained nucleus and a relatively small amount of pale basophilic, non-granular cytoplasm. The amount of cytoplasm varies with the state of activity of the lymphocyte, and in circulating blood there is a predominance of 'small' lymphocytes; however, 'medium' and 'large' lymphocytes are also seen in peripheral blood. Micrograph (a) illustrates small and medium lymphocytes. In the medium lymphocyte, the cytoplasm is readily visible but in the small lymphocyte the cytoplasm is almost too sparse to be seen.

Lymphocytes play the central role in all immunological defence mechanisms; these are described in detail in Chapter 11. Blood provides the medium in which lymphocytes circulate between the various lymphoid tissues and all other tissues of the body. Most of the lymphocytes in the circulation are in a relatively inactive metabolic state; this is reflected in their ultrastructural appearance. The nucleus is small, rounded and often slightly indented and the chromatin is moderately condensed; nucleoli are not usually present. The sparse cytoplasm contains a few mitochondria **M**, a rudimentary Golgi apparatus **G**, little or no endoplasmic reticulum and a comparatively large number of free ribosomes accounting for the basophilia of light microscopy. The plasma membrane has a few irregular pseudopodia **P**. When immunologically activated, lymphocytes become highly motile and propel themselves between blood vessels and tissues by amoeboid movement.

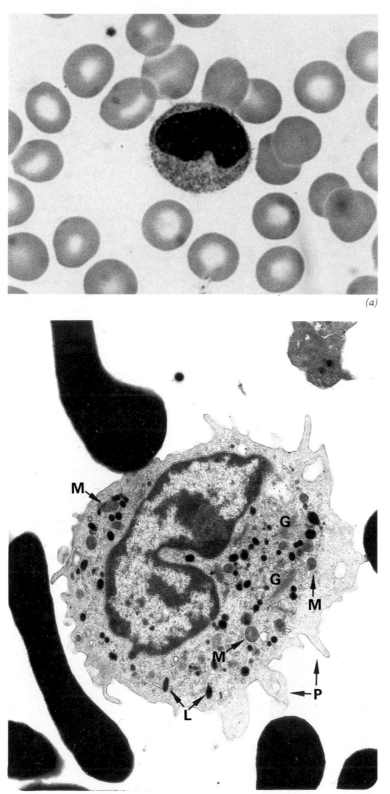

(a)

(b)

Fig. 3.12 Monocytes

(a) Giemsa × 1600 (b) EM × 20 000

Monocytes are the largest members of the white cell series and constitute from 2–10% of leucocytes in peripheral blood. Monocytes are characterised by a large, eccentrically placed nucleus which is stained less intensely than that of other leucocytes. The nucleus is usually indented, a feature which becomes more pronounced as the cell matures, so as to give a horseshoe or even bilobed appearance. Two or more nucleoli may be visible. The extensive cytoplasm is filled with small lysosomes which, in light microscopy, confer a characteristic 'frosted-glass' appearance.

With electron microscopy, lysosomes **L** are prolific, the Golgi apparatus **G** is well developed, rough endoplasmic reticulum is relatively diffuse and mitochondria **M** are more common than in the other leucocytes. Pseudopodia **P** are prominent, reflecting the capacity of monocytes for phagocytosis and ameoboid movement.

In contrast to neutrophils, monocytes are capable of continuous lysosomal activity and regeneration which utilises aerobic and anaerobic metabolic pathways depending on the availability of oxygen in the tissues.

Monocytes appear to have little function in circulating blood. They are highly motile cells and migrate into connective tissues where they are termed *histiocytes* or *tissue fixed macrophages* (see Figs. 4.16 and 4.17).

A major function of macrophages is the destruction of cellular debris arising from normal turnover of cells within the tissues. Macrophages also play an important role in the immune defence system which is described in Chapter 11. The monocytes dispersed throughout the body collectively form the *macrophage-monocyte system*.

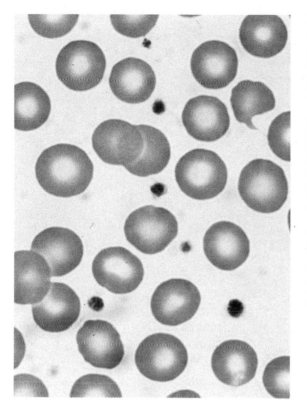

Fig. 3.13 Platelets

(Giemsa × 1600)

Platelets or thrombocytes are small, non-nucleated cells formed in the bone marrow by budding from the cytoplasm of huge cells called *megakaryocytes*. Platelets are present in large numbers in circulating blood, from 150 000–400 000/ml.

Platelets are round or oval, biconvex discs about 2–3 μm in diameter. In blood smears, their shape is not clearly seen and they are often partially clumped together, as in this micrograph. The shape of platelets is maintained by a bundle of microtubules arranged circumferentially around the equator. The cytoplasm has a purple-stained, granular appearance due to a high content of organelles which are concentrated towards the centre of the cell; the peripheral cytoplasm is very poorly stained and therefore barely visible.

Platelets are known to participate in haemostasis in two main ways. Firstly, in normal tissues, platelets clump together to plug small defects which appear continuously in the walls of small blood vessels. Secondly, when blood vessels are injured, platelets contribute to the processes of clot formation and retraction as well as releasing a substance called *serotonin* which reduces blood flow by constricting the damaged vessels.

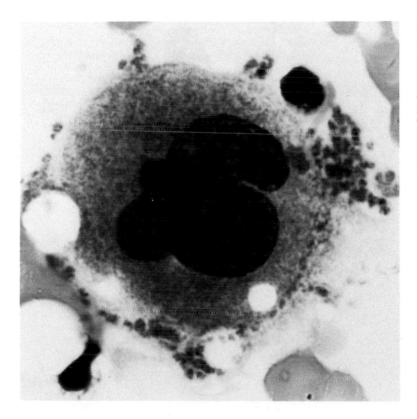

Fig. 3.14 Megakaryocyte

(Giemsa × 1600)

Reflecting its name, the megakaryocyte is a huge cell with a single, highly irregular polyploid nucleus. The extensive cytoplasm appears finely granular due to a profusion of organelles. Megakaryocytes are found in the bone marrow where they are responsible for production of platelets. Platelets are formed by budding from the megakaryocyte cytoplasm.

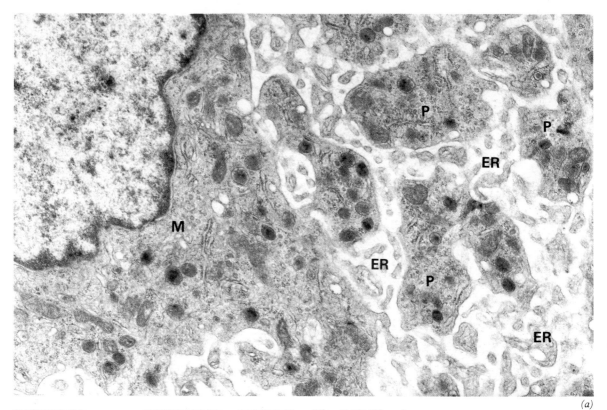

(a)

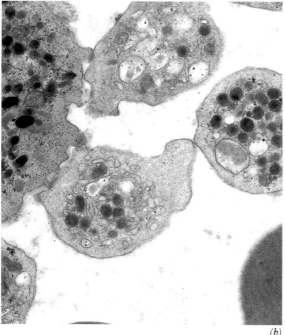

(b)

Fig. 3.15 Platelets

(EM (a) × 22 500 (b) × 22 500)

Micrograph (a) shows newly formed platelets just prior to being shed from a megakaryocyte **M** in the bone marrow. The endoplasmic reticulum **ER** of the megakaryocyte proliferates to form a three-dimensional network which partitions the cytoplasm into areas corresponding to the future platelets **P**. Platelets contain a variety of cytoplasmic organelles derived from the megakaryocyte, including mitochondria, rough endoplasmic reticulum, ribosomes and membrane-bound granules. After release into the general circulation, platelets assume a more regular biconvex disc shape as seen in micrograph (b).

The mature circulating platelets in humans contain membrane-bound granules of two types. One type, the so-called *very dense granules*, are sparse and are known to contain the blood vessel constrictor serotonin (5-hydroxytryptamine), ADP, ATP and calcium. The other type of granules, known as *alpha granules*, are more common and contain hydrolytic enzymes which include acid phosphatase and ß glucuronidase. Biochemical analysis has shown that platelets also contain stores of fibrinogen, a phospholipid called *platelet factor III*, and a protein complex called *thrombosthenin* which is analogous to the actin and myosin contractile complex of skeletal muscle (see Ch. 6).

ADP is thought to promote platelet aggregation during the formation of a platelet plug. Platelet fibrinogen probably supplements plasma fibrinogen during the early stages of haemostasis. Platelet factor III is involved in activating the clotting mechanism. Thrombosthenin may mediate the process of clot retraction thus producing a more stable clot. The function of the other platelet constituents is uncertain.

Haemopoiesis

Haemopoiesis is the process by which mature blood cells develop from precursor cells. In the human adult, haemopoiesis takes place in the marrow of certain bones, mainly the flat bones of the skull, the ribs and sternum, the vertebral column, the pelvis and the proximal ends of some long bones. Before maturity however, haemopoiesis occurs in other sites at different stages in development. In the early embryo, primitive blood cells arise in the yolk sac; a little later, the liver becomes the major site of haemopoiesis, and during further development, the spleen and lymph nodes supplement this activity. As the bones develop during the fourth and fifth months of intra-uterine life, haemopoiesis begins in the marrow cavities and by birth, haemopoiesis is almost exclusively restricted to the bone marrow. From birth to maturity, the number of active sites of haemopoiesis in bone marrow diminishes although all bone marrow retains haemopoietic potential.

The lineage of each blood cell type has been the subject of numerous theories but only one has gained substantial experimental support, the so-called *monophyletic theory*. This theory proposes that all blood cell types are derived from a single primitive stem cell type called a *multipotential stem cell*. The multipotential cells divide at a slow rate to replicate themselves and to give rise to five discrete cell types, each committed to a different developmental fate. Each of the five committed cell types is capable of giving rise to only one of the following cell types: erythrocytes, granulocytes, lymphocytes, monocytes and thrombocytes; thus such stem cells are referred to as *unipotential stem cells*. The unipotential stem cell divides at a rapid rate to provide histologically recognisable precursors of the mature cell type; however, there is no general agreement about the exact histological characteristics of multipotent stem cells. The rate of division of these cells is thought to be modulated by hormones called *poietins*, although only *erythropoietin* has been positively identified.

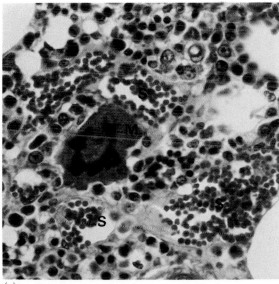

(a)

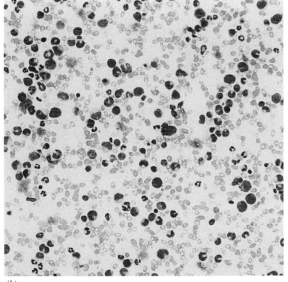

(b)

Fig. 3.16 Bone marrow

(a) Section, H & E × 600 (b) Aspirate, giemsa × 640

These micrographs contrast the appearance of bone marrow in histological section (a) with that of a bone marrow smear (b). In section, bone marrow is seen to consist of a mass of nucleated blood cell precursors pervaded by broad blood sinuses **S**. Specific blood cell precursors are difficult, if not impossible, to identify although megakaryocytes **M** are easily recognisable.

Aspirates of bone marrow are the usual means of studying haemopoiesis since whole unsectioned cells are visible and the cells are disaggregated in the anticoagulated smear.

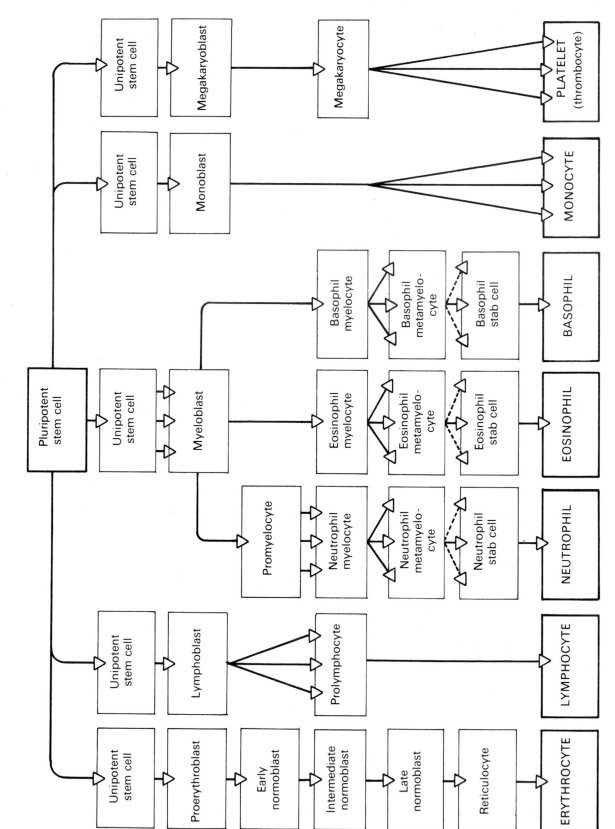

Fig. 3.17 Haemopoiesis (illustration opposite)

This diagram summarises the main recognisable developmental stages in blood cell formation; such a classification is somewhat arbitrary since the process of haemopoiesis is a continuum of proliferation and progressive differentiation from stem cell to the mature form found in circulating blood.

Red cell formation (erythropoiesis): the process of erythropoiesis is directed towards producing a cell devoid of organelles but packed with haemoglobin. The first recognisable erythrocyte precursor is known as the *proerythroblast*, a large cell with numerous cytoplasmic organelles and no haemoglobin. Further stages of differentiation are characterised by three main features:

1. Progressive decrease in cell size
2. Progressive loss of all organelles; the presence of numerous ribosomes at early stages accounts for the marked basophilic (blue) staining property of the cytoplasm which steadily decreases as the number of ribosomes (and rate of haemoglobin synthesis) falls
3. Progressive increase in the cytoplasmic content of haemoglobin; this accounts for the increasing eosinophilia (pink staining) of the cytoplasm towards maturity.

Haemoglobin synthesis begins during the *early normoblast (basophilic erythroblast)* stage and is complete by the end of the reticulocyte stage. Cell division ceases after the early normoblast stage, after which the nucleus progressively condenses and is finally extruded at the *late normoblast (orthochromatic erythroblast)* stage. The early normoblast stage also marks the beginning of the progressive loss of cytoplasmic organelles, only a few remnants of which remain by the reticulocyte stage. This process, accompanied by progressive haemoglobin synthesis, is represented morphologically by the transition from basophilia through polychromasia (intermediate normoblast) to the eosinophilia (*orthochromasia*) of the mature erythrocyte.

The process of erythropoiesis from stem cell to erythrocyte takes about one week. The rate of erythropoiesis is controlled by the hormone erythropoietin secreted by the kidney and by the availability of red cell components particularly iron, folic acid, vitamin B_{12} and protein precursors.

Granulocyte formation (granulopoiesis): the *myeloblast* is the earliest recognisable stage in granulopoiesis. The inappropriate name of myeloblast derives from an outdated view that granulocytes were the only white cells formed in *myeloid tissue* (bone marrow). Myeloblasts give rise to *promyelocytes* which are characterised by their content of azurophilic granules; since the azurophilic granules develop before the specific granules they were referred to as primary granules. As described earlier, the primary granules are merely large lysosomes.

From the promyelocyte stage onwards, the relative proportion of primary granules progressively decreases and the proportion of specific (secondary) granules progressively increases. From the *myelocyte* stage through the *metamyelocyte* stage to the mature granulocyte forms, the nucleus becomes increasingly segmented. The immediate precursors of mature granulocytes tend to have an irregular horseshoe or sometimes ring-shaped nucleus and are termed *stäb cells* or *band forms*.

Granulocytes are normally released from bone marrow only in the mature state but there is a large pool of metamyelocytes, stäb cells and mature granulocytes in the marrow; this pool contains some 15 times more cells than are present in the peripheral circulation. Thus the bone marrow is able to respond to acute inflammation by release of both mature and nearly mature cells into the bloodstream. The immature forms may be distinguished from mature cells not only by their less segmented nuclei but also by their higher content of azurophilic granules.

Lymphocyte formation (lymphopoiesis): only two precursor stages, the *lymphoblast* and the *prolymphocyte*, are recognisable in the development of lymphocytes. The main feature of lymphopoiesis is a progressive diminution in cell size.

Unlike other blood cell types, lymphocytes also proliferate outside the bone marrow. This occurs in the tissues of the immune system in response to specific immunological stimulation (see Ch. 11).

Monocyte formation (monopoiesis): the *monoblast* is the only recognisable precursor of the monocyte. Monopoiesis is characterised by a reduction in cell size and progressive indentation of the nucleus. Mature monocytes circulate in blood for only one or two days before becoming sequestered in the tissues as tissue macrophages.

Platelet formation (thrombopoiesis): platelet formation begins with the development of a large binucleate cell, the *megakaryoblast*. After this stage, fusion of the nuclei occurs and successive duplication of the nuclear material takes place without the formation of separate nuclei and without cell division. The resulting polyploid cell, the *megakaryocyte*, has an enormous volume of cytoplasm and the cell may reach 100 μm in diameter. Ultrastructural studies have shown that areas of cytoplasm representing the future platelets become demarcated by membranes and are eventually shed as platelets; whether the megakaryocyte synthesises further cytoplasm is uncertain.

In bone marrow smears, the earlier phases of haemopoiesis may be recognisable only with great difficulty. The characteristic, detailed features of each stage have been described using techniques of fixation and staining which are rarely applied in routine haematological practice. The recognition of such stages is of little practical value except in certain pathological conditions; under such circumstances the classical characteristics of each cell type are often distorted. Many of the later stages of haemopoiesis are readily recognisable in routine bone marrow smears, several of which are shown in the following micrographs.

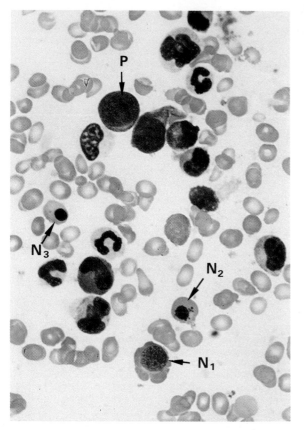

Fig. 3.18 Erythropoiesis

(Giemsa × 1200)

This bone marrow smear illustrates several stages in erythropoiesis. The proerythroblast **P** is the first recognisable erythrocyte precursor; the cell has a large, intensely stained, granular nucleus containing one or more paler nucleoli. The sparse cytoplasm is strongly basophilic due to its high content of RNA and lack of haemoglobin. A narrow, pale zone of cytoplasm close to the nucleus represents the Golgi apparatus.

Three increasingly differentiated normoblast forms can also be distinguished. An early normoblast (basophilic erythroblast) **N₁** is recognised by its basophilic cytoplasm and smaller nucleus with increasingly condensed chromatin. More advanced in the maturation sequence is an intermediate normoblast (polychromatic erythroblast) **N₂**, the cytoplasm of which exhibits both basophilia and eosinophilia (i.e. polychromasia), the latter due to increasing haemoglobin content. The nucleus is also condensed and is accompanied by several small fragments called *Howell-Jolly bodies*, an unusual finding in normal erythropoiesis. With further haemoglobin synthesis and degeneration of cytoplasmic ribosomes, the late normoblast (orthochromatic erythroblast) stage **N₃** is reached and by this time the nucleus is extremely condensed prior to being extruded from the cell.

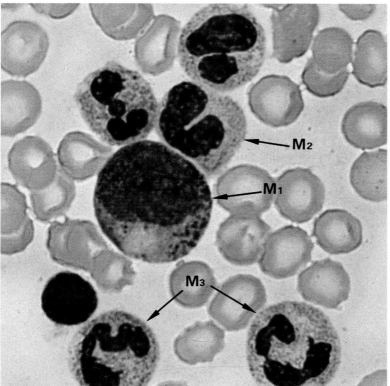

Fig. 3.19 Granulocyte precursors

(Giemsa × 1600)

This micrograph illustrates three phases of neutrophil granulocyte development. A neutrophil myelocyte **M₁** is recognised by a large, eccentrically located nucleus, a prominent Golgi apparatus and cytoplasm containing many azurophilic (primary) granules. The next stage towards maturity, the metamyelocyte **M₂**, is a smaller cell characterised by indentation of the nucleus and loss of prominence of the azurophilic granules. The final stage before maturity, the stäb cell **M₃**, has a more highly segmented nucleus approaching that of the mature neutrophil.

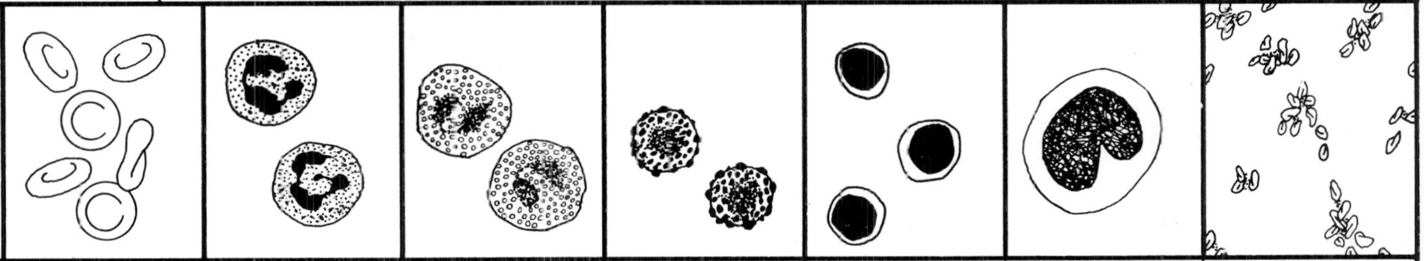

		Erythrocyte	Neutrophil	Eosinophil	Basophil	Lymphocyte	Monocyte	Platelets
Cell type		Erythrocyte	Neutrophil	Eosinophil	Basophil	Lymphocyte	Monocyte	Platelets
Size		6.7-7.7 μm	12-14 μm	16 μm	14-16 μm	9-16 μm	16-20 μm	2-3 μm
Number per litre		$3.9 - 6.5 \times 10^{12}$	$2.0 - 7.5 \times 10^{9}$	$1.3 - 3.5 \times 10^{9}$	$0 - 0.44 \times 10^{9}$	$0 - 0.1 \times 10^{9}$	$0.2 - 0.8 \times 10^{9}$	$150 - 400 \times 10^{9}$
Differential leucocyte count		—	40–75%	1–6%	<1%	20–45%	2–6%	—
Duration of development		5–7 days	6–9 days	6–9 days	3–7 days	1–2 days	2–3 days	4–5 days
Lifespan of mature cell		120 days	6 hours to a few days	8–12 days	?	?	months to years	8–12 days

Fig. 3.20 Mature cell types in the circulating blood of human adults

4. Connective tissue

Introduction

Connective tissue is the term applied to a basic type of tissue of mesodermal origin which provides structural and metabolic support for other tissues and organs throughout the body. Connective tissues carry blood vessels and mediate the exchange of nutrients, metabolites and waste products between tissues and the circulatory system. Connective tissues occur in many different forms with diverse physical properties. In most organs, loose connective tissues act as a biological packing material between other tissues with more specific functions; dense connective tissue provides tough support in the skin. Cartilage and bone, the major skeletal components, are rigid forms of connective tissue. Connective tissue has important metabolic roles such as the storage of fat, as in adipose tissue, while connective tissue elements constitute a major part of the body's defence mechanisms against pathogenic microorganisms. The processes of tissue repair are largely a function of connective tissues.

All connective tissues have two major constituents, *cells* and *extracellular material*. Extracellular material is the constituent which determines the physical properties of each type of connective tissue. Extracellular material consists of a matrix of organic material called *ground substance* within which are embedded a variety of *fibres*.

The cells of connective tissue

The cells of connective tissue may be divided into three types according to their basic function:

1. Cells responsible for synthesis and maintenance of the extracellular material. These cells are termed *fibroblasts*, and are derived from precursor cells in primitive connective tissue which is called *mesenchyme*.

2. Cells responsible for the storage and metabolism of fat. These cells are individually known as *adipocytes* and may collectively form *adipose connective tissue*.

3. Cells with defence and immune functions.

Ground substance

Ground substance is an amorphous transparent material which has the properties of a semi-fluid gel. Tissue fluid is loosely bound to ground substance, thereby forming the medium for passage of materials throughout connective tissues and for the exchange of metabolites with the circulatory system.

Ground substance consists of a mixture of long, unbranched polysaccharide chains of seven different types, each composed of repeating disaccharide units. One of the disaccharide units is always an amino sugar, either N-acetyl glucosamine or N-acetyl galactosamine, thus giving rise to the modern descriptive term *glycosaminoglycans* (formerly called *mucopolysaccarides*); the glycosaminoglycans are acidic (negatively-charged) due to the presence of hydroxyl, carboxyl and sulphate side groups on the disaccharide units. *Hyaluronic acid* is the predominant glycosaminoglycan in the loose connective tissues and is the only one without sulphate side groups; the other glycosaminoglycans (*chondroitin-4-sulphate, chondroitin-6-sulphate, dermatan sulphate, heparan sulphate, heparin sulphate* and *keratan sulphate*) differ from hyaluronic acid in that they are covalently linked to a variety of protein molecules to form *proteoglycans* (formerly known as *mucoproteins*); these proteoglycans are huge molecules consisting of 90–95% carbohydrate. Further, the proteoglycans may form non-covalent links with hyaluronic acid chains to form even larger molecular complexes.

Unlike many proteins, glycosaminoglycan molecules are not flexible enough to form globular aggregates but remain in an expanded form, thus occupying a huge volume for relatively small mass. In addition, their highly charged side groups render them extremely hydrophilic thus attracting a large volume of water and positive ions, particularly sodium, which constitute extracellular fluid. The extracellular fluid imparts the characteristic turgor of connective tissue.

Thus, ground substance is basically composed of glycosaminoglycans in the form of hyaluronic acid and proteoglycans, these huge molecules being entangled and electrostatically linked to one another and their water of hydration, to form a flexible gel through which metabolites may diffuse. The mechanical properties of ground substance are reinforced by the fibrous proteins of the extracellular tissue to which the components of ground substance are also bound. Ground substance, due to its physical nature, is an important barrier to the spread of microorganisms; it is noteworthy that some pathogenic bacteria produce the enzyme hyaluronidase to facilitate their spread.

The fibres of connective tissue

The fibrous components of connective tissue are of three main types; *collagen* (including *reticulin* which was formerly considered a separate fibre type), *elastin* and *structural glycoproteins*.

1. **Collagen** is the principal fibre type found in the extracellular matrix of most connective tissues and is the most abundant protein in the human body. Collagen is secreted into the extracellular matrix in the form of *tropocollagen* which consists of three polypeptide chains bound together to form a helical structure 260 nm long and 1.5 nm in diameter. In the extracellular matrix, the tropocollagen molecules polymerise to form collagen of five different types designated I to V on the basis of morphology, amino acid composition and physical properties.

Type I *collagen* constitutes about 90% of the total collagen in the body and is found in fibrous connective tissue, skin, tendon, ligaments and bone, in a variable arrangement from loose to dense according to the mechanical support required. The tropocollagen molecules are aggregated to form fibres strengthened by numerous intermolecular bonds. Parallel collagen fibres are further arranged into strong bundles which confer great tensile strength to the connective tissue; these bundles are visible in the light microscope. *Type* II *collagen* is found in hyaline cartilage and consists of fine fibrils which are dispersed in the ground substance. *Type* III *collagen* makes up the fibre type known as reticulin which was previously thought to represent a separate species of fibre because of its affinity for silver salts by which it is stained black. Reticulin fibres form the delicate 'reticular' supporting meshwork in highly cellular tissues such as the liver and lymphoid organs. *Collagen types* IV and V do not form fibrils; type IV collagen is present in basement membranes (see Fig. 5.20) and type V collagen is found in small amounts in most connective tissues but its structure and function are as yet poorly understood.

2. **Elastin** is a rubber-like material which is arranged as fibres and discontinuous sheets in the extracellular matrix particularly of skin, lung and blood vessels. Like collagen, elastin is synthesised by fibroblasts in a precursor form known as *tropoelastin* which undergoes polymerisation in the extracellular tissues. Polymerisation requires the presence of glycoprotein microfibrils which become incorporated in the final fibres or sheets.

3. The **structural glycoproteins**, only recently identified, are a group of fibre-forming molecules composed principally of protein chains bound to branched polysaccharides. The structural glycoproteins which include *fibronectin* and *laminin* (which is found in epithelial basement membranes) are known to be associated with cell surface membranes where they appear to play a role in cell-to-cell interactions.

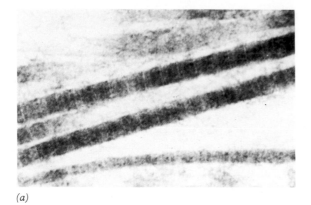

(a)

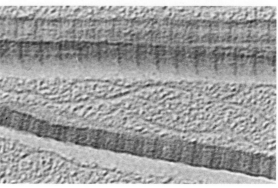

(b)

Fig. 4.1 Collagen

(EM × 124 000 (a) Section (b) Teased preparation)

The typical appearance of Type I collagen, the commonest variety, is shown in these specimens. The characteristic feature is a pattern of cross-banding with a periodicity of approximately 64 nm which results from the polymerisation of tropocollagen molecules (260 nm in length) such that each molecule overlaps the next by approximately one-quarter of its length.

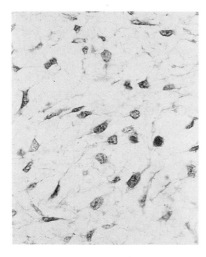

Fig. 4.2 Primitive mesenchyme

(H & E × 320)

Primitive mesenchyme is the embryological tissue from which all types of connective tissue, including that of the skeleton, are derived. Mesenchymal cells are relatively unspecialised and are believed to be capable of differentiation into all the cell types found in mature connective tissue. Some mesenchymal cells remain in fully mature connective tissue and provide a pluripotential source of cells as the need arises for replacement or repair of connective tissues.

Primitive mesenchymal cells have an irregular, stellate shape with delicate branching cytoplasmic extensions which form an interlacing network throughout the tissue. The oval nuclei have dispersed chromatin and prominent nucleoli. The extracellular material consists almost exclusively of ground substance and does not contain mature fibres. In this respect, mesenchyme forms a very loose variant of connective tissue which, in the well developed fetus, is referred to as *mucous connective tissue*. The circulatory system of the embryo is poorly developed until a late stage; mesenchyme thus constitutes an important medium for the diffusion of metabolites to and from developing tissues.

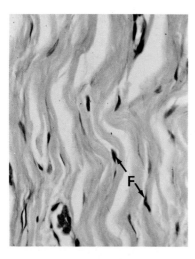

Fig. 4.3 Mature fibroblasts

(H & E × 320)

This micrograph demonstrates the typical histological appearance of mature fibroblasts in loose connective tissue; collagen fibres are stained pink in this preparation. The fibroblast nuclei **F** are condensed and elongated in the direction of the extracellular fibres. The cytoplasm is reduced and spindle-shaped, with long cytoplasmic processes extending into the matrix to meet up with those of other fibroblasts; the cytoplasmic extensions are usually difficult to see with the light microscope. The main function of fibroblasts is to maintain the integrity of connective tissues by continuous slow turnover of the extracellular elements.

It is customary to describe a precursor or immature cell by the suffix 'blast' as in erythroblast (see Fig. 3.17) and the mature form by the suffix 'cyte' as in erythrocyte. This convention, however, is not commonly used to describe fibroblasts, where the term 'fibrocyte' might be more appropriate for the mature form.

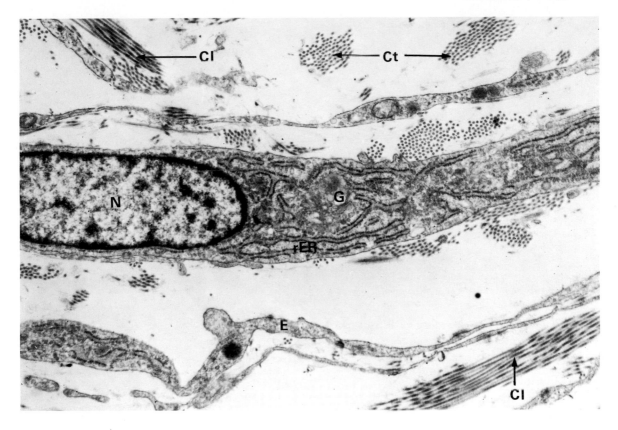

Fig. 4.4 Fibroblast

(EM × 12 000)

This micrograph illustrates the body of a mature fibroblast within loose, collagenous connective tissue. Fine tapering cytoplasmic extensions **E** of adjacent fibroblasts can be seen on either side of the central fibroblast. Bundles of collagen fibres are seen in transverse **Ct** and longitudinal section **Cl** in the extracellular matrix. The nucleus **N** is moderately condensed, and nucleoli are not a prominent feature. The small quantity of cytoplasm contains a relatively sparse network of rough endoplasmic reticulum **rER**; the Golgi apparatus **G** is poorly developed and few mitochondria are present. During active synthesis of extracellular fibres, both the rough endoplasmic reticulum and Golgi apparatus become prominent features of a much more extensive cytoplasm. Fibroblasts synthesise and secrete the precursors of collagen, elastin, the glycosaminoglycans and all other extracellular constituents. In the mature, non-active fibroblast, relatively few secretory vesicles are found within the cytoplasm.

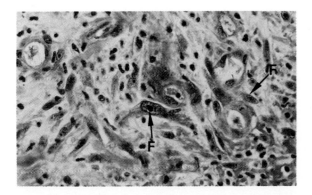

Fig. 4.5 Active fibroblasts: healing wound

(H & E × 400)

Active fibroblasts **F** are readily demonstrated in healing wounds, as in this micrograph. The nuclei are large and rounded in shape with prominent nucleoli suggesting active protein synthesis. The cytoplasm is extensive and its strongly stained, granular appearance is evidence of an extensive system of rough endoplasmic reticulum involved in protein synthesis. The relative absence of formed fibres in the extracellular matrix reveals the fine meshwork of cytoplasmic extensions between fibroblasts.

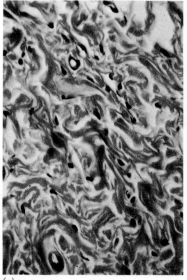
(a)

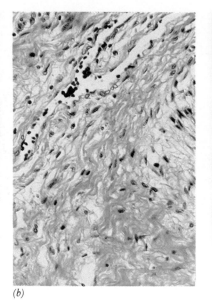
(b)

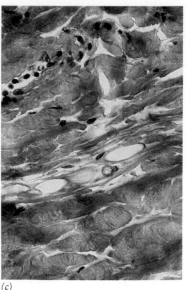
(c)

Fig. 4.6 Dense irregular connective tissue

(a) H & E × 320 (b) Masson's trichrome × 320 (c) Azan × 320

These micrographs all illustrate collagen fibres in dense irregular connective tissue stained by three common histological methods. Collagen is acidophilic due to its positively-charged side groups, thus in standard H & E preparations collagen is eosinophilic (i.e. pink-stained), with the trichrome stain, collagen stains green or blue depending on the variant of the stain used, and with the Azan staining method, collagen is deep blue.

Dense irregular connective tissue is typically found in the skin where the collagen fibres are arranged in coarse irregular interwoven bundles which confer great tensile strength. The fibroblasts are inactive with highly condensed nuclei and minimal cytoplasm.

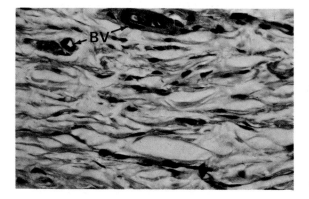

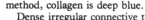

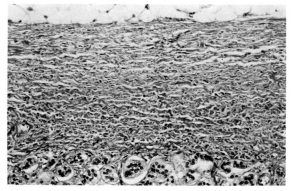

Fig. 4.7 Loose (areolar) connective tissue

(H & E × 320)

Loose collagenous connective tissue supports the epithelial linings of the gastrointestinal, respiratory and urinary tracts, forms the deeper layers of the skin and occurs as a loose interstitial packing in many other organs. The collagen fibres are loosely arranged and have a wavy appearance in unstretched preparations. The open *(areolar)* spaces between collagen fibres are filled with ground substance which is not stained in this type of preparation since it is dissolved away during tissue processing.

The relatively inactive fibroblasts are recognised by their densely stained and elongated nuclei. Several small blood vessels **BV** are seen.

Fig. 4.8 Dense regular connective tissue

(H & E × 128)

This micrograph of the capsule of the adrenal gland shows the typical dense arrangement of collagen fibres where mechanical support is the primary function. The collagen fibres are elongated and arranged in a regular manner to provide a well organised and robust enveloping capsule. Fibroblast nuclei are elongated in the direction of the collagen fibres.

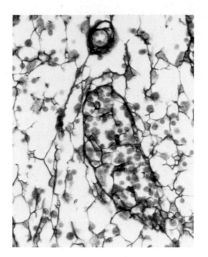

Fig. 4.9 Reticulin fibres

(Silver impregnation method/Haemotoxylin × 800)

Reticular connective tissue forms a delicate supporting framework for many highly cellular organs such as endocrine glands, lymph nodes and the liver. In such organs, a fine network of branching fibres ramifies throughout the parenchyma usually anchored to a dense, collagenous capsule and septae which traverse the tissue. Reticulin is a non-banded form of collagen designated collagen Type III.

Reticulin fibres are usually poorly stained in common preparations but are able to absorb metallic silver and are thus stained black with silver nitrate solutions under appropriate conditions. This phenomenon led early histologists to believe that reticulin had a completely different chemical composition from that of collagen. Reticulin is the earliest type of collagen fibre to be produced during the development of all connective tissues and is also present in varying quantities in most mature connective tissues.

This micrograph shows the fine reticular architecture of part of a lymph node; this framework provides a loose support for lymphoid cells, the nuclei of which have been counterstained blue.

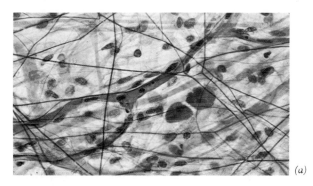

(a)

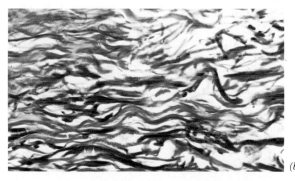

(b)

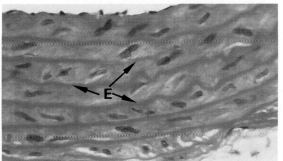

(c)

Fig. 4.10 Elastin fibres

(a) Areolar spread, Elastin/H & E × 320 (b) Elastic van Gieson × 320 (c) H & E × 400

Elastin is a protein found in varying proportions in most connective tissues where it confers elastic properties which enable recovery of tissue shape following normal physiological deformation or stretching. Elastin is thus present in large amounts in tissues such as lung, skin and bladder. In most tissues, elastin occurs as short branching fibres which form an irregular network throughout the tissue. This three-dimensional network is not easily seen in sections but is better demonstrated in spread preparations. In the spread of areolar connective tissue shown in micrograph (a) the elastin fibres are stained black, collagen fibres are stained pink and nuclei are stained blue.

Elastin is synthesised and secreted by fibroblasts as the precursor form *tropoelastin* which polymerises in the extracellular matrix to form fibres.

As mentioned above, elastin fibres are difficult to demonstrate in histological sections. In large arteries however, elastin is disposed in fenestrated sheets and these are thick enough to be visible with light microscopy.

Micrograph (b) shows a histological section of the wall of a large artery stained specifically for elastin; with this method, elastin is stained black, collagen is stained red and smooth muscle cells are stained yellow.

Micrograph (c) shows a similar specimen stained by the standard H & E method. Like the collagen and smooth muscle cytoplasm, the elastin E is eosinophilic and it is only recognisable in this situation because the elastin sheets are so thick and because the elastin has a relaxed wavy conformation, the vessel wall being collapsed.

Adipose tissue

Most connective tissues contain cells which are adapted for the storage of fat; these cells, called *adipocytes*, are derived from primitive mesenchyme. Adipocytes are found in isolation or in clumps throughout loose connective tissue, or may constitute the main cell type as in adipose tissue.

Stored fat within adipocytes is derived from three main sources: dietary fat circulating in the blood stream as chylomicrons, triglycerides synthesised in the liver and transported in blood, and triglycerides synthesised from glucose within adipocytes. Adipose tissue is often regarded as an inactive energy store, however it is an extremely important participant in general metabolic processes in that it acts as a temporary store of substrate for the energy-deriving processes of almost all tissues. Adipose tissue, therefore, generally has a rich blood supply. The rate of fat deposition and utilisation within adipose tissue is largely determined by dietary intake and energy expenditure, but a number of hormones and the sympathetic nervous system profoundly influence the fat metabolism of adipocytes.

There are two main types of adipose tissue, *white* and *brown adipose tissue:*

1. **White adipose tissue:** this type of adipose tissue comprises up to 20% of total body weight in normal, well-nourished male adults and up to 25% in females. It is distributed throughout the body particularly in the deep layers of the skin (see Ch. 9). In addition to being an important energy store, white adipose tissue acts as a thermal insulator under the skin and functions as a cushion against mechanical shock in such sites as around the kidneys.

2. **Brown adipose tissue:** this highly specialised type of adipose tissue is found in newborn mammals and some hibernating animals, where it plays an important part in body temperature regulation. Only small amounts of brown adipose tissue are found in human adults and, although previously thought to contribute little to thermoregulation, there is now increasing evidence that, at least in some individuals, brown adipose tissue may play a role in burning off excess energy thus preventing obesity.

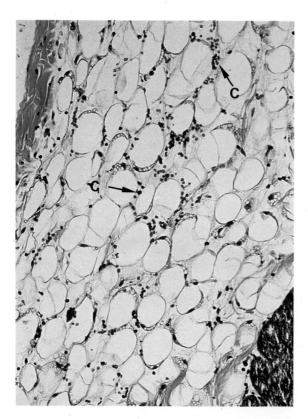

Fig. 4.11 White adipose tissue
(Masson's trichrome × 480)

The typical appearance of white adipose tissue is illustrated in this micrograph. Fat stored in adipocytes accumulates as lipid droplets which fuse to form a single large droplet which distends and occupies most of the cytoplasm. The adipocyte nucleus is compressed and displaced to one side of the stored lipid droplet and the cytoplasm is reduced to a small rim around the periphery. In commonly used, routine histological sections, the lipid content of adipocytes is extracted during tissue processing leaving a large, unstained space within each cell.

Ultrastructural studies have shown that the cytoplasm of white adipocytes contains the usual organelles; the single lipid droplet is not bounded by a membrane and new lipid droplets entering the cell readily fuse with the major droplet which is highly accessible to the enzymes responsible for triglyceride breakdown when the need arises.

Note the minute dimensions of capillaries C compared with the size of the surrounding adipocytes.

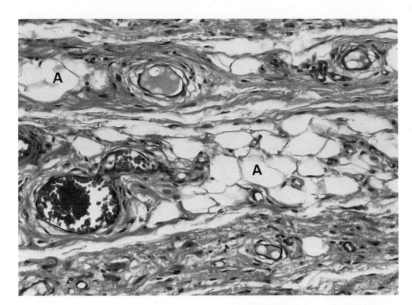

Fig. 4.12 Fibrofatty connective tissue

(H & E × 200)

This micrograph demonstrates the typical appearance of adipocytes **A** distributed amongst loose, collagenous connective tissue. Adipocytes occur either singly or in groups in loose connective tissues, particularly those supporting the gastrointestinal tract lining. Like the adipocytes of white adipose tissue, the size of adipocytes in loose connective tissue depends on the equilibrium between dietary fat intake and energy expenditure.

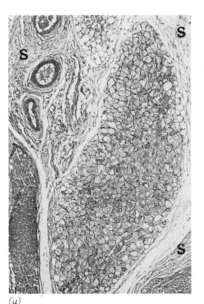

(a)

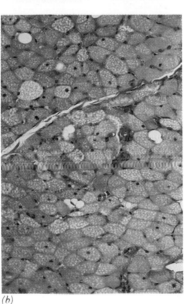

(b)

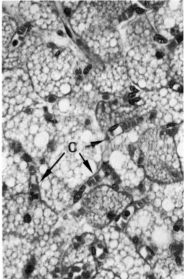

(c)

Fig. 4.13 Brown adipose tissue

(H & E (a) × 100 (b) × 200 (c) × 320)

These micrographs demonstrate the typical histological appearance of brown adipose tissue. Brown adipose tissue may be differentiated from white adipose tissue on the basis of the following features. Firstly, lipid is stored in the form of multiple, small vesicles rather than a single, large droplet; this gives the cytoplasm of brown adipocytes a vacuolated appearance. Secondly, brown adipocytes have a relatively large amount of cytoplasm which is strongly stained due to a high content of mitochondria. Thirdly, brown adipose tissue is extremely vascular. Fourthly, brown adipose tissue is arranged in lobules separated by connective tissue septae **S** which convey blood vessels and sympathetic nerve fibres. These characteristics have led some histologists to compare the appearance of brown adipose tissue to that of steroid-secreting endocrine glands (see Ch. 16) and indeed the discrete adipose tissue of hibernating mammals has been inappropriately named the 'hibernating gland'.

At high magnification in micrograph (c), the nuclei of brown adipocytes are seen to be eccentrically located within the cell, but unlike the nuclei of white adipocytes, the nuclei are plump and surrounded by a significant quantity of strongly eosinophilic cytoplasm. The stored lipid is contained within multiple droplets, all of which have been dissolved away during tissue processing; a frozen section of brown adipose tissue stained for lipid is shown in Figure 1.25(b). Note also the rich network of capillaries **C** between the brown adipocytes.

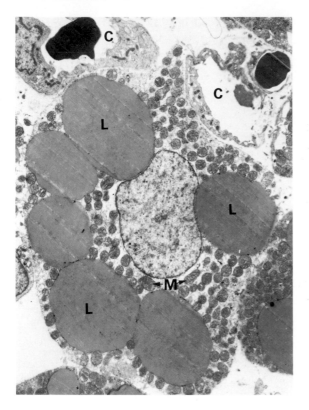

Fig. 4.14 Brown adipocyte

(Rabbit: EM × 4070)

The multilocular nature of stored lipid **L** within brown adipocytes is seen in this electron micrograph of brown adipose tissue taken from a newborn rabbit. The cytoplasm of brown adipocytes is crammed with mitochondria **M** which have numerous, closely packed cristae. These mitochondria are extremely rich in cytochromes, molecules involved in oxidative energy production; this accounts for the brown colour of brown adipose tissue when examined macroscopically.

Unlike the metabolism of other tissues, in brown adipose cells the process of electron transport is readily uncoupled from the phosphorylation of ADP to form ATP. The energy derived from oxidation of lipids, and energy released by electron transport in the uncoupled state, is dissipated as heat; this is rapidly conducted to the rest of the body by the rich vascular network of brown adipose tissue. Note the intimate association of capillaries **C** with the brown adipocyte in this micrograph.

Using these metabolic processes, neonatal humans and other mammals utilise brown adipose tissue to generate body heat during the vulnerable period after birth. Brown adipose tissue undergoes involution in early infancy and in adult humans is found only in odd sites such as around the adrenal gland and great vessels. The production of heat by brown adipose tissue is controlled directly by the sympathetic nervous system.

The defence cells of connective tissue

The basic connective tissues not only contain cells responsible for synthesis, maintenance and metabolic activity, but also contain a variety of cells with defence and immune functions. Traditonally, these cells have been divided into two categories: fixed (intrinsic) cells and wandering (extrinsic) cells. The fixed category included *tissue macrophages (histiocytes)* and *mast cells*. Tissue macrophages are now generally believed to be derived from circulating monocytes (see Fig. 3.12) which have become at least temporarily resident in connective tissues. Mast cells are functionally analogous to basophils (see Fig. 3.10) but there are structural differences which suggest that mast cells are not merely basophils resident in connective tissues. The wandering category of defence and immune cells includes all the remaining members of the white blood cell series (see Ch. 3). Although leucocytes are usually considered as a constituent of blood, their principal site of activity is outside the blood circulation, particularly within loose connective tissues. Leucocytes are normally found only in relatively small numbers within connective tissues but in response to inflammation and other disease processes their numbers increase greatly. The connective tissues of those regions of the body which are subject to the constant threat of pathogenic invasion, such as the gastrointestinal and respiratory tracts, contain a large population of leucocytes, even in the absence of overt disease.

The reticulo-endothelial concept

The term *reticulo-endothelial system* has long been used to describe a diverse group of cells found in many tissues but in particular the bone marrow, liver, spleen, lymph nodes and thymus. The principal functional charactaristic of such cells is their ability to phagocytise particulate matter and effete (worn out or dead) cells, e.g. old blood cells. Such phagocytic cells are found lining certain blood and lymph-filled spaces, such as the sinusoids of the liver (see Fig. 15.8), bone marrow (see Fig. 10.17) and spleen (see Fig. 11.18), and in this context they have some features in common with the endothelial cells which line all blood and lymphatic vessels (see Ch. 8).

Certain highly cellular tissues, such as lymph nodes (see Fig. 11.6) and the haemopoeitic cords of bone marrow, have a supporting framework of reticulin fibres (see Fig. 4.9) upon which are draped cells with long cytoplasmic processes morphologically similar to primitive mesenchymal cells (see Fig. 4.2); these cells are traditionally described as *reticulum cells*. Some if not all of the cells are probably responsible for synthesis of the reticulin framework, being thus analogous to fibroblasts, and many of these cells, if not all, may exhibit considerable phagocytic activity.

Because of the close structural and functional association of these cell types with the haemopoietic, macrophage-monocyte (see Fig. 3.12) and immune systems, they were thought to represent some common functional denominator. Consequently, 'reticulo-endothelial' and related terms became widely and often indiscriminately applied to tissues and cells within these systems. Scientific advances have rendered the concept so imprecise as to serve little purpose and it should now be considered of historical interest only.

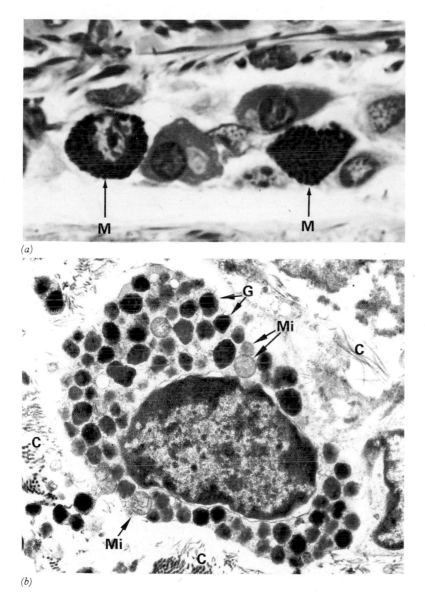

(a)

(b)

Fig. 4.15 Mast cells

(a) Thin section, toluidine blue × 1200
(b) EM × 5250

Mast cells are found in connective tissues, particularly in association with blood vessels.

Mast cells are not readily identified in routine histological preparations; with suitable staining, however, the characteristic feature of mast cells is an extensive cytoplasm packed with large granules. When stained with certain blue basic dyes such as toluidine blue, the granules bind to the dye changing its colour to red. This property is known as *metachromasia*. In mast cells, metachromasia is thought to be due to the presence of a highly acidic sulphated glycosaminoglycan called *heparin*, which is a potent blood anticoagulant. Mast cell granules also contain histamine, one of the chemical mediators of inflammation, which causes dilatation of small vessels and increases capillary permeability. It is proposed, therefore, that mast cells are primarily involved in inflammatory and immune mechanisms.

Mast cell granules are similar in composition to basophil granules, but there is no evidence that mast cells are merely basophils resident in connective tissues, although both cell types appear to have similar actions and may degranulate in response to similar stimuli as described with Fig. 3.10.

This micrograph of the connective tissue underlying the tracheal surface demonstrates two mast cells **M**. A pale nucleus can be seen in one cell but the plane of section is outside the nucleus of the other. Note the large, densely packed granules which exhibit metachromasia.

With electron microscopy in micrograph (b) mast cell granules **G** are seen to be membrane-bound and to contain a dense amorphous material. The granules are liberated from the cell by exocytosis when stimulated during an inflammatory or allergic response. The cytoplasm contains several rounded mitochondria **Mi**, but little rough endoplasmic reticulum. Note also the collagen fibrils **C** in the extracellular matrix.

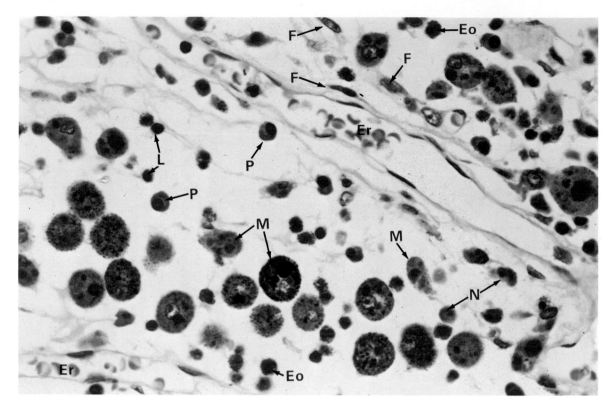

Fig. 4.16 Leucocytes in loose connective tissue

(H & E × 640)

The appearance of leucocytes within sections of connective and other tissues differs greatly from the appearance seen in blood smears (see Ch. 3). In this micrograph, a variety of leucocytes are seen in the loose connective tissue supporting the lining of the large intestine, a site which is normally rich in such cells even in the absence of inflammation.

Fibroblasts **F**, are identified by their relatively large, elongated nuclei. Erythrocytes **Er** within small blood vessels are intensely eosinophilic (red stained); the presence of erythrocytes (approximate diameter 7 μm) provides a reference for the size of other cells. Of the granulocyte series (see Ch. 3), neutrophils are only rarely seen in tissues except in acute or chronic inflammation. Neutrophils **N** are recognised by their multilobed nuclei and poorly stained cytoplasm. Eosinophils **Eo** are present in large numbers in normal connective tissues and are recognised by their bilobed nuclei and strongly eosinophilic cytoplasmic granules. Basophils, and their analogues mast cells, are poorly stained in H & E preparations and are therefore difficult to recognise.

Lymphocytes **L** are easily recognised by their small, densely-stained nuclei and a thin halo of poorly stained cytoplasm. Plasma cells **P**, immunologically activated lymphocytes responsible for antibody synthesis (see Ch. 11), are recognised by their large granular nuclei and extensive basophilic (blue-stained) cytoplasm containing a pale stained peri-nuclear area which represents a well-developed and active Golgi apparatus. The basophilia of plasma cells is largely attributable to profuse rough endoplasmic reticulum, involved in the synthesis of antibody molecules.

Large mononuclear phagocytes, analogous to the monocytes of blood, are distributed throughout all connective tissues where they may exhibit intense phagocytic activity; these cells are also known as macrophages, tissue-fixed macrophages, and histiocytes when present in connective tissue. The macrophages of connective tissue drape themselves on the fibres of the matrix when inactive; actively phagocytic macrophages, however, may move in an amoeboid manner through the ground substance. Macrophages and monocytes have a common origin in primitive mesenchymal cells of bone marrow. Recent evidence suggests that monocytes and all macrophages should be considered as members of a single functional unit, *the macrophage-monocyte system* (see also Fig. 3.12). Inactive macrophages are often difficult to visualise in histological sections, but when actively phagocytic, macrophages may be easily recognised by their large size and content of engulfed material; note, however, that active macrophages have an extremely variable appearance, depending on the nature of their phagocytic activity. Most of the cytoplasmic detail of the macrophages **M** shown in this preparation is obscured by engulfed material which appears brown. For comparison, a different example of the appearance of active macrophages is seen in Figure 11.7 (b).

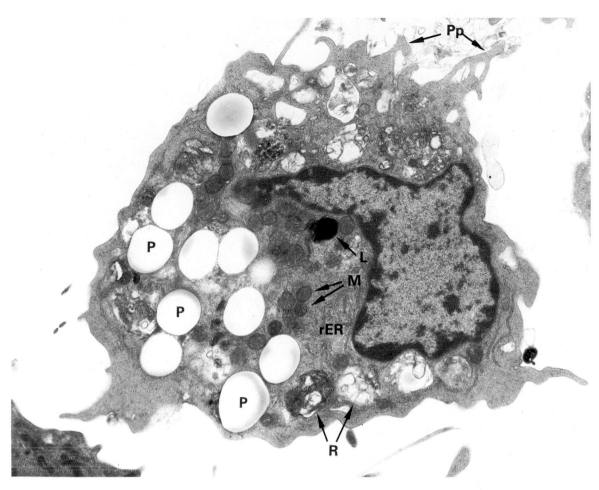

Fig. 4.17 Macrophage

(EM × 11 600)

The ultrastructural features of macrophages vary widely according to their state of activity and tissue location. This micrograph shows an active macrophage obtained from the peritoneum of a rat which had previously been injected intra-peritoneally with latex particles; a number of particles **P** have been engulfed by the macrophage.

The macrophage nucleus is irregular with heterochromatin typically clumped around the nuclear envelope. The cytoplasm contains a few mitochondria **M** and a variable amount of free ribosomes and rough endoplasmic reticulum **rER**. In quiescent macrophages, lysosomes **L** are abundant but their number is much reduced in actively phagocytic cells; lysosomes are later regenerated by the Golgi apparatus. The macrophage cytoplasm contains an assortment of phagosomes and residual bodies **R**. Residual material may be released from the macrophage by exocytosis; such material may remain sequestered in the tissues, as occurs with the dyes used in tattooing of the skin, or the material may be returned to the circulation for excretion or re-use in biosynthetic processes. Actively phagocytic cells exhibit irregular cytoplasmic projections or pseudopodia **Pp** which are involved in amoeboid movement and phagocytosis.

In addition to their role as tissue scavengers, macrophages play an important role in immune mechanisms (see Ch. 11) since they are often the first cells to make contact with antigens. Macrophages process antigenic material in some way before presenting it to lymphocytes; lymphocytes are then stimulated to undergo specific immune responses. As a result of various immune mechanisms, antigenic material may become combined or coated with substances such as antibodies and complement which are then collectively known as *opsonins*. Opsonins greatly enhance the phagocytic ability of macrophages and other phagocytes such as neutrophils (see Ch. 3), a process which is known as *opsonisation*. Other substances such as lymphokines, which are released during the immune response, act directly upon macrophages to increase greatly their metabolic and phagocytic activity.

5. Epithelial tissues

Introduction

The epithelia are a diverse group of tissues which, with rare exceptions, line all body surfaces, cavities and tubes. Epithelia thus function as interfaces between biological compartments. Epithelial interfaces are involved in a wide range of activities such as absorption, secretion and protection and all these major functions may be exhibited at a single epithelial surface. For example, the epithelial lining of the small intestine is primarily involved in absorption of the products of digestion, but the epithelium also protects itself from noxious intestinal contents by the secretion of a surface coating of mucus.

Surface epithelia consist of one or more layers of cells separated by a minute quantity of intercellular material which may represent the fused glycocalyces of adjacent cells (see Ch. 1). Epithelial cells are closely bound to one another by a variety of specialisations of the cell membrane which may also allow exchange of 'information' and metabolites (see Fig. 5.24).

All epithelia are supported by a *basement membrane* of variable thickness. Basement membranes separate epithelia from underlying connective tissues and are never penetrated by blood vessels; epithelia are thus dependent on the diffusion of oxygen and metabolites from underlying tissues. Basement membranes consist of a condensation of ground substance reinforced by fibres which merge with those of the underlying connective tissue; both epithelial and connective tissue cells are thought to participate in the formation of basement membranes (see Fig. 5.20).

Classification of epithelia

Epithelia are classified according to three morphological characteristics:

1. The number of cell layers: a single layer of epithelial cells is termed *simple epithelium*, whereas epithelia composed of more than one layer are termed *stratified epithelia*.

2. The shape of the component cells when seen in sections taken at right angles to the epithelial surface: in stratified epithelia the shape of the outermost layer of cells determines the descriptive classification. Cellular outlines are often difficult to distinguish, but the shape of epithelial cells is usually reflected in the shape of their nuclei.

3. The presence of surface specialisations such as cilia and keratin: an example is the epithelial surface of skin which is classified as 'stratified squamous keratinising epithelium' since it consists of many layers of cells, the surface cells of which are flattened (squamous) in shape and covered by an outer layer of the proteinaceous material, keratin (see Fig. 5.14).

Epithelia may be derived from ectoderm, mesoderm or endoderm although in the past it was thought that true epithelia were only of ectodermal or endodermal origin; two types of epithelia derived from mesoderm, the lining of blood and lymphatic vessels and the linings of the serous body cavities, were not considered to be epithelia and were termed *endothelium* and *mesothelium* respectively. By both morphological and functional criteria, such distinction has little practical value, nevertheless, the terms endothelium and mesothelium are still used to describe these types of epithelium.

Glandular epithelia

Epithelium which is primarily involved in secretion is often arranged into structures called *glands*. Glands are merely invaginations of epithelial surfaces which are formed during embryonic development by proliferation of epithelium into the underlying connective tissues. Those glands which maintain their continuity with the epithelial surface via a duct are called *exocrine glands* and secrete onto the free surface. In some cases, the duct degenerates during development to leave isolated islands of epithelial secretory tissue deep within other tissues. These glands, known as *endocrine* or *ductless glands*, secrete directly into the bloodstream and their secretions are known as hormones (see Ch. 17); in addition, some endocrine glands develop by migration of epithelial cells into connective tissues, without the formation of a duct.

Simple epithelia

Simple epithelia are defined as surface epithelia consisting of a single layer of cells. Simple epithelia are almost always found on absorptive or secretory surfaces; they provide little protetion against mechanical abrasion and thus are almost never found on surfaces subject to such stresses. The cells comprising simple epithelia range in shape from extremely flattened to tall columnar, depending on their function. For example, flattened simple epithelia present little barrier to passive diffusion and are therefore found in sites such as the lung alveoli and the lining of blood vessels. In contrast, highly active epithelial cells, such as the cells lining the small intestine, are generally tall since they must accommodate the appropriate organelles. Simple epithelia may exhibit a variety of surface specialisations, such as microvilli and cilia, which facilitate their specific surface functions.

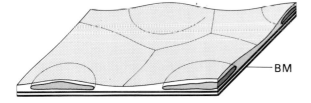

Fig. 5.1 Simple squamous epithelium

Simple squamous epithelium is composed of flattened, irregularly-shaped cells forming a continuous surface which is often referred to as *pavemented epithelium*. Like all epithelia, this delicate lining is supported by an underlying basement membrane **BM**.

Simple squamous epithelium is often found lining surfaces involved in passive transport of either gases, such as in the lungs, or fluids, such as in the walls of blood capillaries. Simple squamous epithelium also forms a delicate lining to the pleural, pericardial and peritoneal cavities where it permits passage of tissue fluid into and out of these cavities; the simple squamous epithelium of these sites is traditionally known as mesothelium.

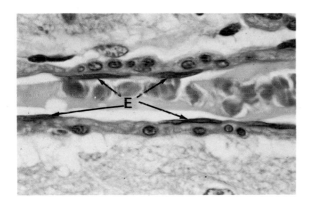

Fig. 5.2 Simple squamous epithelium

(H & E × 800)

This micrograph of a small blood vessel illustrates the typical appearance of simple squamous epithelium in section; the epithelial lining cells **E** (known as endothelium in the circulatory system) are so flattened that they can only be recognised by their nuclei which bulge into the vessel lumen. The supporting basement membrane is thin and, in haematoxylin and eosin stained preparations, has similar staining properties to the endothelial cell cytoplasm; hence the basement membrane cannot be seen in this micrograph.

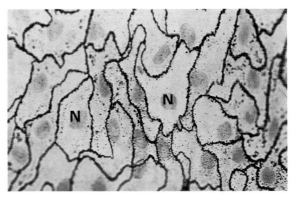

Fig. 5.3 Simple squamous epithelium

(Spread preparation, silver method × 320)

In this preparation, the mesothelial lining of the peritoneal cavity has been stripped from the underlying connective tissues and spread onto a slide thus permitting a surface view of simple squamous epithelium. The intercellular substance has been stained with silver thereby outlining the closely interdigitating cell boundaries; the nuclei **N** have been stained with the dye, neutral red.

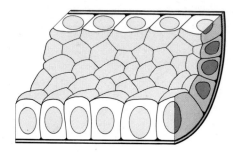

Fig. 5.4 Simple cuboidal epithelium

Simple cuboidal epithelium represents an intermediate form between simple squamous and simple columnar epithelium; the distinction between tall cuboidal and low columnar is often arbitrary and is of descriptive value only. In section perpendicular to the basement membrane, the epithelial cells appear square, leading to its traditional description as cuboidal epithelium; on surface view, however, the cells are actually polygonal in shape.

Simple cuboidal epithelium usually lines small ducts and tubules which may have excretory, secretory or absorptive functions; examples are the small collecting ducts of the kidney, salivary glands and pancreas.

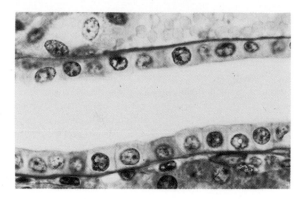

Fig. 5.5 Simple cuboidal epithelium
(Azan × 400)

This micrograph of the cells lining a small collecting tubule in the kidney shows simple cuboidal epithelium in section. Although the boundaries between individual cells are indistinct, the nuclear shape provides an approximate indication of the cell size and shape. The underlying basement membrane appears as a prominent blue line with this staining method.

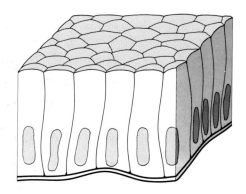

Fig. 5.6 Simple columnar epithelium

Simple columnar epithelium is similar to simple cuboidal epithelium except that the cells are taller and appear columnar in sections at right angles to the basement membrane. The height of the cells may vary from low to tall columnar depending on the site and/or degree of functional activity. The nuclei are elongated and may be located towards the base, the centre or occasionally the apex of the cytoplasm. Simple columnar epithelium is most often found on highly absorptive surfaces such as in the small intestine, although it may constitute the lining of highly secretory surfaces such as that of the stomach.

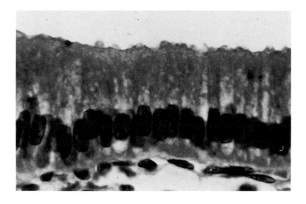

Fig. 5.7 Simple columnar epithelium
(H & E × 800)

This example of simple columnar epithelium is unusually tall and is taken from the lining of the gall bladder where it has the function of absorbing water, thus concentrating bile. The luminal plasma membranes of highly absorptive epithelial cells are often arranged into numerous, minute, finger-like projections called *microvilli* which greatly increase the surface area of the absorptive interface. Microvilli are usually too small to be resolved individually by light microscopy although they may collectively give the appearance of a *striated* or *brush border* at the luminal surface (see Fig. 5.22).

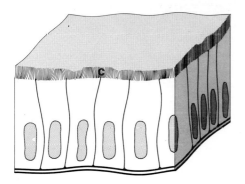

Fig. 5.8 Simple columnar ciliated epithelium

This type of simple columnar epithelium is traditionally described as a separate entity because of the presence of cilia C, surface specialisations which are readily visible with the light microscope. Cilia, which are much larger than microvilli, are motile projections from the luminal surface (see also Fig. 5.21). The action of cilia generates a current which propels fluid or minute particles over the epithelial surface. *Simple columnar ciliated epithelium* is not common in humans except in the female reproductive tract.

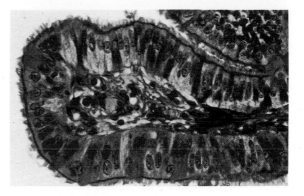

Fig. 5.9 Simple columnar ciliated epithelium

(Azan × 320)

This micrograph shows part of the highly folded epithelial lining of the oviduct. The predominant cell type in this epithelium is tall columnar and ciliated; the less numerous, blue-stained cells are not ciliated and have a secretory function. The cilia of the oviduct are believed to generate a current of fluid which helps to transport the ovum from the ovary to the uterus. As in this preparation, cilia are often stuck together in clumps by surface secretions or they may become flattened during tissue processing and therefore difficult to distinguish.

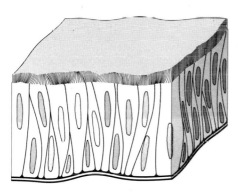

Fig. 5.10 Pseudostratified columnar ciliated epithelium

Another variant of simple columnar epithelium is described in which the cells are also usually ciliated. The term *pseudostratified* is derived from the appearance of this epithelium in section which conveys the erroneous impression that there is more than one layer of cells. This, however, is a true simple epithelium since all the cells rest on the basement membrane, although not all the cells extend to the luminal surface. The nuclei of these cells are disposed at different levels, thus creating the illusion of cellular stratification. Pseudostratified epithelium is almost exclusively confined to the larger airways of the respiratory system in mammals and is therefore often referred to as *respiratory epithelium*. The functional significance of pseudostratification has never been satisfactorily explained.

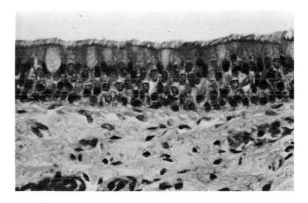

Fig. 5.11 Pseudostratified columnar ciliated epithelium

(H & E × 320)

The pseudostratified columnar ciliated epithelium shown in this micrograph is from the trachea. Pseudostratified columnar ciliated epithelium may be distinguished from true stratified epithelia by two characteristics. Firstly, the individual cells of the pseudostratified epithelium exhibit polarity, that is the apical cytoplasm does not contain nuclei. Secondly, cilia are never present on stratified epithelia. The cilia of respiratory epithelium continuously propel a surface coat of mucus containing entrapped particles towards the pharynx.

Stratified epithelia

Stratified epithelia are defined as epithelia consisting of two or more layers of cells. In contrast to simple epithelia, stratified epithelia primarily have a protective function and the degree and nature of the stratification is related to the kinds of physical stresses to which the surface is exposed. In general, stratified epithelia are poorly suited for the functions of absorption and secretion by virtue of their thickness, although some stratified surfaces are moderately permeable to water and other small molecules. The classification of the various stratified epithelia usually relates to the structure of the surface layer since cells of the basal layer are, in general, cuboidal in shape.

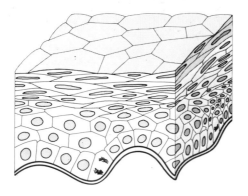

Fig. 5.12 Stratified squamous epithelium

Stratified squamous epithelium consists of a variable number of cell layers which undergo morphological and functional transition from the cuboidal basal layer to the extremely flattened surface layers. The basal cells undergo regular mitotic division giving rise to a succession of cells which are progressively pushed towards the free surface. During migration to the surface the cells undergo first maturation, then degeneration, as they become increasingly distant from the source of nutrition provided by the underlying connective tissue. Towards the surface, the cells show overt signs of degeneration particularly in the nuclei which become progressively condensed *(pyknotic)* and flattened, before ultimately disintegrating. The degenerate surface cells are continuously sloughed off and replaced from the deeper layers. The rate of mitosis in the basal layer normally approximates to the rate of surface loss.

Stratified squamous epithelium is well adapted to withstand moderate abrasion since loss of surface cells does not compromise the underlying connective tissue; stratified squamous epithelium is, however, poorly adapted to withstand desiccation. This type of epithelium constitutes the lining of the oral cavity, pharynx, oesophagus, anal canal and vagina; such sites are normally subject to moderate mechanical abrasion and are kept moist by local glandular secretions.

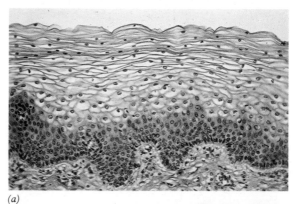

(a)

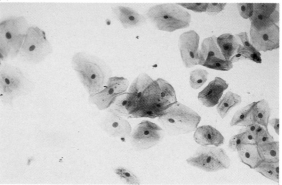

(b)

Fig. 5.13 Stratified squamous epithelium

(a) H & E × 128 (b) Papanicolou × 400

The vaginal epithelium demonstrated in micrograph (a) is a typical example of stratified squamous epithelium. Note the highly cellular basal layer and the transformation through the large polygonal cells of the intermediate layers to the degenerate superficial squamous cells. The junction between epithelium and underlying connective tissue is usually irregular, a feature which may enhance the adhesion of the epithelium to the underlying tissues. Note that, as in all epithelia, blood vessels do not extend beyond the basement membrane.

Micrograph (b) shows a smear made from cells scraped from the surface of the stratified squamous epithelium lining the uterine cervix as it projects into the vagina. The degenerate, scaly superficial cells stain pink with this staining method, the living cells from deeper layers staining blue.

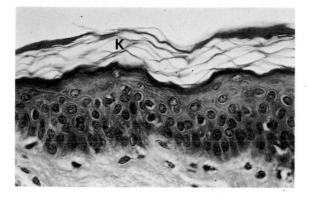

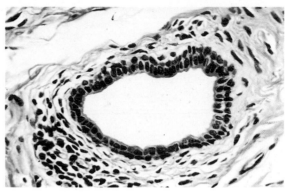

Fig. 5.14 Stratified squamous keratinising epithelium

(H & E × 320)

This specialised form of stratified squamous epithelium constitutes the epithelial surface of the skin and is adapted to withstand the constant abrasion and desiccation to which the body surface is exposed. During maturation, the epithelial cells undergo a process called *keratinisation* resulting in the formation of a tough, non-cellular surface layer consisting of the protein, *keratin* **K**, and the remnants of degenerate epithelial cells. Keratinisation may be induced in normally non-keratinising stratified squamous epithelium such as that of the oral cavity when exposed to excessive abrasion or desiccation. The process is described in detail in Chapter 9.

Fig. 5.15 Stratified cuboidal epithelium

(H & E × 320)

Stratified cuboidal epithelium is a thin, stratified epithelium which usually consists of only two or three layers of cuboidal or low columnar cells. This type of epithelium is usually confined to the lining of the larger excretory ducts of exocrine glands such as the salivary glands (as shown in this micrograph), the pancreas and sweat glands. Stratified cuboidal epithelium is probably not involved in significant absorptive or secretory activity but merely provides a more robust lining than would be afforded by a simple epithelium.

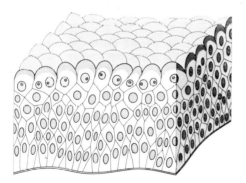

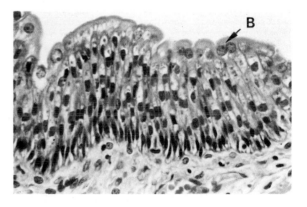

Fig. 5.16 Transitional epithelium

Transitional epithelium is a form of stratified epithelium almost exclusively confined to the urinary tract in mammals where it is highly specialised to accommodate a great degree of stretch and to withstand the toxicity of urine. This epithelial type is so named because it has some features which are intermediate between stratified cuboidal and stratified squamous epithelium. In the relaxed state, transitional epithelium appears to be about four to five cell layers thick; the basal cells are roughly cuboidal, the intermediate cells are polygonal and the surface cells are large and rounded and may contain two nuclei. In the stretched state, transitional epithelium often appears only two or three cells thick (although the actual number of layers remains constant) and the intermediate and surface layers are extremely flattened.

Fig. 5.17 Transitional epithelium

(H & E × 320)

This micrograph shows the appearance of transitional epithelium from the lining of a relaxed bladder. The shape and apparent size of the basal and intermediate cells vary considerably depending on the degree of distension, but the cells of the surface layer usually retain several characteristic features. Firstly, the surface cells are large and pale-stained and present a scalloped surface outline. Secondly, the luminal surface of the cells appears thickened and more densely stained. Thirdly, the nuclei of the surface cells are large and round, and often exhibit prominent nucleoli; some surface cells are binucleate **B**.

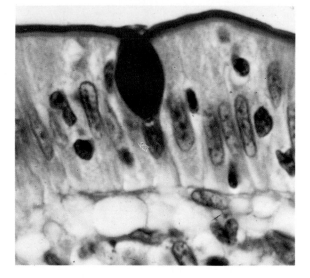

Fig. 5.18 Goblet cell
(PAS/Haematoxylin × 800)

Goblet cells are modified columnar epithelial cells which synthesise and secrete mucus. In man, goblet cells are scattered amongst the cells of many simple epithelial linings, particularly those of the respiratory and gastrointestinal tracts. Goblet cells are so named because of their resemblance to drinking goblets. The distended apical cytoplasm contains a dense aggregation of *mucigen* granules which, when released by exocytosis, combine with water to form the viscid secretion called mucus. Mucigen is composed of a mixture of neutral and acidic mucopolysaccharides (proteoglycans) and therefore can be readily demonstrated by the PAS method which stains carbohydrates magenta. The 'stem' of the goblet cell is occupied by a condensed, basal nucleus and is crammed with other organelles involved in mucigen synthesis. Note in this example from the lining of the small intestine, the tall columnar nature of the surrounding absorptive cells.

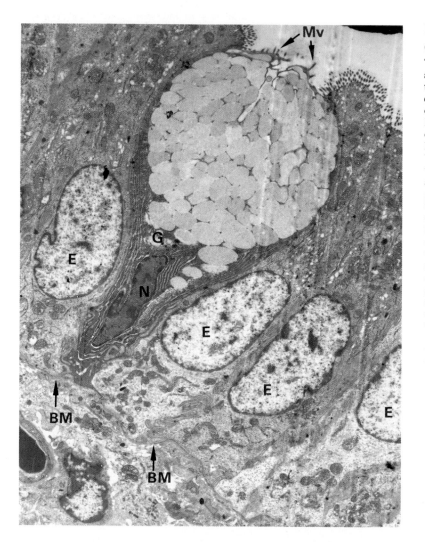

Fig. 5.19 Goblet cell
(EM × 4300)

This micrograph shows a goblet cell amongst columnar absorptive cells **E** of the small intestine. Although not always evident with light microscopy, goblet cells rest on the basement membrane **BM**. The base of the goblet cell contains an elongated nucleus **N** which has moderately condensed euchromatin. The surrounding cytoplasm is packed with rough endoplasmic reticulum and a few mitochondria are present; a prominent Golgi apparatus **G** is found in the supranuclear region. The protein component of mucigen is synthesised by the rough endoplasmic reticulum and passed to the Golgi apparatus where it is combined with carbohydrate and packaged into membrane bound, secretory vacuoles called mucigen granules. Goblet cells secrete at a steady basal rate but they may be stimulated by local irritation to release their entire mucigen contents. Sparse microvilli **Mv** are seen at the surface of the goblet cell and may be associated with the secretory process.

Membrane specialisations of epithelia

The basal, luminal and intercellular surfaces of epithelial cells have a variety of specialisations.

1. **Basal surfaces:** the interface between all epithelia and underlying connective tissues is marked by a non-cellular structure known as the *basement membrane* or *basal lamina*; these terms are often used synonymously but the term 'basal lamina' has a more specific meaning (see Fig. 5.20) and to avoid confusion, the term basement membrane is employed throughout this book. The basement membrane provides structural support for epithelia and constitutes a selective barrier to the passage of materials between the epithelial and connective tissue compartments.

2. **Luminal surfaces:** the luminal surfaces of epithelial cells may exhibit three main types of specialisation: *cilia, microvilli* and *stereocilia*. Cilia are relatively long, motile structures which are easily resolved by light microscopy. In contrast, microvilli are short often extremely numerous projections of the plasma membrane which cannot be individually resolved with the light microscope. Stereocilia are merely extremely long microvilli usually found only singly or in small numbers in odd sites such as the male reproductive tract; stereocilia are not motile and are thus inappropriately named.

3. **Intercellular surfaces:** epithelial cells are bound together by several types of specialisation of their opposed surfaces which permit epithelia to form cohesive, continuous layers and which may serve as points of metabolite or information transfer between cells. Analogous intercellular specialisations are found between cells in some non-epithelial tissues, particularly muscle, where they serve similar general functions.

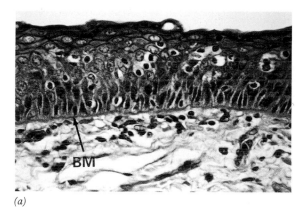

(a)

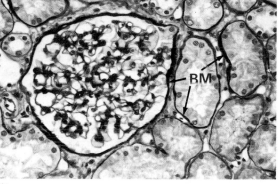

(b)

Fig. 5.20 Basement membranes

(a) *Laryngeal epithelium: PAS × 320 (b) Renal cortex: Jones' methenamine silver × 320*

These micrographs illustrate two methods for the demonstration of basement membranes **BM**. Basement membranes vary widely in thickness in different sites and even the thickest are often difficult to resolve in common haematoxylin and eosin stained preparations.

The structure of basement membranes is not well understood, but the current concept is that they consist of two basic layers. The layer in contact with the epithelial basal plasma membrane is composed of a fine feltwork of fibrils embedded in an amorphous matrix of ground substance. The fibrils are of two types, a species of collagen designated as Type IV collagen and a structural glycoprotein called laminin (see Ch. 4). This layer adjacent to the epithelium is strictly described as the *basal lamina*. Deep to this layer, is a layer consisting mainly of fine reticulin fibres (collagen Type III) also embedded in a ground substance-like matrix. This layer merges with underlying connective tissues.

The PAS staining method is thought to stain specifically the ground substance components and the silver method to stain the reticulin components of basement membranes; other common staining methods empirically differentiate basement membranes (see Fig. 5.5)

Which cells are responsible for elaborating basement membranes is in dispute. There is evidence that the true basal lamina is synthesised by epithelial cells and the reticular layer by the underlying connective tissue; in terms of this concept, the basal lamina may represent an extremely thickened epithelial glycocalyx (see Fig. 1.2).

Basement membranes appear to have much more than a supporting function. They are permeable to small molecules but impermeable to large molecular weight substances. This property is a critical factor in the function of certain organs particularly the kidney where the glomerular basement membrane acts as a highly selective filter (see Ch. 16). The permeability of basement membranes is probably an important but more subtle factor influencing the integrity and proper function of other epithelial tissues. In addition, basement membranes constitute a selective barrier to passage of cells between epithelia and connective tissues. For example, they permit the passage of cells of the immune system but strictly confine epithelial and connective tissue cells to their appropriate domains.

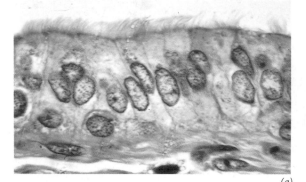

(a)

Fig. 5.21 Cilia

(a) Thin section, toluidine blue × 800 (b) EM × 5600
(c) Schematic diagram

Cilia are motile structures which project in parallel rows
from certain epithelial surfaces, notably in the respiratory
and female reproductive tracts. Cilia beat with a wave-like
synchronous rhythm propelling surface films of mucus or
fluid in a consistent direction over the epithelial surface. In
the airways for example, mucus secreted by goblet cells traps
debris from inspired air and cilia move the mucus upwards
towards the throat where it is swallowed thus keeping the
airways clean. In the oviducts, ciliary action plays a part in
transporting the ovum from the ovary down towards the
uterus.

Cilia measure from about 7–10 μm in length and may
therefore be of the order of half the length of the cell
depending on cell size. A single epithelial cell may have up
to 300 cilia and these are usually of about the same length as
one another.

Micrographs (a) and (b) show ciliated cells lining the
respiratory tract. Note that the cilia are readily visible with
light microscopy although during processing they often
become matted together and flattened making them less
conspicuous. In micrograph (b) their length is seen to be
almost half that of the cell itself. A three-dimensional
surface view of cilia in the respiratory tract is shown in
Figure 12.6.

Each cilium is bounded by an evagination of the luminal
plasma membrane and, as shown diagramatically, contains a
central core called the *axoneme* consisting of 20 microtubules
arranged as a central pair surrounded by nine peripheral
doublets. At its base, the axoneme inserts into a structure
called a *basal body* which has a microtubular arrangement
identical to that of a centriole i.e. nine triplets of
microtubules forming a short cylinder (see Fig. 2.6). Each
peripheral doublet of the cilium axoneme is continuous with
the two inner microtubules of the corresponding triplet of
the basal body. Basal bodies **BB** can be readily identified in
micrograph (b); in micrograph (a), note that evidence of basal
bodies can be seen even with light microscopy.

Each axoneme doublet consists of one tubule, which is
circular in cross-section, closely applied to another
incomplete tubule which is C-shaped in cross-section. From
each complete tubule, pairs of 'arms' consisting of the
protein *dynein*, which has ATP-ase activity, extend towards
the incomplete tubule of the adjacent doublet. It is believed
that ciliary action results from longitudinal movement of the
doublets relative to one another, energy for the process
being provided in the form of ATP by mitochondria which
crowd the subjacent cytoplasm as seen in micrograph (b). It
is not yet clear whether basal bodies arise *de novo* or by
repeated division of centrioles.

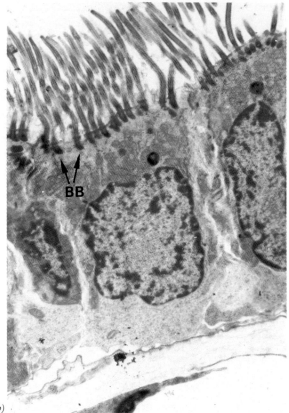

(b)

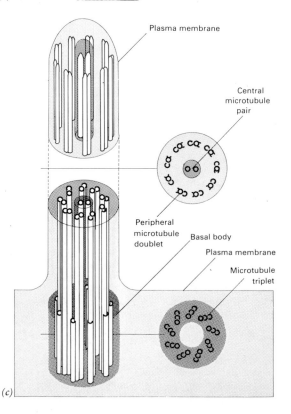

Plasma membrane

Central
microtubule
pair

Peripheral
microtubule
doublet

Basal body

Plasma membrane

Microtubule
triplet

(c)

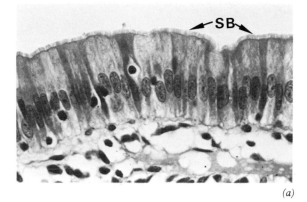

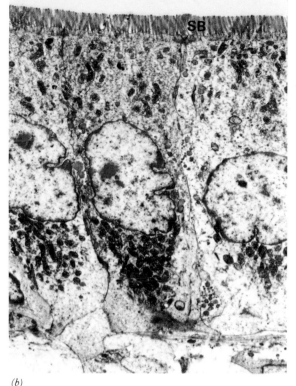

(a)

Fig. 5.22 Microvilli

(a) H & E × 320 (b) EM × 4750 (c) EM × 28 000

Microvilli are minute finger-like projections of the luminal plasma membrane found in many epithelia particularly those specialised for absorption where their presence may increase the surface area for absorption by as much as 30 times. Microvilli are only 0.5–1.0 μm in length and are thus very short in relation to the size of the cell, a feature contrasting markedly with cilia (see Fig. 5.21). Furthermore, individual microvilli are too small to be resolved by light microscopy.

Some epithelia have only a small number of irregular microvilli. However, epithelia in such highly absorptive sites as in the small intestine and proximal renal tubules have up to 3000 regular microvilli per cell; collectively these can be seen with the light microscope as so-called *striated* and *brush borders* respectively. Micrographs (a) and (b) illustrate the typical features of microvilli constituting the striated border **SB** of cells lining the small intestine.

As seen at very high magnification in micrograph (c), the cytoplasmic core of each microvillus contains fine protein filaments which insert into the terminal webb **TW**, a specialisation of the cytoskeleton lying immediately beneath the cell surface; at the tip of the microvillus, the filaments attach to an electron-dense part of the plasma membrane. The filaments, of which the principal constituent is actin, maintain stability of microvilli and may also mediate some contraction and elongation of the microvilli.

(b)

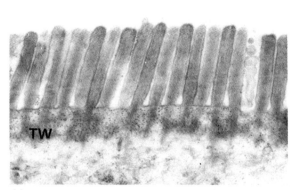

(c)

Fig. 5.23 Stereocilia

(H & E × 320)

Extremely long microvilli, readily visible with light microscopy, are found in small numbers in parts of the male reproductive tract such as the epididymis, shown in this micrograph, and other odd sites. Originally, these structures were thought to be an unusual form of cilia and were termed stereocilia; however, electron microscopy has shown that they do not have the internal structure of cilia but merely a filamentous skeleton like that of microvilli. Stereocilia **S** are thought to facilitate absorptive processes in the epididymis but the reason for their unusual form is not known.

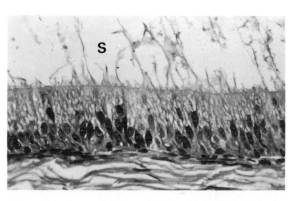

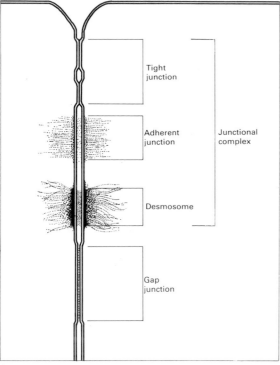

(a)

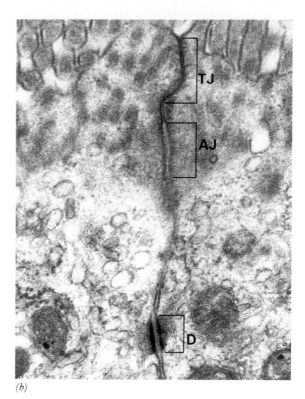

(b)

Fig. 5.24 Cell junctions and junctional complexes

(a) Schematic diagram (b) Junctional complex: EM × 59 400

Before the advent of electron microscopy, epithelial cells were thought to be bound together by an intercellular adhesive which was called *intercellular cement*. It is now known that epithelial cells are bound together by several types of plasma membrane specialisations to which a variety of somewhat confusing names have been applied. The commonest type of cell junction is the *desmosome (macula adherens)*. Desmosomes are found scattered throughout intercellular interfaces where they provide strong points of cohesion between cells and act as anchorage points for the cytoskeleton of each cell. Another widely distributed type of cell junction is the *gap junction* or *nexus* which not only functions as an adherent zone but also permits transfer of information and metabolites between adjacent cells.

Between the cells of simple cuboidal and simple columnar epithelia, the intercellular membranes exhibit specialisations called *junctional complexes* which encircle the cells preventing access of luminal contents to the intercellular spaces. Junctional complexes begin immediately below the luminal surface and are made up of three components, one of which is the desmosome; the other two components are called *tight junctions (zonula occludentes)* and *adherent junctions (zonula adherentes)*.

This electron micrograph of a typical junctional complex between two columnar intestinal epithelial cells illustrates tight and adherent junctions and a desmosome; the principal features of these junctions and of a gap junction are shown in the schematic diagram.

1. **Tight junctions:** tight junctions **TJ** begin just below the luminal surface and consist of small areas where the outer lamina of opposing plasma membranes are fused with one another. Between these areas of fusion are areas which are not fused. The tight junction forms a complete circumferential belt around each cell thus sealing the intercellular space from the lumen.

2. **Adherent junctions:** adherent junctions **AJ** are found deep to the tight junctions and are areas where the opposing plasma membranes diverge; no structures are evident between the opposing cell membranes. On the cytoplasmic aspect of these junctions, there is a fine mat of filamentous material which merges with the filaments of the terminal web (see Fig. 5.22). Like tight junctions, adherent junctions also form a circumferential band around each cell.

3. **Desmosomes:** desmosomes **D** form the third component of junctional complexes but also occur singly at many other intercellular sites. At the desmosome, the opposing plasma membranes are separated by a gap in which many fine, transverse filaments or a dense, longitudinal lamina may be seen. At the cytoplasmic aspect of each plasma membrane there is a closely applied electron-dense layer into which fibrillar elements of the cytoskeleton appear to converge. Desmosomes always appear as the paired structures just described, except at the interface of stratified squamous epithelia and the basement membrane where half desmosomes *(hemi-desmosomes)* can be found.

4. **Gap junctions:** gap junctions are broad areas of closely opposed plasma membranes, but there is no fusion of the plasma membranes and a narrow gap remains. Although this type of junction is a site of intercellular adhesion, gap junctions also permit passage of ions and other molecules between adjacent cells; that is, they are sites of intercellular information exchange.

Exocrine glands

Exocrine glands are glands which discharge their secretory product via a duct onto an epithelial surface. The cells of which they are composed are highly specialised epithelial cells, the internal structure of the cells reflecting the nature of the secretory product and the mode of secretion (see Ch. 1).

Endocrine glands may be classified according to two major characteristics:

1. The morphology of the gland: exocrine glands may be broadly divided into simple and compound glands. *Simple glands* are defined as those with a single, unbranched duct. The secretory portions of simple glands have two main forms, tubular or acinar, which may be coiled and/or branched. *Compound glands* have a branched duct system and their secretory portions have similar morphological forms to those of the simple glands.

2. The means of discharge of secretory products from the cells:

(a) *Merocrine.* Merocrine secretion (also called eccrine secretion) involves the process of exocytosis and is the most common form of secretion; proteins are usually the major secretory product.

(b) *Apocrine.* Apocrine secretion involves the discharge of free, unbroken, membrane-bound vesicles containing secretory products and is an unusual means of secretion of lipid products in such glands as the breasts and some sweat glands.

(c) *Holocrine.* This is another unusual form of secretion which involves the discharge of whole secretory cells with subsequent disintegration of the cells to release the secretory product. Holocrine secretion occurs principally in sebaceous glands.

In general, all glands have a basal rate of secretion which is modulated by nervous and hormonal influences. The secretory portions of some exocrine glands are embraced by contractile cells which lie between the secretory cells and the basement membrane. The contractile mechanism of these cells is thought to be similar to that of muscle cells and has given rise to the term *myoepithelial cells*.

Fig. 5.25 Exocrine gland types

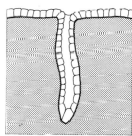
Simple tubular

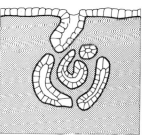
Simple coiled tubular

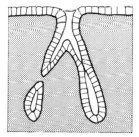
Simple branched tubular

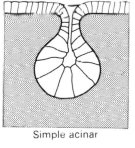
Simple acinar

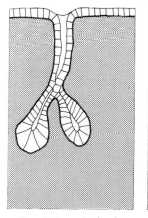
Simple branched acinar

Compound branched tubular

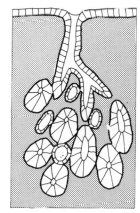
Compound acinar

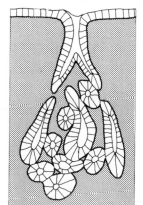
Compound tubulo-acinar

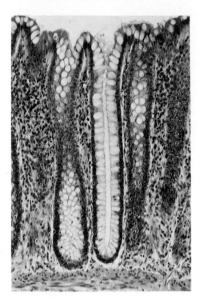

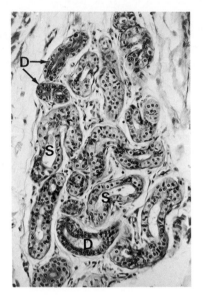

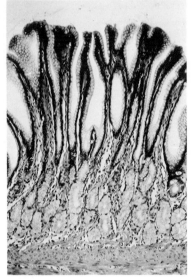

Fig. 5.26 Simple tubular glands

(H & E × 50)

This example of *simple tubular glands* is taken from the large intestine; this type of gland has a single, straight tubular lumen into which the secretory products are discharged. In this example, the entire duct is lined by secretory cells; the secretory cells are goblet cells. In other sites mucus is secreted by columnar cells which do not have the classical goblet shape but nonetheless function in a similar manner.

Fig. 5.27 Simple coiled tubular glands

(H & E × 80)

Sweat glands are almost the only example of *simple coiled tubular glands.* Each consists of a single tube which is tightly coiled in three dimensions; portions of the gland are thus seen in various planes of section. Sweat glands have a terminal secretory portion **S** lined by simple epithelium which gives way to a non-secretory (excretory) duct **D** lined by stratified cuboidal epithelium.

Fig. 5.28 Simple branched tubular glands

(H & E × 50)

Simple branched tubular glands are found mainly in the stomach; the mucous glands of the pyloric stomach are shown in this example. Each gland consists of several tubular secretory portions which converge onto a single, unbranched duct which, in this case, is also lined by mucus-secreting cells. Unlike those of the large intestine (see Fig. 5.26), these mucous cells do not have a goblet shape.

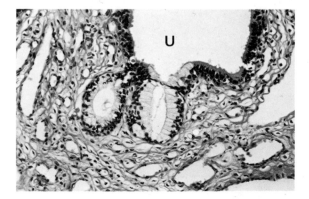

Fig. 5.29 Simple acinar glands

(H & E × 128)

Simple acinar glands occur as pockets in epithelial surfaces and are lined by secretory cells; in this example of the mucus-secreting glands of the penile urethra, the secretory cells are pale stained compared to the non-secretory cells lining the urethra **U**. Note that the term *acinus* can be used to describe any rounded exocrine secretory unit.

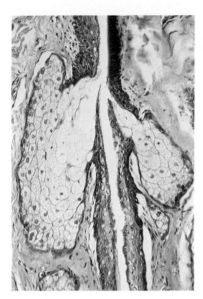

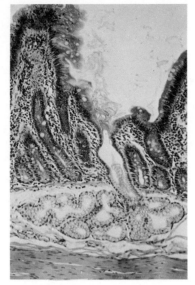

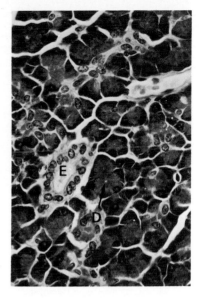

Fig. 5.30 Simple branched acinar gland

(Masson's trichrome × 80)

Sebaceous glands provide a good example of *simple branched acinar glands*. Each gland consists of several secretory acini which empty into a single excretory duct; the excretory duct is formed by the stratified epithelium surrounding the hair shaft. The mode of secretion of sebaceous glands is holocrine; the secretory product, sebum, accumulates within the secretory cells and is discharged by degeneration of the cells.

Fig. 5.31 Compound tubular gland

(H & E × 20)

Brunner's glands of the duodenum, as shown in this example, are described as *compound tubular glands*. The duct system is branched, thus defining the gland as a compound gland; the secretory portions have a tubular form which is branched and coiled.

Fig. 5.32 Compound acinar gland

(Chrome alum haematoxylin/ Phloxine × 320)

Compound acinar glands are those in which the secretory units are acinar in form and drain into a branched duct system. The pancreas shown in this micrograph consists of numerous acini, each of which drains into a minute duct. These minute ducts **D**, which are just discernible in the centre of some acini, drain into a system of branched excretory ducts of increasing diameter; a small excretory duct **E** lined by simple cuboidal epithelium is seen in the centre of the field.

Fig. 5.33 Compound tubulo-acinar gland

(H & E × 200)

Compound tubulo-acinar glands have secretory units which consist of branched tubular components, branched acinar components, and branched tubular components with acinar end-pieces called *demilunes*. The submandibular salivary gland, which is the classical example and which is shown in this micrograph, has two types of secretory cells, mucous cells (poorly stained) and serous cells (strongly stained). Generally, the mucous cells form tubular components **T** whereas the serous cells form acinar components **A** and demilunes **D**. Excretory ducts **E** of two different sizes are seen in this field.

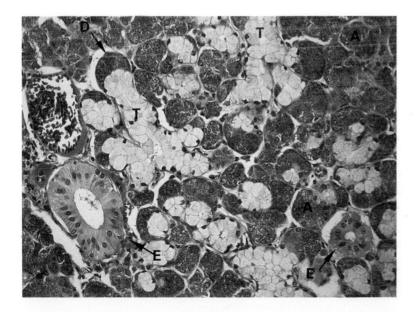

Endocrine glands

Endocrine glands are ductless glands, the secretory products diffusing directly into the bloodstream. The secretory products are known as hormones and control the activity of cells and tissues usually far removed from the site of secretion.

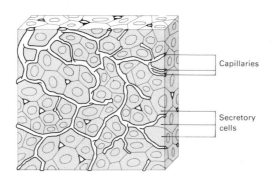

Fig. 5.34 Endocrine gland

Most endocrine glands consist of clumps or cords of secretory cells surrounded by a rich network of small blood vessels. Each clump of endocrine cells is surrounded by a basement membrane, reflecting its epithelial origin. Endocrine cells release hormones into the intercellular spaces from which they diffuse rapidly into surrounding blood vessels.

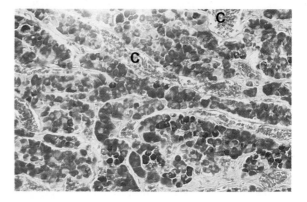

Fig. 5.35 Endocrine gland
(Isamine blue/Eosin × 128)

This micrograph of the pituitary gland shows the features typical of most endocrine glands. The secretory cells are arranged in cords and clumps and are surrounded by a rich network of broad capillaries **C** in a fine supporting connective tissue. The basement membrane surrounding each clump of cells is not visible at this magnification. Like many other endocrine glands, the secretory cells of the pituitary are of several different types and thus may have different staining properties.

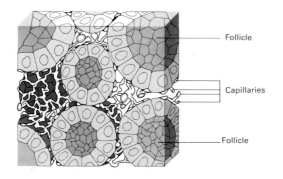

Fig. 5.36 Follicular endocrine gland

The thyroid gland is an unusual endocrine gland which stores hormone within spheroidal cavities enclosed by secretory cells; these spheroidal units are called follicles. Secretion of stored hormone involves reabsorption of hormone from the follicular lumen, release into the surrounding interstitial spaces, and thence diffusion into the rich capillary network which embraces each follicle.

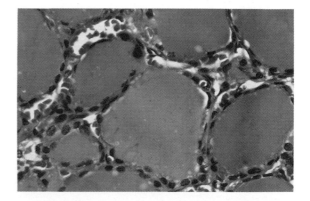

Fig. 5.37 Follicular endocrine gland
(H & E × 320)

The follicular nature of the thyroid gland is evident from this micrograph. The secretory cells lining the follicles are flattened cuboidal in shape. Stored thyroid hormone is bound to a glycoprotein which is strongly eosinophilic. The relatively sparse interfollicular connective tissue is mainly occupied by capillaries.

6. Muscle

Introduction

Contractility is an inherent property of all cells which is necessary for the performance of basic functions involving movement such as phagocytosis and cell division, and more specialised functions such as motility as in white blood cells.

In multicellular organisms, some cells are specialised to enable movement of tissues or organs. These cells may function as single contractile units, such as the myoepithelial cells surrounding the acini of some exocrine glands, or may be aggregated to form muscles for the movement of large structures. Recent evidence, partly based on the study of the contractile mechanisms of some unicellular organisms, suggests that there is a homologous contractile mechanism in all cells. This mechanism consists of fibrillar proteins arranged in an organised manner in the cytoplasm, and linked by intermolecular bonds. Contraction results from the rearrangement of the intermolecular bonds with the utilisation of chemical energy.

There are three types of muscle tissue:

1. Skeletal muscle: this is responsible for the movement of the skeleton and organs such as the globe of the eye and the tongue. Skeletal muscle is often referred to as *voluntary muscle* since it may be controlled voluntarily. The arrangement of the contractile proteins gives rise to the appearance of prominent cross-striations in some histological preparations and hence the name *striated muscle* is often applied to skeletal muscle.

2. Visceral muscle: this type of muscle forms the muscular component of visceral structures, such as blood vessels, the gastrointestinal tract, the uterus and the urinary bladder. Since visceral muscle is under inherent, autonomic and hormonal control, it is described as *involuntary muscle*. As the arrangement of contractile proteins does not give the histological appearance of cross-striations, the name *smooth muscle* is also commonly applied

3. Cardiac muscle: cardiac muscle has many structural and functional characteristics, intermediate between those of skeletal and visceral muscle, which provide for the continuous, rhythmic contractility of the heart. Although striated in appearance, cardiac muscle is readily distinguishable from skeletal muscle.

The highly specialised functions of the cytoplasmic organelles of muscle cells has led to the use of a special terminology for some muscle cell components: plasma membrane or plasmalemma=*sarcolemma*; cytoplasm—*sarcoplasm*; endoplasmic reticulum=*sarcoplasmic reticulum*; mitochondria=*sarcosomes*.

Skeletal muscle

Skeletal muscles have a wide variety of morphological forms and modes of action, nevertheless all have the same basic structure being composed of extremely elongated, multinucleate cells, often described as *muscle fibres*, bound together by connective tissue. Individual muscle fibres range considerably in diameter from 10–100 μm and may extend throughout the whole length of a muscle reaching up to 35 cm in length.

Skeletal muscle contraction is controlled by large motor nerves, individual nerve fibres branching within the muscle to supply a group of muscle fibres, collectively described as a *motor unit*; excitation of any one motor nerve results in simultaneous contraction of all the muscle fibres of the corresponding motor unit. The structure of neuromuscular junctions is described in Figure 7.13. The vitality of skeletal muscle fibres is dependent on the maintenance of their nerve supply which if damaged, results in atrophy of the fibres. Skeletal muscle contains highly specialised stretch receptors known as neuromuscular spindles which are shown in Figure 7.29.

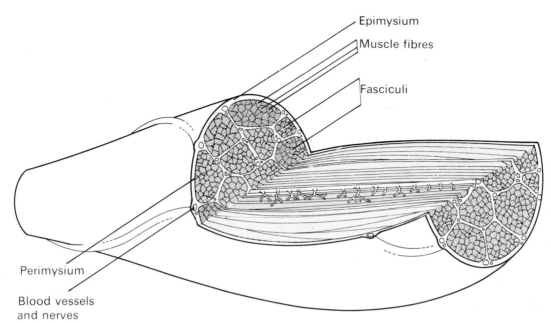

Fig. 6.1 Skeletal muscle

This diagram illustrates the arrangement of the basic components which make up a typical skeletal muscle.

The individual muscle cells (muscle fibres) are grouped together into elongated bundles called *fasciculi* with delicate connective tissue called *endomysium* occupying the spaces between individual muscle fibres.

The fasciculi are surrounded by loose collagenous connective tissue called *perimysium*. Most muscles are made up of many fasciculi and the whole muscle mass is invested in a dense, outer connective tissue sheath called the *epimysium*. Large blood vessels and nerves enter the epimysium and divide to ramify throughout the muscle in the perimysium and endomysium.

The size of the fasciculi reflects the function of the particular muscle concerned. Muscles responsible for fine, highly controlled movements, e.g. the external muscles of the eye, have small fasciculi and a relatively greater proportion of perimysial connective tissue. In contrast, muscles responsible for gross movements only, e.g. the muscles of the buttocks, have large fasciculi and relatively little perimysial connective tissue. Within each muscle, the connective tissue component contains both collagen and elastic fibres acting as a flexible skeleton to which individual muscle fibres and fasciculi are anchored. This connective tissue becomes continuous with that of the tendons and muscle attachments (see Ch. 10) which distribute and direct the motive forces of the muscle to bone, skin etc. as appropriate.

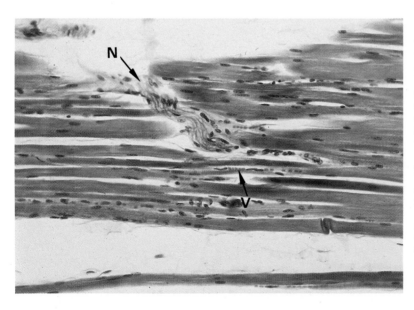

Fig. 6.2 Skeletal muscle

(Masson's trichrome × 150)

This micrograph shows part of a fasciculus of skeletal muscle at high magnification. The individual red-stained muscle cells (fibres) are highly elongated and arranged in parallel, the spaces between them being occupied by small amounts of endomysial connective tissue. The endomysium, which consists mainly of reticulin fibres (unstained) and a small amount of collagen (stained blue in this preparation), conveys numerous small blood vessels and nerves throughout the muscle. In this micrograph, a small nerve bundle **N** is seen and the tiny blood vessels **V** can only be identified by the rows of erythrocytes contained within them.

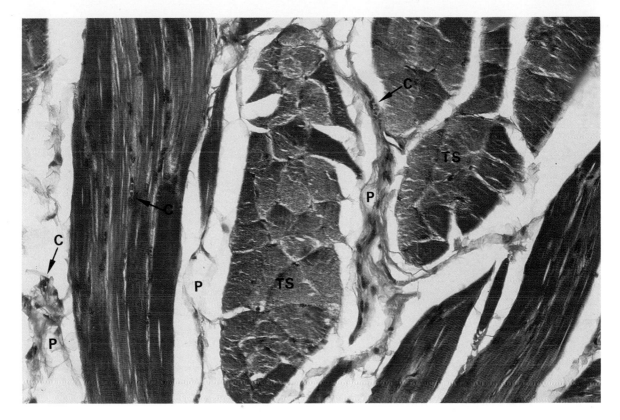

Fig. 6.3 Skeletal muscle

(Masson's trichrome × 300)

This micrograph shows the skeletal muscle of the tongue which is made up of numerous small fasciculi oriented in various different directions. This staining method clearly distinguishes skeletal muscle cells, stained red, from connective tissue, the collagen of which is stained blue.

In the centre and at the upper left of the field are fasciculi cut in transverse section **TS**, the remaining fasciculi being cut longitudinally. The spaces between the fasciculi are filled with loose collagenous connective tissue, the perimysium **P**, which is continuous with the delicate endomysium, separating individual muscle fibres making up the fasciculi. The connective tissue of skeletal muscle also contains elastin fibres which are most numerous in muscles attached to soft tissues as in the tongue and face. Note the rich network of capillaries C in the endomysium and perimysium.

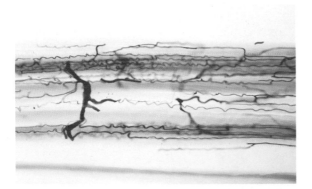

Fig. 6.4 Skeletal muscle blood supply

(Perfusion method × 128)

This specimen was prepared by perfusing the blood supply of a skeletal muscle with a red dye; the muscle fibres were then teased apart to reveal the endomysial capillary bed.

Large blood vessels enter the epimysium and divide to ramify throughout the muscle in the perimysium. Fine branches arise from the perimysial arteries and pass between the muscle fibres transversely to their long axes. These give rise to numerous capillaries which run longitudinally through the endomysium. Frequent transverse anastomoses between the capillaries result in a fine, elongated capillary network surrounding each muscle fibre.

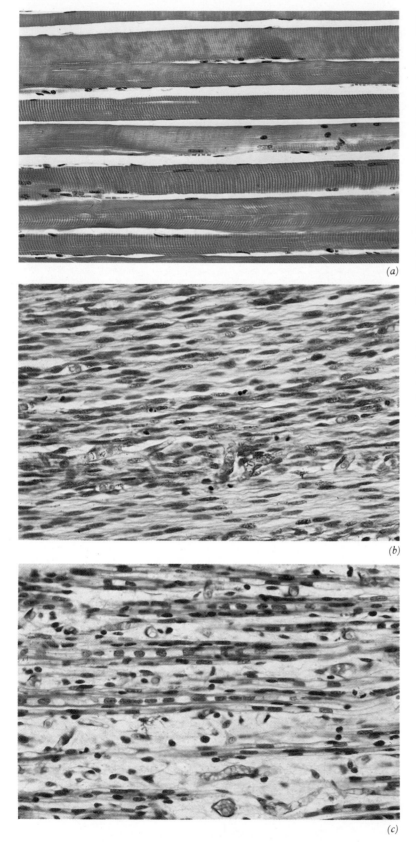

(a)

(b)

(c)

Fig. 6.5 Skeletal muscle and its embryogenesis

(H & E (a) Mature skeletal muscle × 320 (b) Myoblasts × 150 (c) Myotubes × 150)

Micrograph (a) demonstrates the characteristic histological features of skeletal muscle fibres in longitudinal section. Skeletal muscle fibres are extremely elongated, unbranched cylindrical cells with numerous flattened nuclei located at fairly regular intervals just beneath the sarcolemma.

During embryological development, myotomal mesenchymal cells differentiate into long, mononuclear skeletal muscle precursors called *myoblasts* which then proliferate by mitosis; this is shown in micrograph (b). Subsequently, the myoblasts fuse end to end forming progressively elongated multinucleate cells called *myotubes*, seen in micrograph (c), which may eventually contain up to 100 nuclei.

Synthesis of the contractile proteins begins after myoblast fusion, the proteins being laid down initially in the central axis of the myotube, the nuclei being displaced peripherally as more contractile protein is formed. Most of the process of muscle development is completed by the time of birth along with the process of nervous innervation. Thereafter, growth occurs by increase in bulk of the muscle cell cytoplasm.

Mature muscle cells are highly differentiated and, if damaged, have very limited capacity for repair and regeneration; nevertheless, a few myoblasts persist after maturity and appear to play some part in rejoining severed muscle cells after injury.

Regular cross-striations are the characteristic feature of skeletal muscle fibres and can be seen in longitudinal sections as in micrograph (a). The cross-striations result from the arrangement of the contractile proteins as described later.

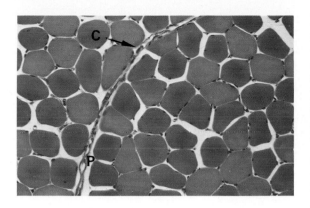

Fig. 6.6 Skeletal muscle

(TS: H & E × 320)

This micrograph of skeletal muscle cut in transverse section shows the extreme peripheral location of the nuclei of skeletal muscle fibres. In unfixed tissue, the fibres appear oval or round; however, in the more commonly used fixed preparations such as this, the fibres appear artefactually irregular and polyhedral. Similarly, the wide endomysial spaces seen between the muscle fibres result from shrinkage during tissue preparation.

In the endomysial spaces, note the numerous minute capillaries **C** recognisable by the eosinophilic erythrocytes contained within them. Compare the huge diameter of the muscle fibres with respect to that of the capillaries, the latter being approximately 7 μm across. Note also a strand of perimysial connective tissue **P** cutting across the field separating two fasciculi from one another.

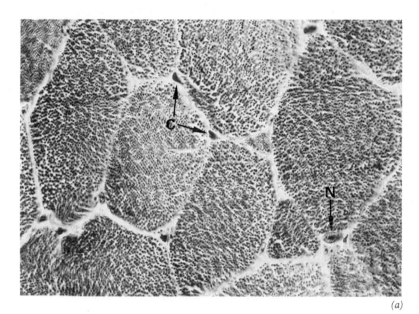

(a)

Fig. 6.7 Skeletal muscle

(a) TS: Iron haematoxylin × 1200 (b) Schematic diagram

Micrograph (a) shows a transverse section through several skeletal muscle fibres at a magnification close to the limit of resolution of the light microscope. The plane of section includes only one skeletal muscle nucleus **N**. Note the presence of erythrocytes in endomysial capillaries **C**.

In some preparations such as this, the transversely-sectioned muscle fibres are seen to be packed with numerous small dark dots. These represent the cut ends of *myofibrils*, elongated cylindrical structures which lie parallel to one another in the sarcoplasm.

As shown diagramatically in (b), each myofibril is made up of contractile proteins arranged in a highly ordered fashion which results in the myofibril appearing longitudinally cross-striated; this can only be seen with electron microscopy (see Fig. 6.8). Furthermore, the parallel myofibrils are arranged with their cross-striations in register so as to give rise to the light microscopical appearance of regular cross-striations along the whole length of the muscle fibre.

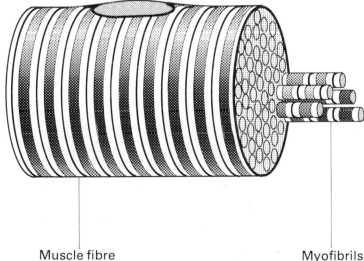

Muscle fibre   Myofibrils

(b)

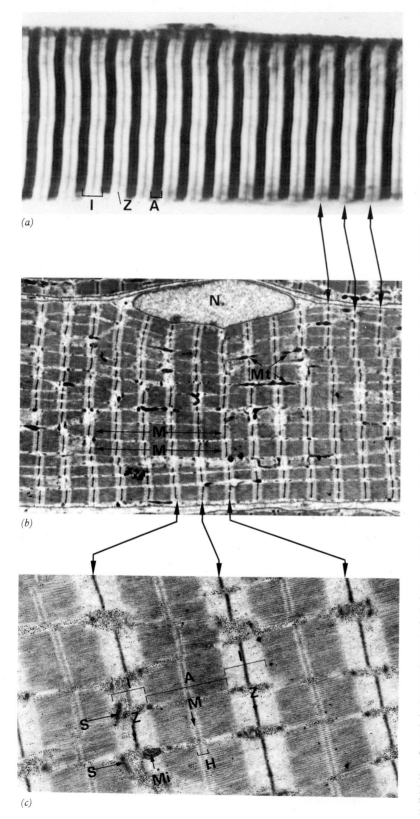

(a)

(b)

(c)

Fig. 6.8 Skeletal muscle

(a) Heidenhain's haematoxylin × 1200 (b) EM × 2860 (c) EM × 18 700

This series of micrographs at increasing degrees of magnification demonstrates the arrangement of the contractile proteins within skeletal muscle and explains the striations seen with light microscopy.

Micrograph (a) shows the striations of a skeletal muscle fibre at a magnification close to the limit of resolution of the light microscope. The striations are composed of alternating broad light I bands (isotropic in polarised light) and dark A bands (anisotropic in polarised light). Fine dark lines called Z bands (Zwischenscheiben) can be seen bisecting the light I bands. Note also the nucleus N at the extreme periphery of the cell.

Micrograph (b) shows the electron microscopic appearance of a similar muscle cell at the same magnification and with a nucleus N situated in a similar position immediately beneath the sarcolemma. The sarcoplasm is filled with myofibrils M oriented in parallel to the long axis of the cell. The myofibrils are separated by a small amount of sarcoplasm containing rows of mitochrondria Mt which are oriented with their long axes parallel to the myofibrils.

Each myofibril has prominent regular cross-striations which correspond to the I, A and Z bands seen in light microscopy due to the fact that the myofibrils are arranged with their cross-striations in register.

The Z bands are the most electron-dense bands in the myofibril and divide each myofibril into numerous contractile units, called *sarcomeres*, arranged end to end. With further magnification in micrograph (c), the arrangement of the contractile proteins or *myofilaments* may be seen in each sarcomere. Within the sarcomere, the dark A band is bisected by a broad lighter band, the H (heller) band, which is further bisected by a more dense M (Mittelscheibe) band. Irrespective of the degree of contraction of the muscle fibre, the A band remains constant in width. In contrast, the I bands and H bands narrow during contraction and the Z bands are drawn closer together. These findings are explained by the *sliding filament theory* of muscle contraction described in Figure 6.9.

Note the mitochondria Mi and numerous glycogen granules which provide a rich energy source in the scanty cytoplasm between the parallel myofibrils. The mature muscle cell contains little rough endoplasmic reticulum; it contains, however, a smooth membranous system S which conducts contractile stimuli to the myofibrils (see Figs. 6.10 and 6.11).

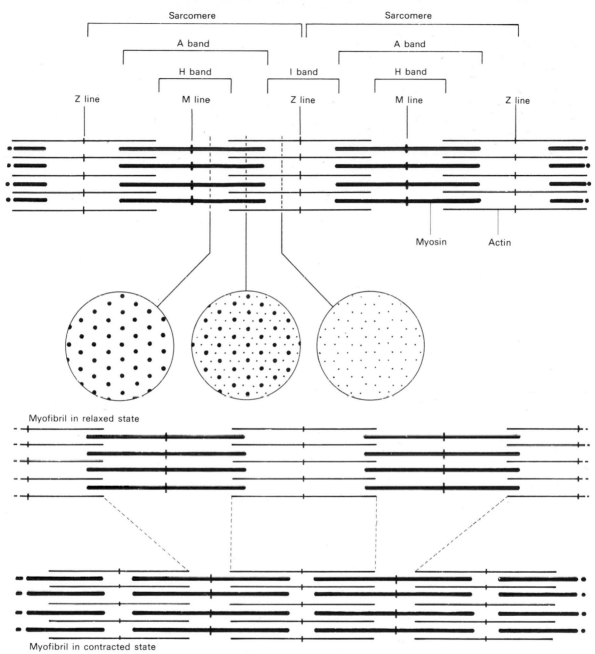

Fig. 6.9 The arrangement of myofilaments in the sarcomere

The sarcomere consists of two types of myofilaments, *thick filaments* and *thin filaments*. Each type remains constant in length irrespective of the state of contraction of the muscle. The filaments are arranged in a symmetrical interdigitating manner parallel to the long axis of the myofibril.

The thick filaments, which are composed mainly of the protein *myosin*, are maintained in parallel by their attachment to a disc-like zone represented by the M band. Similarly the thin filaments, which are composed mainly of

the protein *actin*, are united in a disc-like zone represented by the Z band. The I and H bands, both areas of low electron-density, represent areas where the thick and thin filaments do not overlap one another.

The widely accepted sliding filament theory proposes that under the influence of energy released from ATP, the thick and thin filaments slide over one another, thus causing contraction in the length of the sarcomere.

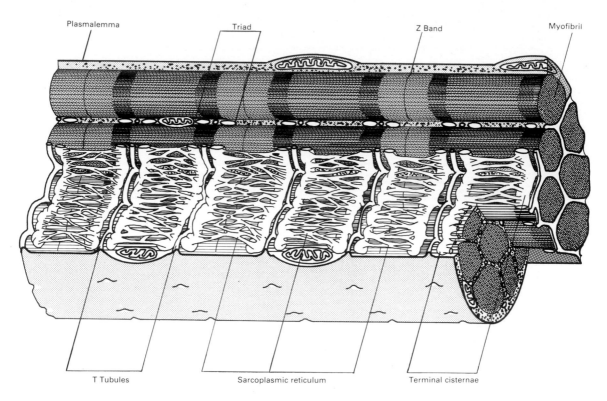

Plasmalemma Triad Z Band Myofibril

T Tubules Sarcoplasmic reticulum Terminal cisternae

Fig. 6.10 The conducting system for contractile stimuli

To permit the synchronous contraction of all sarcomeres in the muscle fibre, a system of tubular extensions of the muscle cell plasma membrane or sarcolemma extends transversely into the muscle cell to surround each myofibril at the region of the junction of the A and I bands (in mammals). Thus, throughout the muscle fibre, there is a tubular system, the *T system*, the lumen of which is continuous with the extracellular space.

Closely associated with, but not interconnected with, each T tubule system there are two complementary membrane systems derived from smooth endoplasmic reticulum; these are called *sarcoplasmic reticulum*. The sarcoplasmic reticulum ramifies to form a membranous network which embraces each myofibril. Each T tubule, with its pair of associated sarcoplasmic reticulum elements called *terminal cisternae*, forms a *triad* near the junction of the I and A bands of each sarcomere.

Calcium ions are concentrated within the lumen of the sarcoplasmic reticulum. Excitation of the sarcolemma of the muscle fibre is rapidly disseminated throughout the sarcoplasm by the T tubule system. This promotes the release of calcium ions from the sarcoplasmic reticulum into the sarcoplasm surrounding the myofilaments. Calcium ions activate the sliding filament mechanism resulting in muscle contraction.

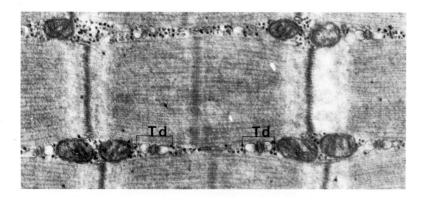

Fig. 6.11 Skeletal muscle

(EM × 38 000)

This electron micrograph of mammalian skeletal muscle demonstrates triads **Td** of the conducting system, each comprising a tubule of the T system and a pair of terminal cisternae of the sarcoplasmic reticulum. In mammals the position of the triads approximates to the junction of the A and I bands; during contraction, these junctions move in relation to the triads.

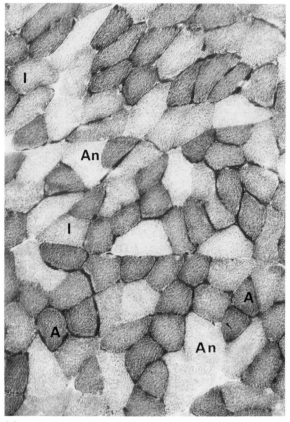

(a)

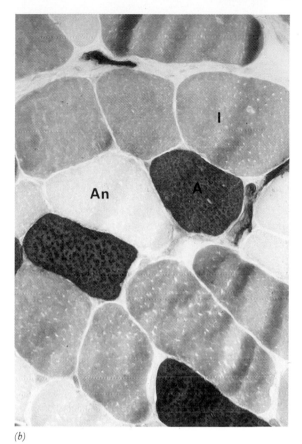

(b)

Fig. 6.12 Skeletal muscle

(TS: Histochemical techniques (a) Succinate dehydrogenase × 200 (b) ATP-ase × 600)

The mode of activity of skeletal muscle varies from one part of the body to another, some muscles such as those involved in the maintenance of posture, being required to contract almost continuously, whilst others such as the extra-ocular muscles, make rapid short-lived movements. In humans, distinction between these types cannot be made on gross examination of the muscle. However, in domestic poultry the extremes are easily identified by a difference in colours; for example, leg muscles are red and flight muscles are white.

Correspondingly, 'slow-twitch' and 'fast-twitch' muscles fibre types can be demonstrated by nerve stimulation studies. The metabolic requirements of each fibre type differ markedly, the slow red fibres mainly relying on aerobic metabolism and the fast white fibres being predominantly anaerobic. Most muscles actually contain a mixture of these extreme fibre types as well as an intermediate type.

Aerobic (*type* I) muscle fibres are small in cross section and contain abundant cytochromes and mitochondria. They also contain a large content of *myoglobin*, an oxygen-storage molecule analogous to haemoglobin, which accounts for the red colour of such fibres. In addition these fibres have a rich blood supply.

In contrast, anaerobic (*type* II) muscle fibres are large in cross-section, contain few mitochondria and cytochromes and relatively little myoglobin; they also have a relatively

poor blood supply. These muscle fibres are, however, rich in glycogen and glycolytic enzymes. These characteristics account for the 'white' colour of such fibres. Anaerobic fibres predominate in muscles responsible for intense but sporadic contraction such as the biceps and triceps of the arms.

The activity of the specific mitochondrial enzyme *succinate dehydrogenase*, which catalyses one of the stages of Krebs' cycle, demonstrates the relative proportions of mitochondria within the muscle fibres. In micrograph (a), note the presence of intensely stained small-diameter aerobic fibres **A**, poorly stained large-diameter anaerobic fibres **An** and intermediate fibres **I**.

Similarly, the amount of ATP-ase activity can be used to determine the relative proportion of different fibre types as in micrograph (b). The small aerobic fibres **A** have the greatest activity and stain strongly, whilst the anaerobic fibres **An** show little ATP-ase activity; intermediate fibres **I** predominate in this specimen. The type of metabolism of each fibre is determined by the frequency of impulses in its motor nerve supply. Any one motor nerve supplies fibres of one type only and all the fibres of a particular motor unit are of the same metabolic type. Indeed, if the motor nerve supply to one type of fibre is experimentally transplanted to supply another fibre type, this fibre type will become converted to the metabolic pattern of the former.

Visceral muscle

In contrast to skeletal muscle, which is specialised for relatively forceful contractions of short duration and under fine voluntary control, visceral muscle is specialised for continuous contractions of relatively low force producing diffuse movements resulting in contraction of the whole muscle mass rather than contraction of individual motor units. Contractility is an inherent property of visceral muscle, occurring independently of neurological innervation often in a rhythmic or wave-like fashion. Superimposed on this inherent contractility are the activities of the autonomic nervous system, hormones and local metabolites which modulate contractility to accommodate changing functional demands. For example, the smooth muscle of the intestinal wall undergoes continuous rhythmic contractions which result in waves of constriction passing along the bowel, propelling the luminal contents distally. This activity is enhanced by parasympathetic stimulation and influenced by a variety of hormones released in response to changes in the nature and volume of the gut contents. The structure of autonomic neuromuscular junctions is described in Chapter 7.

The cells of visceral muscle are relatively small with only a single nucleus. The fibres are bound together in irregular branching fasciculi, the arrangement varying considerably from one organ to another according to functional requirements.

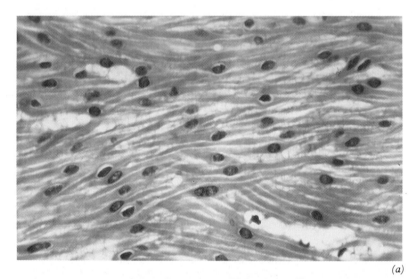

(a)

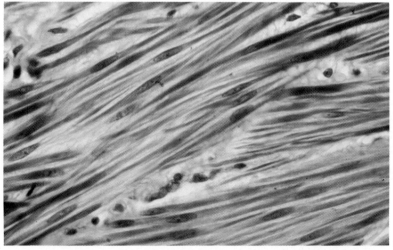

(b)

Fig. 6.13 Visceral muscle

(LS (a) H & E × 480 (b) Masson's trichrome × 480)

As seen in these micrographs, visceral muscle fibres are elongated, spindle-shaped cells with pointed ends which may be occasionally bifurcated. Visceral muscle fibres are generally much shorter than skeletal muscle fibres and contain only one nucleus which is elongated and centrally located in the cytoplasm at the widest part of the cell; however, depending on the contractile state of the fibres at fixation, the nuclei may sometimes appear to be spiral-shaped.

Visceral muscle fibres are bound together in irregular, branching fasciculi and these fasciculi, rather than individual fibres, are the functional contractile units. Within the fasciculi, individual muscle fibres are arranged roughly parallel to one another with the thickest part of one cell lying against the thin parts of adjacent cells.

The contractile proteins of visceral muscle are not arranged in myofibrils as in skeletal and cardiac muscle, thus visceral muscle cells are not striated, giving rise to the common name of smooth muscle.

Between individual muscle fibres and between fasciculi is a supporting network of connective tissue which is well demonstrated in micrograph (b) in which the collagen is stained blue.

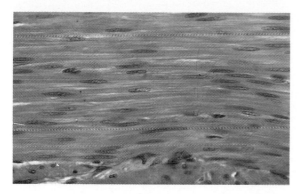

Fig. 6.14 Visceral muscle

(LS. H & E × 320)

This micrograph illustrates smooth muscle from the bowel wall cut in longitudinal section. In this case, the fibres are arranged in a highly regular manner and packed so closely that it is difficult to identify individual cell outlines although cell shape can be deduced from that of the nuclei.

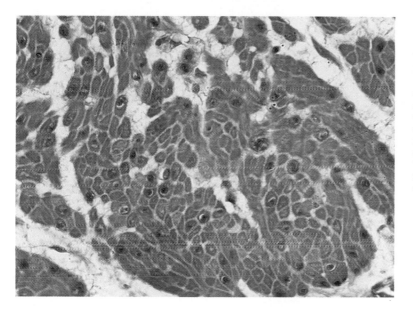

Fig. 6.15 Visceral muscle

(TS: H & E × 600)

This micrograph shows smooth muscle in transverse section at very high magnification. The spindle-shaped cells are sectioned at various different points along their length which gives the erroneous impression that they are of differing diameters. Nuclei are only included in the plane of section where fibres have been cut through their widest diameter. Note the plump nuclear shape and central location of nuclei within the cytoplasm.

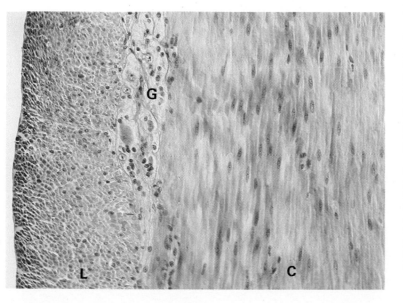

Fig. 6.16 Visceral muscle

(Masson's trichrome × 150)

In many tubular visceral structures such as the ileum seen in this micrograph, smooth muscle is disposed in layers with the cells of one layer arranged at right angles to those of the adjacent layer. This arrangement permits a wave of contraction to pass down the tube propelling the contents forward; this action is called *peristalsis.*

Typically, the longitudinal smooth muscle layer **L** is closely applied to the circular layer **C** with only a minimal amount of connective tissue between; in this specimen the connective tissue collagen is stained blue. The connective tissue is usually seen to contain clumps of large cells with pale nuclei which represent parasympathetic ganglia **G** (see Fig. 7.21).

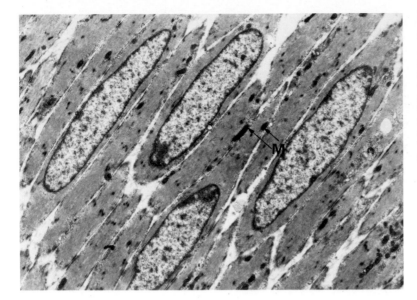

Fig. 6.17 Visceral muscle
(LS: EM × 5500)

At low magnification, electron microscopy demonstrates the spindle shape and elongated, central nuclei of visceral muscle cells. Note the relative sparsity of mitochondria **M** and other intracellular organelles. Most of the cytoplasm is occupied by fibrillar contractile protein, the organisation of which does not give rise to the appearance of cross-striations.

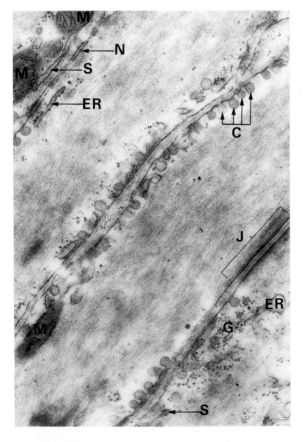

Fig. 6.18 Visceral muscle
(EM × 32 400)

At high magnification, details of the plasma membrane and endomembrane system can be seen.

The plasma membrane contains numerous flask-shaped invaginations. In some areas these are irregular in shape and size and may be involved in pinocytosis. In other areas, the invaginations are regular in shape and distribution, and are called *caveolae* **C**.

The endomembrane system contains some elements which appear to represent a poorly developed Golgi and endoplasmic reticulum system **ER**. Other vesicular and tubular structures **S** are seen near the plasma membrane, often in association with caveolae. This has led to the theory that these structures constitute a system which is analogous to the sarcoplasmic reticulum of skeletal muscle and that the caveolae are analogous to the T tubule system.

At this magnification, parallel myofilaments are seen to occupy most of the cytoplasm. These are believed to be analogous to the thin (actin) filaments of skeletal muscle. Recently, thick (myosin) filaments have also been demonstrated in visceral muscle cells using special techniques. The mechanism of smooth muscle contractility is therefore believed to be basically similar to that of skeletal muscle. Note also mitochondria **M** and glycogen granules **G** throughout the cytoplasm.

The narrow intercellular spaces are of almost uniform width but at numerous sites the plasma membranes of adjacent cells closely approximate to each other. Some of these intercellular contact areas **N** are believed to facilitate spread of excitation throughout visceral muscle and may be considered as nexus-like junctions (see Fig. 5.24). Other contacts may bind adjacent cells and provide anchorage points for contractile proteins; such junctions **J** bear a resemblance to the desmosomes of epithelia (see Fig. 5.24).

Cardiac muscle

Cardiac muscle exhibits many structural and functional characteristics intermediate between those of skeletal and visceral muscle. Like the former, its contractions are strong and utilise a great deal of energy, and like the latter the contractions are continuous and initiated by inherent mechanisms though modulated by external autonomic and hormonal stimuli.

Cardiac muscle fibres are essentially long, cylindrical cells with one or at most two nuclei, centrally located within the cell. The ends of the fibres are split longitudinally into a small number of branches the ends of which abut onto similar branches of adjacent cells giving the impression of a continuous three-dimensional cytoplasmic network; this was formerly described as a *syncytium* before the discrete intercellular boundaries were recognised.

Between the muscle fibres, delicate connective tissue analogous to the endomysium of skeletal muscle supports the extremely rich capillary network necessary to meet the high metabolic demands of strong continuous activity.

Cardiac muscle fibres have a similar arrangement of contractile proteins to that of skeletal muscle and are consequently striated in a similar manner. However, this is often difficult to visualise in cardiac muscle due to the irregular branching shape of the cells and their myofibrils. Cardiac muscle fibres also have a system of T tubules and sarcoplasmic reticulum analogous to that of skeletal muscles. In the case of cardiac muscle, however, there is a slow leak of calcium ions into the cytoplasm from the sarcoplasmic reticulum after recovery from the preceding contraction; this causes a succession of automatic contractions independent of external stimuli. The rate of this inherent rhythm is then modulated by external autonomic and hormonal stimuli.

Between the ends of adjacent cardiac muscle cells are specialised intercellular junctions called *intercalated discs* which not only provide points of anchorage for the myofibrils but permit extremely rapid spread of contractile stimuli from one cell to another. Thus, adjacent fibres are caused to contract almost simultaneously, thereby acting as a functional syncytium. In addition, a system of highly modified cardiac muscle cells constitute the pacemaker regions of the heart and ramify throughout the organ as the Purkinje system thus co-ordinating contraction of the myocardium as a whole in each cardiac cycle (see Ch. 8).

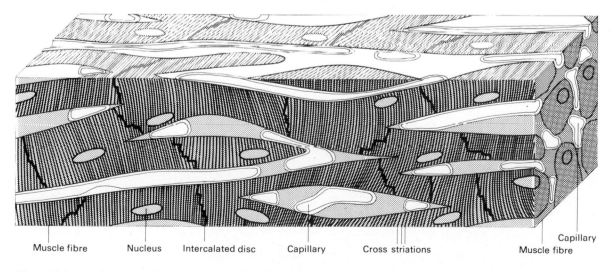

Muscle fibre   Nucleus   Intercalated disc   Capillary   Cross striations   Capillary / Muscle fibre

Fig. 6.19 Cardiac muscle

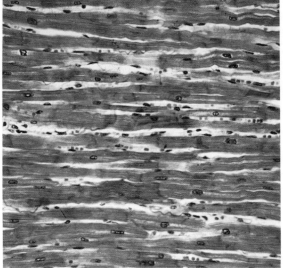

(a)

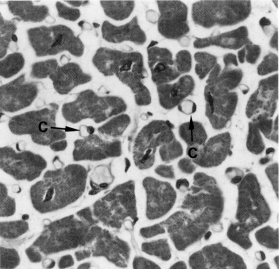

(b)

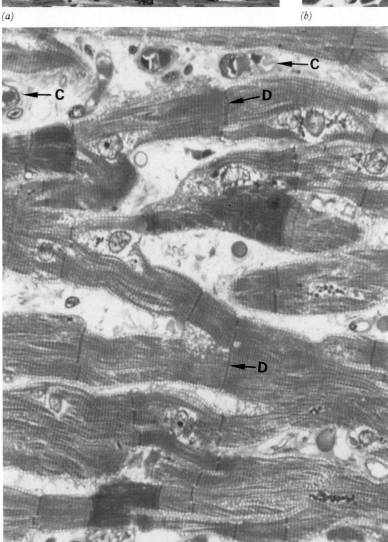

(c)

Fig. 6.20 Cardiac muscle

(a) *LS: H & E × 198*
(b) *TS: H & E × 480*
(c) *Thin section, toluidine blue × 640*

In longitudinal section in micrograph (a), cardiac muscle cells are seen to contain one or two nuclei and an extensive cytoplasm which branches to give the appearance of a continuous three-dimensional network. In routine H & E preparation such as this, the cross striations are not readily visible. The elongated nuclei are mainly centrally located, a characteristic well demonstrated in transverse section as in micrograph (b).

Micrograph (c) illustrates an extremely thin resin section at very high magnification. The branching cytoplasmic network is readily seen with prominent intercalated discs **D** marking the intercellular boundaries. Note the typical cross-striations.

In each of these specimens, note the delicate connective tissue, extremely rich in blood capillaries **C**, filling the intercellular spaces.

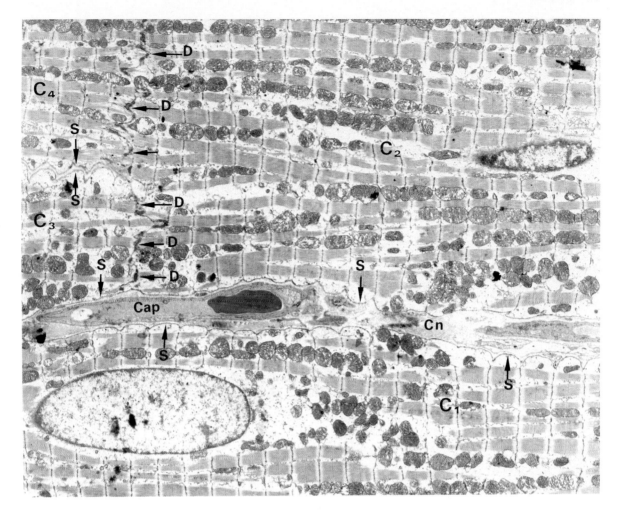

Fig. 6.21 Cardiac muscle

(EM × 4500)

This electron micrograph illustrates portions of four cardiac muscle cells C_1, C_2, C_3, and C_4 the outlines of which can be demarcated by following the sarcolemma **S** (i.e. plasma membranes). The nuclei of two cells C_1 and C_2 are included in the plane of section and are characteristically located deep to the sarcolemma. The intercellular space between cells C_1, C_2 and C_3 are occupied by capillaries **Cap** and collagen fibres **Cn**. The cell junctions between C_4 and C_2 and between C_3 and C_2 are defined by a single intercalated disc **D**.

The sarcomeres of cardiac muscle have an identical banding pattern to that of skeletal muscle. The sarcomeres are not, however, arranged into single columns making up cylindrical myofibrils as in skeletal muscle, but form a branching myofibrilar network continuous in three dimensions throughout the cytoplasm. The branching columns of sarcomeres are separated by sarcoplasm containing rows of mitochondria and sarcoplasmic reticulum. The great abundance of mitochondria in cardiac muscle, compared with skeletal muscle, reflects the enormous metabolic demands of continuous cardiac muscle activity.

Conduction of excitatory stimuli to the sarcomeres of cardiac muscle is mediated by a system of T tubules and sarcoplasmic reticulum essentially similar in arrangement to that of skeletal muscle. The T tubules, however, ramify throughout the cardiac muscle cytoplasm at the Z lines and their origins are seen as indentations in the sarcolemma which thus has a somewhat scalloped outline.

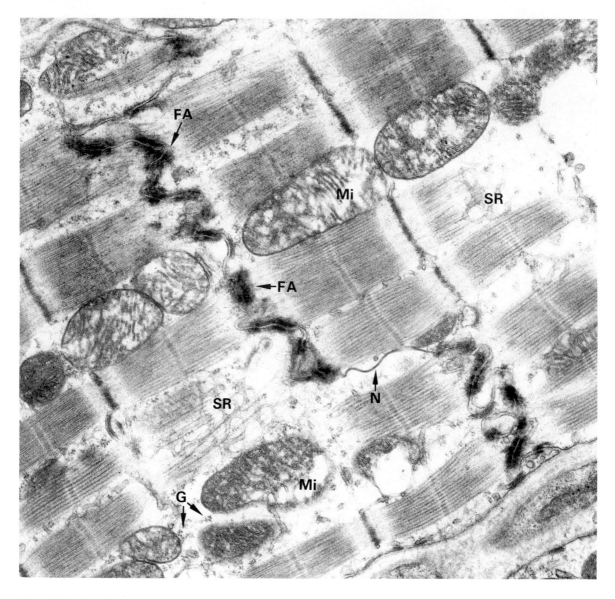

Fig. 6.22 Cardiac muscle: intercalated disc

(EM × 29 000)

Intercalated discs are specialised transverse junctions between cardiac muscle cells at sites where they meet end to end. Intercalated discs always coincide with the Z lines. Intercalated discs bind the cells, transmit forces of contraction and provide areas of low electrical resistance for the rapid spread of excitation throughout the myocardium.

The intercalated disc is an interdigitating junction, the entire surface of which consists of three types of membrane to membrane contacts. The predominant type of contact, the *fascia adherens* FA resembles the zona adherens of epithelial junctional complexes (see Fig. 5.24) but is more extensive and less regular. The ends of terminal sarcomeres insert into *fasciae adherentes* and thereby transmit contractile forces from cell to cell. Desmosomes occur less frequently and provide additional intercellular adhesion. Gap junctions or nexuses N occur in some longitudinal portions of the interdigitations and are believed to be sites of low electrical resistance through which excitation passes from cell to cell.

Note the similarity of the sarcomeres of cardiac and skeletal muscle (see Fig. 6.8). The mitochondria Mi of cardiac muscle are elongated or spheroidal and have abundant closely packed cristae rich in oxidative enzyme systems. The sarcoplasm within and between the sarcomeres is rich in glycogen granules G.

The T tubule and sarcoplasmic reticulum system form triads at the Z lines. The sarcoplasmic reticulum SR is less extensive than that of skeletal muscle and does not form dilated terminal cisternae; its lace-like form is well demonstrated in this micrograph.

7. Nervous tissues

Introduction

The function of the nervous system is to receive stimuli from both the internal and external environments; these are then analysed and integrated to produce appropriate, co-ordinated responses in various effector organs. The nervous system is composed of an intercommunicating network of specialised cells called *neurones* which constitute most sensory receptors, the conducting pathways, and the sites of integration and analysis.

The functions of the nervous system depend on a fundamental property of neurones called *excitability*. As in all cells, the resting neurone maintains an ionic gradient across its plasma membrane thereby creating an electrical potential. Excitability involves a change in membrane permeability in response to appropriate stimuli such that the ionic gradient is reversed and the plasma membrane becomes *depolarised*; a wave of depolarisation, known as an *action potential*, then spreads along the plasma membrane. This is followed by the process of *repolarisation* in which the membrane rapidly re-establishes its resting potential. At *synapses*, the sites of intercommunication between adjacent neurones, depolarisation of one neurone causes it to release chemical transmitter substances, *neurotransmitters*, which initiate an action potential in the adjacent neurone.

Within the nervous system, neurones are arranged to form pathways for the conduction of action potentials from receptors to effector organs via integrating neurones. Neurotransmitters not only mediate neurone-to-neurone transmission but also act as chemical intermediates between the nervous system and effector organs which also exhibit the property of excitability. The effector organs of voluntary nervous pathways are generally skeletal muscle, and those of involuntary pathways are usually smooth muscle, cardiac muscle and muscle-like epithelial cells (myoepithelial cells) within some exocrine glands.

The nervous system is divided anatomically into the *central nervous system* (CNS) comprising the brain and spinal cord, and the *peripheral nervous system* (PNS) which constitutes all nervous tissue outside the CNS. Functionally, the nervous system is divided into the *somatic nervous system* which is involved in voluntary functions, and the *autonomic nervous system* which exerts control over many involuntary functions. Histologically, however, the entire nervous system merely consists of variations in the arrangement of neurones and their supporting tissues.

This chapter covers the cell and tissue types found in the nervous system and includes the structure of the elements of the peripheral nervous system and simple types of sensory receptor. Details of the arrangement of nervous tissue in the central nervous system is the subject of Chapter 20 whilst the structure of the highly specialised organs of sensory reception e.g. eye and ear is shown in Chapter 21.

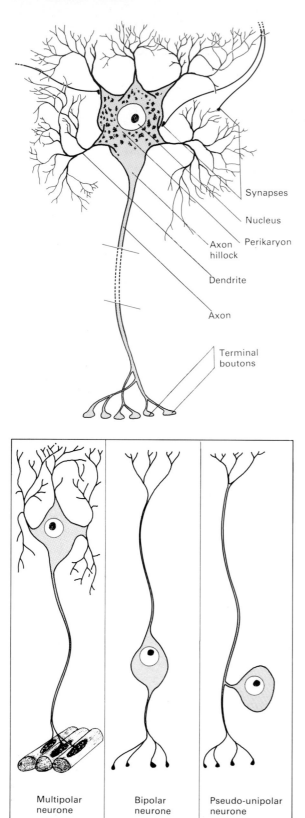

Synapses

Nucleus

Axon
hillock Perikaryon

Dendrite

Axon

Terminal
boutons

Multipolar
neurone

Bipolar
neurone

Pseudo-unipolar
neurone

Fig. 7.1 The neurone

Despite great variation in size and shape in different parts of the nervous system, all neurones have the same basic structure as shown in this idealised diagram. The neurone consists of a large *cell body* containing the nucleus surrounded by cytoplasm known as the *perikaryon*. Processes of two types extend from the cell body: a single *axon* and one or more *dendrites*.

Dendrites are highly branched, tapering processes which either end in specialised sensory receptors, as in primary sensory neurones, or form synapses with neighbouring neurones from which they receive stimuli. In general, dendrites function as the major sites of information input into the neurone.

Each neurone has a single axon arising from a cone-shaped portion of the cell body called the *axon hillock*. The axon extends as a cylindrical process of variable length terminating on other neurones or effector organs by a variable number of small branches which end in small swellings called *terminal boutons*.

Action potentials arise in the cell body as a result of integration of afferent stimuli; action potentials are then conducted along the axon to influence other neurones or effector organs. Axons are commonly referred to as *nerve fibres*.

In general, the cell bodies of all neurones are located in the central nervous system with the exception of the cell bodies of most primary sensory neurones and the terminal effector neurones of the autonomic nervous system in which case the cell bodies lie in aggregations called *ganglia* in peripheral sites.

Fig. 7.2 Basic neurone types

Throughout the nervous system, neurones have a wide variety of shapes which fall into three main patterns according to the arrangement of the axon and dendrites with respect to the cell body.

The most common form is the *multipolar neurone* in which numerous dendrites project from the cell body; the dendrites may all arise from one pole of the cell body or may extend from all parts of the cell body. In general, intermediate, integratory and motor neurones conform to this pattern.

Bipolar neurones have only a single dendrite which arises from the pole of the cell body opposite to the origin of the axon. These unusual neurones act as receptor neurones for the senses of smell, sight and balance.

Most other primary sensory neurones are described as *pseudo-unipolar neurones* since a single dendrite and the axon arise from a common stem of the cell body; this stem is formed by the fusion of the first part of the dendrite and axon of a bipolar type of neurone during embryological development.

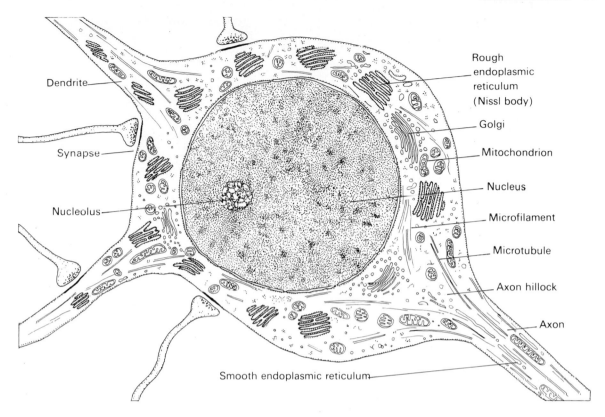

Dendrite

Synapse

Nucleolus

Rough
endoplasmic
reticulum
(Nissl body)

Golgi

Mitochondrion

Nucleus

Microfilament

Microtubule

Axon hillock

Axon

Smooth endoplasmic reticulum

Fig. 7.3 Ultrastructure of the neurone

This diagram illustrates the main ultrastructural features of
the neurone. The nucleus is large, round or ovoid and
usually centrally located within the perikaryon, reflecting
intense activity of the neurone, the chromatin is completely
dispersed and the nucleolus is a conspicuous feature.

The cytoplasm of the cell body contains large aggregations
of rough endoplasmic reticulum which correspond to the
Nissl substance of light microscopy (see Fig. 7.4); the rough
endoplasmic reticulum extends into the dendrites but not
into the axon hillock or axon. Rough endoplasmic reticulum
is a much more prominent feature in large neurones, such as
somatic motor neurones, than in smaller neurones such as
those of the autonomic nervous system. A diffuse Golgi
apparatus is found adjacent to the nucleus; smooth
endoplasmic reticulum is not a prominent feature of the
perikaryon but tubules, cisternae and vesicles are prominent
in the axon and dendrites. The mitochondria of the
perikaryon have the usual rod like appearance, but those of
the axon are extremely slender and elongated.

Neurones are highly metabolically active cells and expend
much energy in maintaining ionic gradients across the
plasma membrane. Neurones synthesise neurotransmitter
substances or their precursors in the perikaryon from where
they are transported along the axon to the synapse to be
released when appropriately stimulated.

Numerous microfilaments and microtubules are arranged
in parallel bundles throughout the perikaryon and along the
length of the axon and dendrites. These elements form the
neuronal cytoskeleton providing structural support as well as
being involved in axonal transport of neurotransmitter
substances, enzymes, membrane and other cellular
constituents.

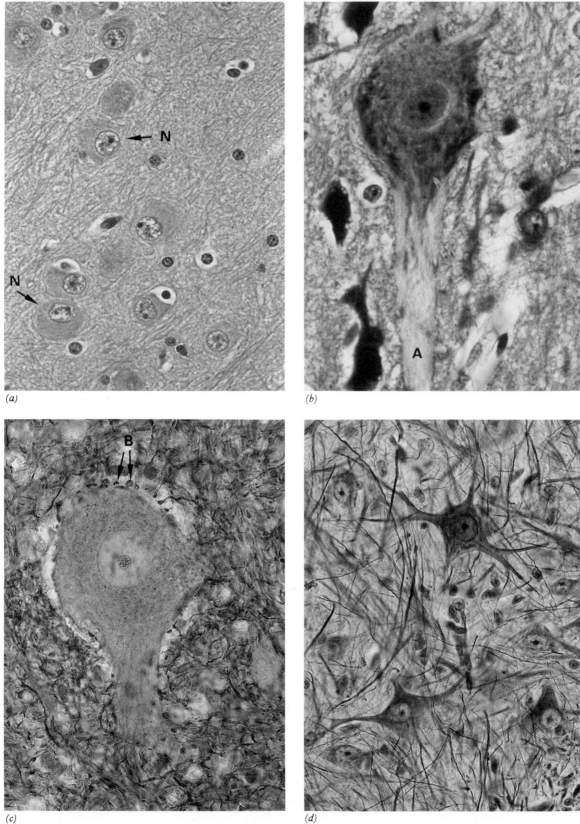

(a)

(b)

(c)

(d)

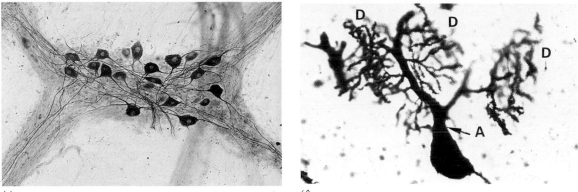

(e)   (f)

Fig. 7.4 Neurones and methods of study *(micrographs (a)–(d) opposite)*

(a) H & E × 480 (b) Nissl × 1200 (c) Gold method × 1200 (d) Gold toluidine blue × 600 (e) Spread preparation, Gold method × 62320 (f) Golgi-Cox × 320

The large size and complex morphology of neurones, the extreme elongation of axons, and the need to study neuronal interconnections has resulted in an extensive range of techniques being employed in neurohistology.

Methods which demonstrate nuclei, cell bodies and their cytoplasmic contents include routine stains such as H & E and more specific techniques for demonstrating particular cytoplasmic elements such as the Nissl method for RNA; however, these methods are of limited use in the study of axons and dendrites.

Heavy metal impregnation techniques with gold and silver are valuable in the study of neurone morphology including axons and dendrites and were widely employed by the pioneers of neuro-anatomy such as Cajal and Golgi from whom they take their names. Thick sections are often used with such methods as there is then a much greater chance of whole cells being included in the plane of section. Likewise, spread preparations often permit the examination of complete neurones and their cytoplasmic processes. Heavy metals are also deposited in the neuronal microtubules thus permitting study of the cytoskeleton.

Micrograph (a), stained with H & E, shows neurones **N** in the brain; the nuclei are huge in comparison with those of surrounding support cells; dispersed chromatin and prominent nucleoli reflect a high level of protein (enzyme) synthesis. The extensive cytoplasm is basophilic (blue-stained) due to extensive ribosomal RNA. No detail can be seen of cytoplasmic processes.

In micrograph (b), the Nissl method stains ribosomes (Nissl substance) dark blue giving the neuronal cytoplasm a granular appearance; DNA in the nucleus and nucleoli has similar staining properties. In this specimen, note the axon **A** which is devoid of Nissl substance beyond the axon hillock.

An almost identical neurone is shown in micrograph (c) using a heavy metal technique. Virtually the only intracellular detail that can be seen is the cytoskeleton and a negative image of the nucleus. Note the numerous axons with tiny terminal boutons **B** making synapses with the cell body.

Micrograph (d) employs another gold method which provides excellent detail of neuronal shape and shows the presence of the cytoskeleton in the dendrites and axons; the blue counter-stain demonstrates the nuclei of surrounding support cells. Note that detail of neuronal processes is lost when these pass out of the plane of section.

Spread preparations, as shown in micrograph (e), overcome this problem to a certain extent. This example shows neurones in a small peripheral ganglion, their cytoplasmic processes being very clearly delineated.

Finally, micrograph (f) illustrates a very thick section stained by a silver method which shows a Purkinje cell in the cerebellar cortex. These cells have a single small axon **A** at one pole and an extraordinary, finely branching dendritic tree **D** at the other pole.

Myelinated and non-myelinated nerve fibres

In the peripheral nervous system, all axons are enveloped by specialised cells called *Schwann cells* which provide both structural and metabolic support. In general, small diameter axons, for example those of the autonomic nervous system and small pain fibres, are simply enveloped by the cytoplasm of Schwann cells; these nerve fibres are said to be *non-myelinated*. Large-diameter fibres are wrapped by a variable number of concentric layers of the Schwann cell plasma membrane forming the so-called *myelin sheath*; such nerve fibres are said to be *myelinated*. Within the central nervous system, myelination is similar to that in the peripheral nervous system except that the myelin sheaths are formed by cells called *oligodendrocytes* (see Fig. 7.22). All non-myelinated fibres in the CNS have no specific cellular support but are indirectly supported by the mass of surrounding tissue.

In all nerve fibres, the rate of conduction of action potentials is proportional to the diameter of the axon; myelination greatly increases axon conduction velocity compared with that of a non-myelinated fibre of the same diameter.

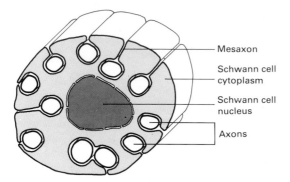

Fig. 7.5 Non-myelinated nerve fibres

The relationship of non-myelinated fibres and their supporting Schwann cell is illustrated in this diagram. One or more nerve fibres become longitudinally invaginated into the cytoplasm of a Schwann cell so that each fibre is embedded in a groove in the Schwann cell cytoplasm. The Schwann cell plasma membrane fuses along the opening of the groove, thus effectively sealing the nerve fibre within an extracellular compartment within the Schwann cell. The site of fusion of the Schwann cell membrane is called the *mesaxon*. Each Schwann cell extends for only a short distance along the nerve tract and at its termination its role is supplanted by another Schwann cell with which it interdigitates closely.

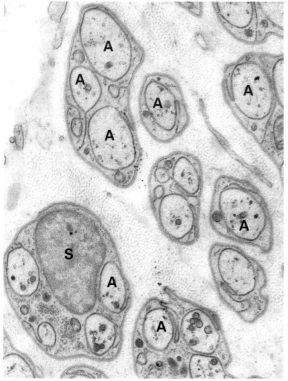

(a)

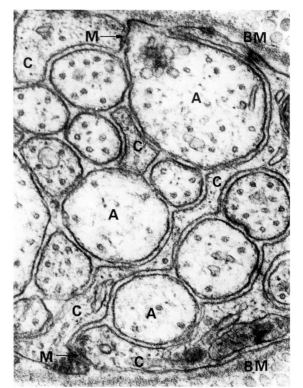

(b)

Fig. 7.6 Non-myelinated nerve fibres

(EM (a) × 9450 (b) × 75 600)

At low magnification, non-myelinated axons **A** of various sizes are seen embedded in Schwann cells; one of the Schwann cells has been sectioned transversely through its nucleus **S**. Note the variable number of fibres enclosed by each Schwann cell.

At high magnification, part of the cytoplasm of a Schwann cell **C** is shown enveloping several axons **A**; axons are readily identified by their content of tubules of smooth endoplasmic reticulum and microtubules, seen in cross-section. Two mesaxons **M** can be seen. Note that more than one nerve fibre may occupy a single groove within the Schwann cell. The external surface of the Schwann cell is bounded by a condensation of extracellular material forming a basement membrane **BM**.

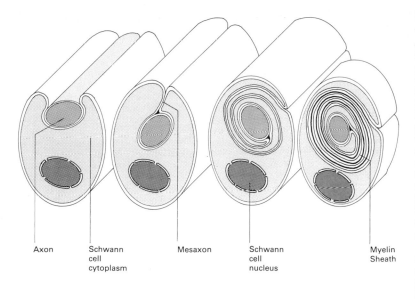

Axon   Schwann
cell
cytoplasm

Mesaxon   Schwann
cell
nucleus

Myelin
Sheath

Fig. 7.7 Myelination

The process of myelination starts during fetal development and continues for a considerable time after birth. In peripheral nerves, myelination begins with the invagination of a single nerve fibre into a Schwann cell; a mesaxon, like that of unmyelinated fibres, is then formed (see Fig. 7.5). As myelination proceeds, the mesaxon wraps around the axon thereby enveloping the axon in a spiral layer of Schwann cell cytoplasm. As this process continues, the cytoplasm is excluded; by maturity, the inner layers of plasma membrane fuse with each other so that the axon becomes surrounded by several layers of modified membranes which together constitute the myelin sheath.

In the CNS, oligodendrocytes are responsible for the process of myelination which follows a similar pattern; a single oligodendrocyte, however, forms the myelin sheaths of several axons (see Fig. 7.22).

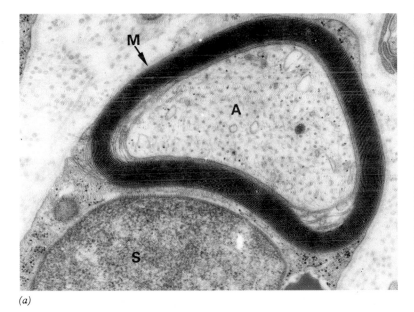

(a)

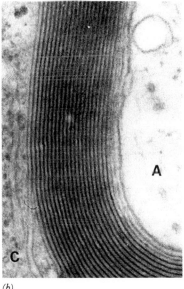

(b)

Fig. 7.8 Myelinated nerve fibre

(EM (a) × 17 000 (b) × 75 250)

At low magnification, a myelinated nerve fibre is seen sectioned transversely at the level of the nucleus of an associated Schwann cell **S**. A single large axon **A** is enveloped by many spiral layers of fused, Schwann cell plasma membrane forming a thick myelin sheath **M**. At higher magnification, it can be seen that Schwann cell cytoplasm is completely absent from the myelin sheath and

that the sheath consists merely of many regular layers of plasma membrane material. These successive layers of predominantly lipid material are thought to insulate the axon from the extracellular environment thus preventing ion fluxes across the plasma membrane of the nerve axon. The Schwann cell cytoplasm **C** encircles the myelin sheath and has no unusual ultrastructural features.

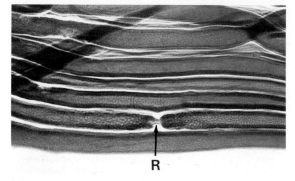

(a)

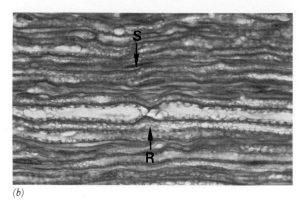

(b)

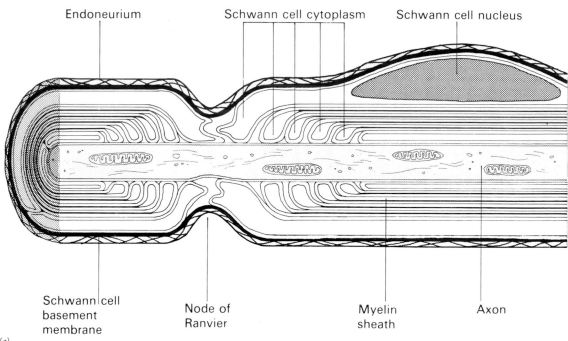

Endoneurium   Schwann cell cytoplasm   Schwann cell nucleus

Schwann cell basement membrane   Node of Ranvier   Myelin sheath   Axon

(c)

Fig. 7.9 Node of Ranvier

(a) Teased preparation, Sudan black × 320 (b) H & E × 320 (c) Schematic diagram

The myelin sheath of an individual axon is provided by many Schwann cells (oligodendrocytes in the CNS), each Schwann cell covering only a segment of the axon. Between the Schwann cells there are short intervals at which the axon is not covered by a myelin sheath; these points are known as *nodes of Ranvier*.

In the teased preparation of myelinated axons shown in micrograph (a), a node of Ranvier **R** is seen, representing a site where the continuity of the myelin sheath is interrupted. With this method, only the lipid of the myelin has been stained, thus Schwann cell nuclei are not seen.

Micrograph (b) shows axons in longitudinal section stained with H & E. Due to a fixation artefact, myelin sheaths appear 'bubbly'; the myelin being lipid is mostly dissolved out during preparation and is therefore unstained. A node of Ranvier **R** is identifiable in the large axon in midfield. Scattered Schwann cell nuclei **S** can also be seen.

The diagram illustrates the manner in which Schwann cells terminate at the node of Ranvier, so exposing the axon to the external environment. It is believed that the myelin sheath prevents the nerve action potential from being propagated continuously along the axon and the action potential travels by jumping from node to node. This mode of conduction, known as *saltatory conduction*, is thought to be the mechanism by which myelination greatly enhances the conduction velocity of axons. The internodal distance is proportional to the diameter of the fibre and may be up to one millimetre in the largest fibres.

Synapses and neuromuscular junctions

Synapses are highly specialised intercellular junctions which link the neurones of each nervous pathway, and which link neurones and their effector cells such as muscle fibres; where neurones synapse with skeletal muscle they are referred to as *neuromuscular junctions* or *motor end plates*. Individual neurones intercommunicate via a widely variable number of synapses depending on their location within the nervous system. Classically, the axon of one neurone synapses with the dendrite of another neurone, but axons may synapse with the cell bodies or axons of other neurones; dendrite-to-dendrite and cell body-to-cell body synapses have also been described. For a given synapse, the conduction of an impulse is always in one direction only, but the response may be either excitatory or inhibitory depending on the specific nature of the synapse and its location within the nervous system.

The mechanism of conduction of the nerve impulse is thought to involve the release from one neurone of a chemical transmitter substance, the neurotransmitter, which then diffuses across a narrow intercellular space to induce excitation or inhibition in the other neurone or effector cell of that synapse. Neurotransmitters mediate their effects by interacting with specific receptors incorporated in the opposing plasma membrane.

The chemical nature of neurotransmitters and the morphology of synapses, is highly variable in different parts of the nervous system, but the principles of synaptic transmission and the basic structure of synapses are similar throughout the nervous system.

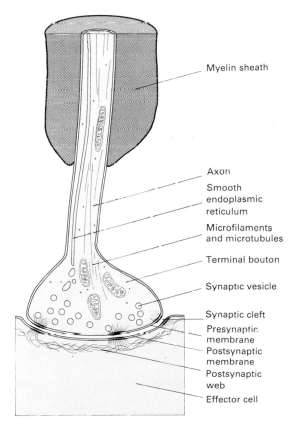

Myelin sheath

Axon

Smooth endoplasmic reticulum

Microfilaments and microtubules

Terminal bouton

Synaptic vesicle

Synaptic cleft

Presynaptic membrane

Postsynaptic membrane

Postsynaptic web

Effector cell

Fig. 7.10 Synapse

This diagram illustrates the general structure of the synapse. The neurone responsible for propagating the stimulus terminates at a swelling or terminal bouton; this is separated from the plasma membrane of the opposed neurone or effector cell by a narrow intercellular gap of uniform width (20–30 nm) called the *synaptic cleft*. The terminal boutons are not myelinated. The boutons contain mitochondria and membrane-bound vesicles of neurotransmitter substance known as *synaptic vesicles*.

Although many types of neurotransmitter substance occur in the CNS, only two types are known in the peripheral nervous system: acetyl choline and noradrenaline (norepinephrine). Acetylcholine precursors, acetate and choline, are synthesised in the perikaryon and transported to the synapse where they are conjugated. Noradrenaline synthesis takes place in both the perikaryon and the terminal bouton. Synaptic vesicles are thought to be derived by budding from the smooth endoplasmic reticulum of the axon.

Synaptic vesicles tend to aggregate towards the *pre-synaptic membrane* and, on arrival of an action potential, are thought to release their contents into the synaptic cleft by exocytosis. The neurotransmitter diffuses across the synaptic cleft to stimulate receptors in the *post-synaptic membrane*. Associated with synapses are a variety of biochemical mechanisms such as hydrolytic and oxidative enzymes which inactivate the released neurotransmitter between successive nerve impulses. The cytoplasm beneath the post-synaptic membrane often contains a feltwork of fine fibrils, the *post-synaptic web*, which may be associated with desmosome-like structures in maintaining the integrity of the synapse.

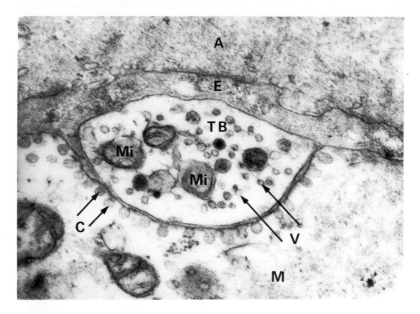

Fig. 7.11 Synapse

(EM × 45 000)

This micrograph illustrates a synapse between a sympathetic nerve and a smooth muscle cell in the vas deferens. The terminal bouton **TB** is recessed into the surface of the effector muscle cell **M** in an area devoid of contractile filaments. Note the uniform width of the synaptic cleft between the pre- and post-synaptic membranes. The terminal bouton contains a few mitochondria **Mi** and numerous synaptic vesicles **V**. The post-synaptic membrane exhibits many flask-like invaginations **C** which may represent caveolae (see Fig. 6.18). Note an adjacent smooth muscle cell **A**, packed with microfilaments, and delicate intervening endomysial connective tissue **E**.

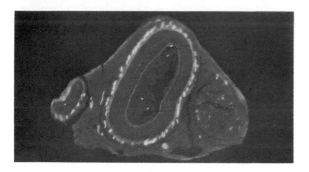

Fig. 7.12 Sympathetic nerve endings

(Formalin-induced fluorescence × 80)

Noradrenaline is the main post-ganglionic neurotransmitter in the sympathetic nervous system. When noradrenaline combines with formalin (and some other compounds) it becomes fluorescent and can be visualised by fluorescence microscopy.

This micrograph illustrates formalin-induced fluorescence in the adventitial layer of large and small arteries, corresponding to the presence of sympathetic noradrenergic nerve endings. Background autofluorescence outlines the general tissue structure; note that the internal elastic lamina is particularly autofluorescent.

Fig. 7.13 Motor end plates *(illustrations opposite)*

(Teased preparations, Gold impregnation method (a) × 320 (b) × 800 (c) Histochemical method for acetylcholinesterase × 320 (d) Schematic diagram)

The motor end plates of skeletal muscle have the same basic structure as other synapses with the addition of several important details. Firstly, one motor neurone may innervate from a few to more than a thousand muscle fibres depending on the precision of movement of the muscle; the motor neurone and the muscle fibres which it supplies together constitute a *motor unit*. At low magnification in micrograph (a), the terminal part of the axon of a motor neurone is seen dividing into several branches, each terminating as a motor endplate on a different skeletal muscle fibre usually near to its mid-point. At high magnification in micrograph (b), a terminal branch is seen to lose its myelin sheath and divides to form a cluster of small bulbous swellings on the muscle fibre surface.

The motor end plate occupies a recess in the muscle cell surface, described as the *sole plate*, and is covered by an extension of the cytoplasm of the last Schwann cell surrounding the axon. The connective tissue covering the nerve (endoneurium) becomes continuous with the endomysium of the muscle fibre.

Each of the terminal swellings of the cluster making up

the motor end plate has the same basic structure as the synapse shown in Figure 7.10 but, as shown in the diagram opposite, the post-synaptic membrane of the neuromuscular junction is deeply folded to form parallel *secondary synaptic clefts*. The overlying presynaptic membrane is also irregular and the cytoplasm immediately adjacent contains numerous synaptic vesicles. The remaining cytoplasm of the terminal bulb contains numerous mitochondria and a considerable amount of rough endoplasmic reticulum. The sole plate of the muscle fibre also contains a concentration of mitochondria and an aggregation of nuclei.

The neurotransmitter of somatic neuromuscular junctions is acetyl choline, the receptors for which are concentrated at the margins of the secondary synaptic clefts. The hydrolytic enzyme acetylcholinesterase is present deeper in the clefts and is involved in deactivation of the neurotransmitter between successive nerve impulses. The histochemical technique shown in micrograph (c) opposite defines the location of motor end plates by demonstrating acetylcholinesterase activity which appears as a brown deposit.

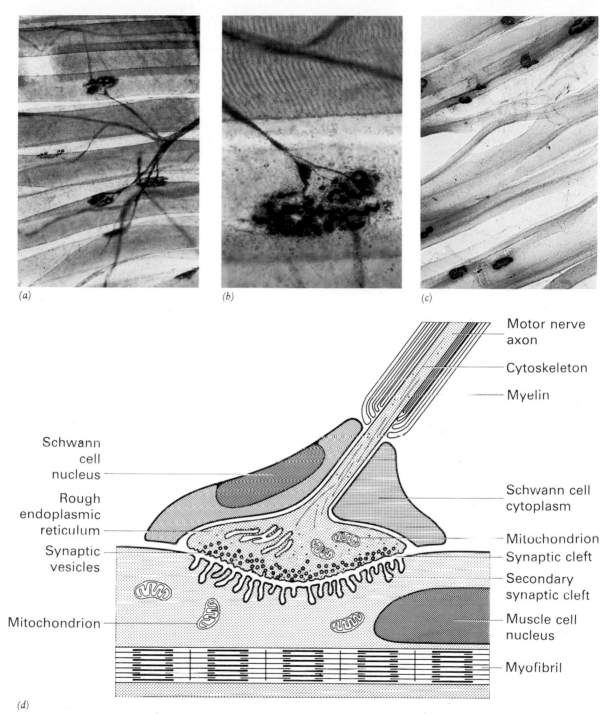

(a)

(b)

(c)

Motor nerve axon

Cytoskeleton

Myelin

Schwann cell nucleus

Rough endoplasmic reticulum

Synaptic vesicles

Mitochondrion

Schwann cell cytoplasm

Mitochondrion

Synaptic cleft

Secondary synaptic cleft

Muscle cell nucleus

Myofibril

(d)

Peripheral nervous tissues

Peripheral nerves are anatomical structures which may contain any combination of afferent or efferent nerve fibres of either the somatic or autonomic nervous systems. The cell bodies of fibres coursing in peripheral nerves are either located in the CNS or in ganglia in peripheral sites.

Each peripheral nerve is composed of one or more bundles or *fascicles* of nerve fibres; within the fascicles, each individual nerve fibre, with its investing Schwann cell, is surrounded by a delicate packing of loose connective tissue called *endoneurium* which contains a few fibroblasts and blood capillaries. Each fascicle is surrounded by a condensed layer of collagenous connective tissue called the *perineurium*. In peripheral nerves consisting of more than one fascicle, a further layer of loose connective tissue called the *epineurium* binds the fascicles together and is condensed peripherally to form a cylindrical sheath. The larger blood vessels supplying the nerve are found within the epineurium. The fibres within a peripheral nerve derive considerable mechanical strength from these three layers of connective tissue.

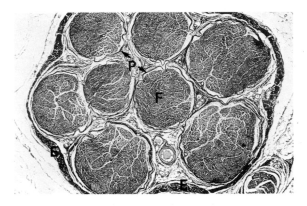

Fig. 7.14 Peripheral nerve

(TS: van Gieson × 20)

This micrograph illustrates the typical appearance of a medium sized peripheral nerve in transverse section. This nerve consists of eight fascicles **F**, each of which contains many nerve fibres. Each fascicle is invested by a condensed connective tissue layer, the perineurium **P**, and the nerve as a whole is encased in a loose connective tissue sheath, the epineurium **E**, which is condensed at its outermost aspect. Blood vessels of various sizes can be seen in the epineurium.

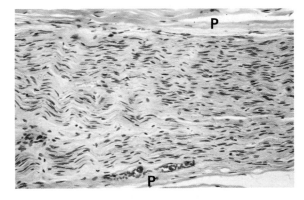

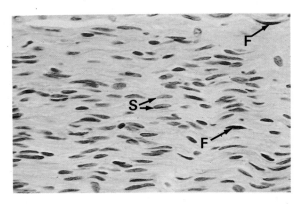

(b)

Fig. 7.15 Peripheral nerve

(LS: H & E (a) × 128 (b) × 320)

The peripheral nerve shown in micrograph (a) consists of a single fascicle invested by dense perineurium **P** containing small blood vessels; a separate epineurium cannot be distinguished. Most of the nuclei seen within the fascicle are those of Schwann cells which mark the course of individual axons; axons are not readily visible in this type of preparation. Fibroblasts of the endoneurium are scattered amongst the much more numerous Schwann cells. A striking feature of peripheral nerves is that the fibres follow a longitudinal zigzag course which permits stretching during movement.

At higher magnification in micrograph (b), Schwann cell nuclei **S** are seen to be elongated in the long axis of the nerve. The relatively sparse fibroblasts **F** are distinguished by their more slender, condensed nuclei.

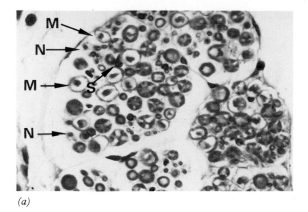

(a)

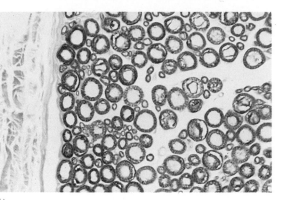

(b)

Fig. 7.16 Peripheral nerve

(TS (a) H & E × 480 (b) Osmium fixation, van Gieson × 800)

In routinely fixed and stained preparations, myelin is poorly preserved since it is largely composed of lipid material. Schwann cell cytoplasm is, however, well-preserved and has eosinophilic staining properties.

Micrograph (a) shows a peripheral nerve stained with H & E; the nerve contains axons of many different types and calibre, some of which are myelinated. Heavily myelinated fibres **M** can be identified by an unstained ring of myelin, the centrally located axon and peripheral rim of Schwann cell cytoplasm being stained pink. In contrast, small non-myelinated fibres **N** can also be easily identified. Between

these extremes are fibres of various sizes with 'bubbly' artefactually distorted myelin sheaths. Note the nuclei of Schwann cells **S** scattered among the nerve fibres. Several flattened fibroblast nuclei are also seen in the perineurium.

In osmium fixed preparations as shown in micrograph (b), the lipid constituents of myelin are well preserved and are stained black. Note the wide variation in axon diameter. The collagen of the delicate endoneurium between the individual nerve fibres and in the condensed perineurium surrounding the fascicle is stained red by the van Gieson method.

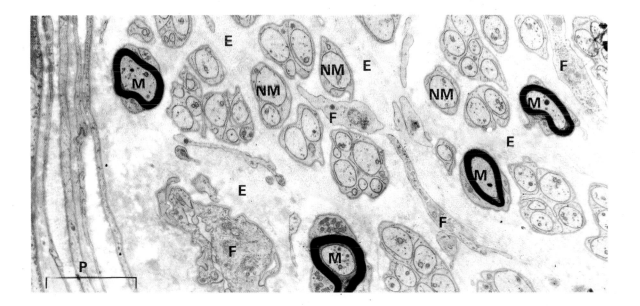

Fig. 7.17 Peripheral nerve

(TS: EM × 5200)

The ultrastructural features of peripheral nerves are seen in this example which contains both myelinated **M** and non-myelinated **NM** fibres. The endoneurium **E** consists of loosely arranged collagen fibres lying parallel to the nerve

fibres. Strands of fibroblast cytoplasm **F** extend throughout the endoneurium. In contrast, the perineurium **P** consists of extremely flattened fibroblasts and more densely packed collagen fibres.

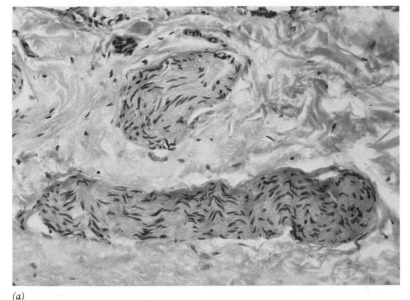

(a)

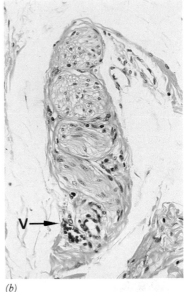

(b)

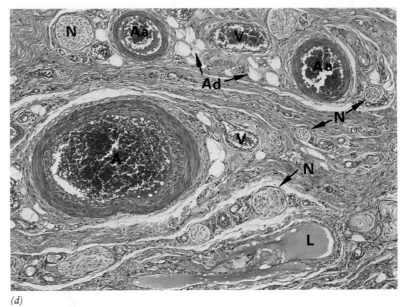

(c)

(d)

Fig. 7.18 Small peripheral nerves

(a) H & E × 480 (b) Masson's trichrome × 320 (c) Masson's trichrome × 100 (d) H & E × 150

These micrographs illustrate the appearance of a variety of small peripheral nerves in the tissues.

Micrograph (a) shows two small nerves in the dermis of the skin, each nerve consisting of a single fascicle of fibres. The nerve at the top of the field is cut in longitudinal section; the wavy shape of the Schwann cell nuclei reflects the course of the axons which are thereby protected from damage when the skin is stretched. The other nerve is cut in oblique section. Note the dense irregular collagenous connective tissue surrounding the nerves in this specimen.

Micrograph (b) shows a very small peripheral nerve in the hypodermis of the skin. In contrast to the first specimen, with this technique collagen is stained blue-green. This nerve runs a zig-zag course in the skin and the plane of section has cut it in such a way as to show it in four transverse-oblique views. Note small associated blood vessels **V** containing red-stained erythrocytes.

Micrograph (c) shows a tiny nerve bundle **N** probably a motor nerve, in skeletal muscle. A nerve bundle of this size would be almost unrecognisable but for its numerous Schwann cell nuclei.

Finally, a neurovascular bundle from the vulva is the subject of micrograph (d). It contains a small artery **A**, arterioles **Aa**, venules **V**, a lymphatic **L**, several small peripheral nerves **N** cut in transverse section and scattered adipocytes **Ad**.

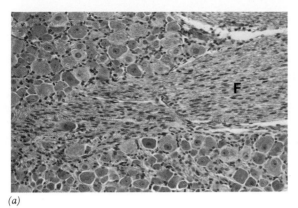

(a)

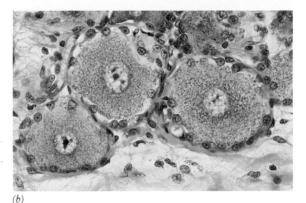

(b)

Fig. 7.19 Spinal ganglion

(H & E (a) × 128 (b) × 800)

Ganglia are discrete aggregations of neurone cell bodies located outside the CNS. The spinal ganglia lie on the posterior nerve roots of the spinal cord as they pass through the intervertebral foramina; they contain the cell bodies of primary sensory neurones which are of the pseudo-unipolar form.

At low magnification in micrograph (a), note the fascicle F of nerve fibres passing to the centre of the ganglion, the ganglion cells being located peripherally. At high magnification in micrograph (b), each cell body is seen to be surrounded by a layer of flattened *satellite cells* which provide structural and metabolic support and have similar embryological origin to the Schwann cells (neural crest).

The whole ganglion is encapsulated by condensed connective tissue which is continuous with the perineurial and epineurial sheaths of the associated peripheral nerve.

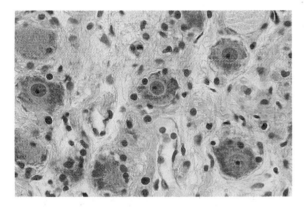

Fig. 7.20 Sympathetic ganglion

(H & E × 400)

The sympathetic ganglia have a similar structure to that of sensory ganglia with a few minor differences. The ganglion cells are multipolar and are thus more widely spaced, being separated by numerous axons and dendrites, many of which pass through the ganglion without being involved in synapses. As seen in this micrograph, the nuclei of the ganglion cells tend to be excentrically located and the peripheral cytoplasm contains a variable quantity of brown-stained lipofuscin granules representing cellular debris sequestered in residual bodies.

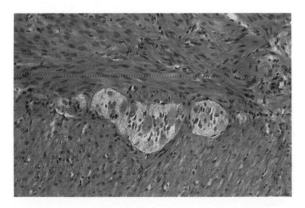

Fig. 7.21 Parasympathetic ganglion

(H·& E × 320)

The cell bodies of the terminal effector neurones of the parasympathetic nervous system are usually located within or near the effector organs. The cell bodies may be aggregated as well-organised ganglia of moderate size (as in the otic ganglion) but more commonly, parasympathetic ganglia merely consist of a few cell bodies clumped together to form minute ganglia scattered in the supporting connective tissue.

This micrograph illustrates a minute ganglion between two smooth muscle layers in the wall of the gastrointestinal tract. Like all neurones, the ganglion cells are recognised by their large nuclei, with dispersed chromatin and prominent nucleoli, and their extensive basophilic cytoplasm. As in other ganglia, the neurones are surrounded by numerous small support cells and afferent and efferent nerve fibres.

Central nervous tissues

The central nervous system consists of the brain and spinal cord, each of which can be divided grossly into areas of so-called *grey matter* and *white matter*; grey matter contains almost all the neurone cell bodies and their associated fibres, whereas white matter consists merely of tracts of nerve fibres. Central nervous tissue consists of a vast number of neurones and their processes embedded in a mass of support cells, collectively known as *neuroglia*; there is little intercellular matrix.

The outer surface of the brain and spinal cord is covered by three specialised connective tissue layers, collectively known as the *meninges*. Although each functional zone of the CNS has its own peculiar histological appearance, the basic organisation of grey and white matter remains consistent throughout; only the principles of organisation are discussed in this section.

Fig. 7.22 Neuroglia *(illustrations opposite)*

(a) Schematic diagram (b) H & E × 480 (c) Cajal method × 400 (d) H & E × 320

The neuroglia comprise all the non-neural cells of the CNS. These highly branched cells, which form almost half the total mass of the CNS, occupy the spaces between neurones and thus the CNS contains little extracellular material. The neuroglia have intimate functional relationships with neurones providing both mechanical and metabolic support.

Four principle types of neuroglia are recognised namely *oligodendrocytes, astrocytes, microglia* and *ependymal* cells which are illustrated schematically opposite.

Common staining methods as employed in micrograph (b) usually permit neurones **N** to be readily distinguished from glial cells which make up the remaining cells seen in this micrograph. Although the size and morphology of neurones varies greatly in different regions of the brain, they are usually recognisable by their large nuclei with prominent nucleoli and extensive basophilic granular cytoplasm, one or more processes of which may be visible.

Neuroglia, particularly oligodendrocytes, have highly variable histological characteristics and are difficult to differentiate by common staining methods, being best identified by metalic impregnation techniques.

1. Oligodendrocytes: Oligodendrocytes (oligodendroglia) are cells of moderate size which were named for their appearance when stained by classical methods with which they appeared to have a small number of short branched processes. It is now known that oligodendrocytes are the cells responsible for myelination of axons in the CNS and the dendrites previously described are the short pedicles that connect the cell body to the myelin sheaths. A single oligodendrocyte may be responsible for the myelination of up to 50 nerve fibres. Oligodendrocytes are the predominant type of neuroglia in white matter. Oligodendrocytes also aggregate closely around neurone cell bodies in the grey matter where they are thought to have a support function analogous to that of the satellite cells which surround neurone cell bodies in peripheral ganglia.

2. Astrocytes: Classical impregnation methods such as that seen in micrograph (c), identify the existence of star shaped neuroglia, the astrocytes. These cells, which are the most numerous glial cells in grey matter, have prolific long, highly-branched processes which occupy most of the interneuronal spaces. In grey matter, many of the astrocyte processes end in terminal expansions upon the basement membranes of capillaries; these are thus called *perivascular feet*. Other processes of the same astrocytes terminate in close apposition to the non-synaptic regions of neurones. Perivascular feet cover most of the capillary basement membranes. On the basis of these observations it has been suggested that astrocytes in grey matter mediate some metabolic exchange between neurones and blood. All astrocytes contain bundles of intracellular microfilaments which are particularly prominent in the astrocytes of white matter where they are known as *fibrous astrocytes*; those of grey matter are called *protoplasmic astrocytes*. Astrocytes contribute considerable structural support to neurones and play an important role in repair of CNS tissue after injury or damage by disease processes.

3. Microglia: Microglia are small cells, relatively few in number, derived from cells of mesenchymal origin which invade the CNS at a late stage of fetal development. Microglia have small irregular nuclei and relatively little cytoplasm which forms fine, highly-branched processes. In response to tissue damage, microglia transform into large amoeboid phagocytic cells and microglia are thus considered to be members of the macrophage-monocyte defence system (see Fig. 3.12).

4. Ependymal cells: Ependymal cells form the simple cuboidal epithelial lining of the ventricles and spinal canal as seen in micrograph (d). The cells are tightly bound together at their luminal surfaces by the usual epithelial junctional complexes. Unlike other epithelia, however, ependymal cells do not rest on a basement membrane but rather, the bases of the cells taper then break up into fine branches which ramify into an underlying layer of processes derived from astrocytes. At the luminal surface, there are a variable number of cilia, which may be involved in propulsion of cerebrospinal fluid within the ventricles, as well as microvilli, which probably have absorptive and secretory functions.

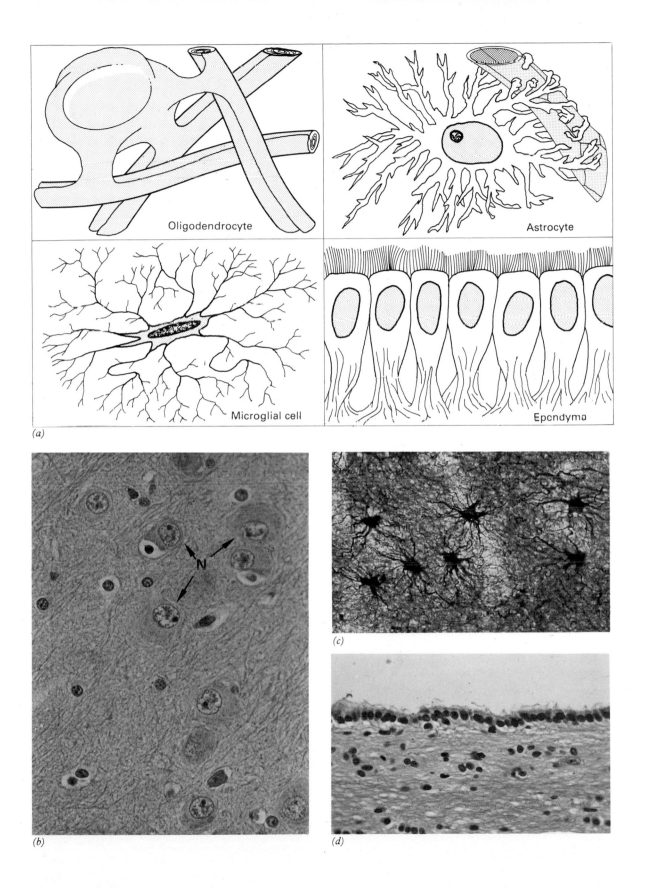

(a)

Oligodendrocyte

Astrocyte

Microglial cell

Epcndyma

(b)

(c)

(d)

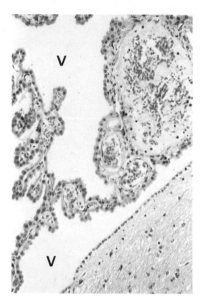

Fig. 7.23 Choroid plexus

(H & E × 128)

The choroid plexus is a vascular structure, arising from the wall of each of the four ventricles of the brain, responsible for the production of cerebro-spinal fluid (CSF). CSF drains from the interconnected ventricular cavities via three channels connecting the fourth ventricle with the subarachnoid space which surrounds the CNS (see Fig. 7.24). CSF is produced at a constant rate and is primarily reabsorbed from the subarachnoid space into the superior sagittal venous sinus via finger-like projections called *arachnoid villi*. Thus the CNS is suspended in a constantly circulating fluid medium which acts as a shock absorber.

Each choroid plexus consists of a mass of capillaries projecting into the ventricle **V** and invested by modified ependymal cells. The choroid epithelial cells are separated from the underlying capillaries and their delicate supporting connective tissue by a basement membrane. Long, bulbous microvilli project from the luminal surfaces of the choroid epithelial cells and the cytoplasm contains numerous mitochondria, features which suggest that the elaboration of CSF is an active process. The capillaries of the choroid plexus are large, thin-walled and sometimes fenestrated. The mode of CSF secretion is thought to involve active secretion of sodium ions by choroid epithelial cells into the CSF, followed by passive movement of water from the choroid capillaries. Small amounts of protein, as well as glucose at the same concentration as that of plasma, are normal constituents of CSF but the mode of their passage into the CSF is unknown.

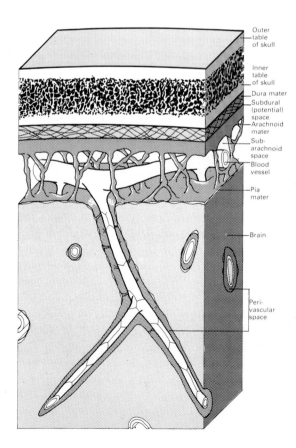

Fig. 7.24 Meninges

The brain and spinal cord are invested by three layers of connective tissue collectively called the meninges. The surface of the nervous tissue is covered by a delicate layer called the *pia mater* containing fibroblasts, collagenous fibres and the processes of underlying astrocytes. Overlying the pia mater is a thicker fibrous layer, the *arachnoid mater*, which derives its name from the presence of web-like strands which connect it to the underlying pia mater; since the pia and arachnoid are structurally continuous, they are often considered as a single unit, the *pia-arachnoid* or *leptomeninges*. The space between the pia and arachnoid layers is called the *subarachnoid space* and in places forms large cisterns. The subarachnoid space is connected with the ventricles by three foramina and CSF circulates continuously from the ventricles into the subarachnoid space. The apposed surfaces of the pia and arachnoid layers, and their interconnecting fibres, are lined by flattened mesothelial cells. The outer surface of the arachnoid mater is also lined by mesothelium.

Arteries and veins passing to and from the CNS pass in the subarachnoid space loosely attached to the pia mater and as the larger vessels extend into the nervous tissue, they are surrounded by a delicate layer of pia mater. Between the penetrating vessels and the pia there is a *perivascular space* which is continuous with the subarachnoid space.

Beyond the arachnoid mater is a dense fibro-elastic layer called the *dura mater* which is lined on its internal surface by mesothelium. The dura is closely applied to, but not connected with, the arachnoid layer and a potential space, the *subdural space*, containing a minute amount of fluid separates the two layers. In the cranium, the dura mater merges with the periosteum of the skull whereas around the spinal cord the dura is suspended from the periosteum of the spinal canal by the so-called *denticulate ligaments*, the intervening *epidural space* being filled with loose, fibro-fatty connective tissue and a venous plexus.

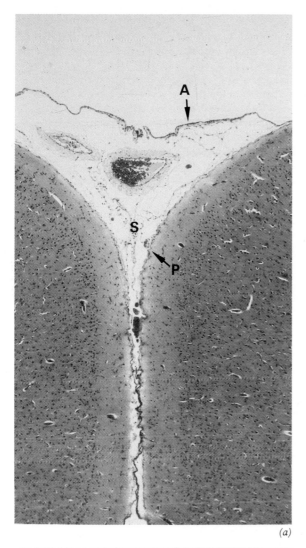

(a)

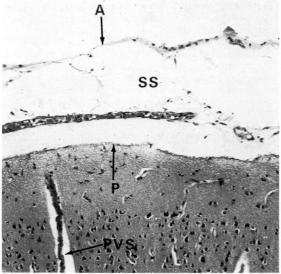

(b)

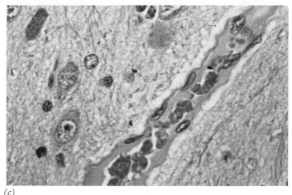

(c)

Fig. 7.25 Meninges

(H & E (a) × 40 (b) × 198 (c) × 480)

The pia and arachnoid layers of the brain meninges are illustrated in micrographs (a) and (b), the dura mater remaining adherent to the skull when the brain is removed from the cranial cavity.

The pia mater **P** is intimately attached to the surface of the brain and, as seen in micrograph (a), continues into the sulci **S** and around the penetrating vessels. The arachnoid mater **A** appears to be a completely separate layer and bridges the sulci. At higher magnification in micrograph (b), delicate fibrous strands can be seen traversing the subarachnoid space **SS** to connect the pia and arachnoid layers. Both these layers consist of delicate connective tissue the surface of which is lined by flattened mesothelium.

The subarachnoid space contains arteries and veins, their branches extending into the brain substance surrounded by a perivascular space **PVS** which is continuous with the subarachnoid space and which is thus filled with CSF. The CNS contains no lymphatics and interstitial fluid is thought to drain outwards from the brain substance to join the subarachnoid CSF via the perivascular spaces.

As seen in micrograph (c), the capillaries of the CNS are similar to those elsewhere in the body with flattened endothelial cells resting on a basement membrane; the endothelial cells are not fenestrated and are bound by tight, intercellular junctions except in the choroid plexus. Externally, the basement membranes are almost completely covered by the perivascular foot processes of astrocytes (see Fig. 7.22). A thin layer of the pia mater extends down into the CNS around smaller arteries and arterioles but is not present around the capillaries of the CNS; the perivascular space is extremely thin although it often appears artefactually wider as in micrograph (c).

Perfusion studies have shown that the CNS capillaries are relatively impermeable to certain plasma constituents especially larger molecules and this has led to the theory that a *blood-brain barrier* exists. Although poorly understood, this barrier probably consists of capillary endothelial cells, the supporting basement membrane and the perivascular feet of astrocytes, the last probably playing the least important role.

Sensory receptors

Sensory receptors are nerve endings or specialised cells which convert (transduce) stimuli from the external or internal environments into afferent nerve impulses; the impulses pass into the CNS where they initiate appropriate voluntary or involuntary responses.

No classification system for sensory receptors has yet been devised which adequately incorporates either functional or morphological features. A widely used functional classification divides sensory receptors into three groups: *exteroceptors, proprioceptors* and *interoceptors*. Exteroceptors are those which respond to stimuli from outside the body and include separate receptors for touch, light pressure, deep pressure, cutaneous pain, temperature, smell, taste, sight and hearing. Proprioceptors are located within the skeletal system and provide conscious and unconscious information about orientation, skeletal position, tension and movement; such receptors include the vestibular apparatus of the ear, tendon organs and neuromuscular spindles. Interoceptors respond to stimuli from the viscera and include the chemoreceptors of blood, vascular baroreceptors, the receptors for the state of distension of hollow viscera such as the gastrointestinal tract and urinary bladder, and receptors for such nebulous senses as visceral pain, hunger, thirst, well-being and malaise.

The nature of the receptors involved in some of these sensory modalities is poorly understood; however, sensory receptors may be classified morphologically into two groups *simple* and *compound*. Simple receptors are merely free, branched or unbranched nerve endings such as those responsible for cutaneous pain and temperature and are rarely visible with the light microscope unless special staining methods are employed. Compound receptors involve organisation of associated non-neural tissues to complement the function of the neural receptors. The degree of organisation may range from mere encapsulation to highly sophisticated arrangements such as in the eye and ear; by tradition, the eye, ear and receptors for the senses of smell and taste are described as the *organs of special sense* and are the subject of Chapter 21.

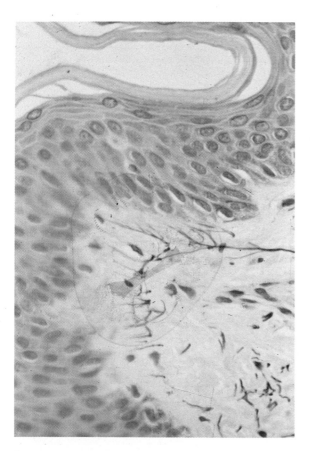

Fig. 7.26 Free nerve endings
(Silver/Haematoxylin × 480)

Free nerve endings are the simplest form of sensory receptor, merely consisting of numerous small terminal branches of afferent nerve fibres. Such free nerve endings are found in connective tissue throughout the body subserving a variety of relatively unsophisticated sensory modalities such as temperature, touch and pain. The afferent fibres are of relatively small diameter with slow rates of conduction and although some of these fibres are myelinated, the nerve endings are devoid of myelin.

In the skin, free nerve endings are found along the dermo-epidermal junction where they are intimately associated with non-neurone cells called Merkel cells scattered in the basal layers of the epidermis (see Fig. 9.4). The adjacent Merkel cell cytoplasm contains vesicles with ultrastructural features similar to those found in synapses but no neurotransmitter has yet been demonstrated. Such free nerve endings are served by large-diameter myelinated fibres and are thought to be responsible for the sensation of touch.

In addition, a variety of different arrangements of free nerve endings are incorporated in the follicles of fine and coarse hairs acting as touch receptors, the most sophisticated type being those associated with the whiskers of animals such as cats and rodents.

This thick section of skin stained by a heavy metal impregnation method shows a nerve fibre with many fine terminal branches extending as free nerve endings into the dermo-epidermal junction; Merkel cells cannot be reliably identified.

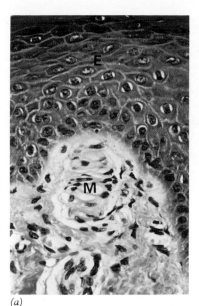 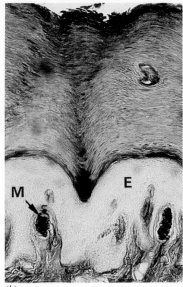

(a) *(b)*

Fig. 7.27 Meissner's corpuscles

(a) H & E × 320 (b) Silver method × 150

Meissner's corpuscles are small, encapsulated, sensory receptors found in the dermis of the skin, particularly of the fingertips, soles of the feet and lips. They are involved in the reception of light discriminatory touch; the degree of discrimination in a given area depends on the proximity of receptors to one another.

As seen in micrograph (a), Meissner's corpuscles **M** are oval in shape and are usually located in the dermal papillae immediately beneath the epidermis **E**. The receptors consist of a delicate connective tissue capsule surrounding a mass of plump, oval cells arranged transversely at the epidermal end. Non-myelinated branches of large myelinated sensory fibres ramify throughout the cell mass as shown by the heavy metal impregnation technique in micrograph (b).

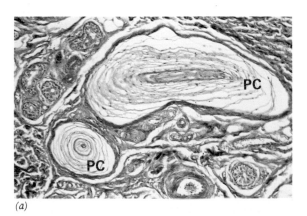

(a)

(b)

Fig. 7.28 Pacinian corpuscles

(a) Masson's trichrome × 80 (b) H & E × 100

Pacinian corpuscles **PC** are large encapsulated sensory receptors responsive to pressure or coarse touch, vibration and tension, and found in the deeper layers of the skin, ligaments and joint capsules, serous membranes, mesenteries, some viscera and in some erogenous areas.

Pacinian corpuscles range from 1–4 mm in length and in section have the appearance of an onion. These organs consist of a delicate capsule enclosing many concentric lamellae of flattened cells separated by interstitial fluid spaces and connective tissue fibres. Towards the centre of the corpuscle the lamellae become closely packed and the core contains a single large unbranched non-myelinated nerve fibre which becomes myelinated as it leaves the corpuscle. Distortion of the Pacinian corpuscle produces an amplified mechanical stimulus in the core which is transduced into an action potential in the sensory neurone.

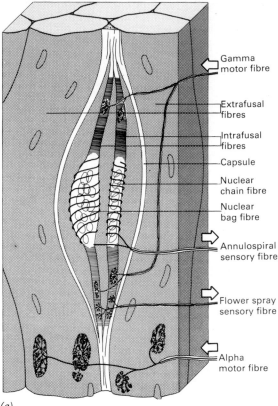

(a)

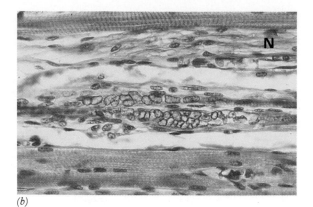

(b)

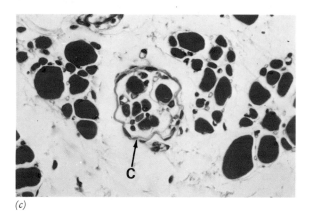

(c)

Gamma
motor fibre

Extrafusal
fibres

Intrafusal
fibres

Capsule

Nuclear
chain fibre

Nuclear
bag fibre

Annulospiral
sensory fibre

Flower spray
sensory fibre

Alpha
motor fibre

Fig. 7.29 Neuromuscular spindle

(a) Schematic diagram (b) LS: H & E × 320 (c) TS: Masson's trichrome × 320

Neuromuscular spindles are stretch receptor organs within skeletal muscles which are responsible for the regulation of muscle tone via the spinal stretch reflex. These receptors are particularly numerous in muscles involved in fine, precision movements such as the intrinsic muscles of the hand and the external muscles of the eye.

Neuromuscular spindles are encapsulated, lymph filled, fusiform structures up to 6 mm long but less than 1 mm in diameter. They lie parallel to the muscle fibres, embedded in endomysium or perimysium. Each spindle contains from 2–10 modified skeletal muscle fibres called *intrafusal fibres* which are much smaller than the skeletal muscle fibres proper, the *extrafusal fibres*. The intrafusal fibres have a central non-striated area in which their nuclei tend to be concentrated. Two types of intrafusal fibres are recognised. In one type, the central nuclear area is dilated, these fibres being known as *nuclear bag fibres*. In the other type, there is no dilatation and the nuclei are arranged in a single row giving rise to the name *nuclear chain fibres*.

Associated with both types of intrafusal fibre are sensory receptors of two types. Firstly, branched, non-myelinated endings of large, myelinated sensory fibres are wrapped around the central non-striated area of the intrafusal fibres forming *annulo-spiral endings*. Secondly, *flower-spray endings* of smaller, myelinated sensory fibres are located on the striated portions of the intrafusal fibres.

Together, these sensory receptors are stimulated by stretching of the intrafusal fibres which occurs when the extrafusal muscle mass is stretched. This stimulus evokes reflex contraction of the extrafusal muscle fibres via large (alpha) motor neurones of a simple two-neurone spinal reflex arc. Contraction of the extrafusal muscle mass thus removes the stretch stimulus from the intrafusal stretch receptors and equilibrium is restored.

The sensitivity of the neuromuscular spindle is modulated by higher centres via small (gamma) motor neurones arising from the extrapyramidal system. These gamma motor neurones innervate the striated portions of the intrafusal fibres thus controlling their state of contraction. Contraction of the intrafusal fibres increases the sensitivity of the intrafusal receptors to stretching of the extrafusal mass.

In any one histological section it is impossible to demonstrate all the structural features of a neuromuscular spindle, but many of the features of the organ are shown in these micrographs. The most easily recognisable features are the discrete capsule C, best seen in micrograph (c) which is continuous with the endomysium of the surrounding muscle, and the small size of the intrafusal muscle fibres compared with the surrounding extrafusal fibres. In micrograph (b), note the small bundle of nerve fibres N passing to and from the spindle.

PART THREE

Organ systems

8. Circulatory system
9. Skin
10. Skeletal tissues
11. Immune system
12. Respiratory system
13. Oral tissues
14. Gastrointestinal tract
15. Liver and pancreas
16. Urinary system
17. The endocrine glands
18. Male reproductive system
19. Female reproductive system
20. Central nervous system
21. Special sense organs

Notes on staining methods

8. Circulatory system

Introduction

The circulatory system mediates the continuous movement of all body fluids; its principal functions are the transport of oxen and nutrients to the tissues and transport of carbon dioxide and other metabolic waste products from the tissues. The circulatory system is also involved in temperature regulation and the distribution of molecules such as hormones, and cells such as those of the immune system. The circulatory system has two functional components: the blood vascular system and the lymph vascular system. The *blood vascular system* constitutes a circuit of vessels through which a flow of blood is maintained by continuous pumping of the heart. The *arterial system* provides a distribution network to the *capillaries* which are the main sites of interchange between the tissues and blood. The *venous system* returns blood from the capillaries to the heart. In contrast, the *lymph vascular system* is merely a passive drainage system for returning excess extravascular fluid called *lymph* to the blood vascular system. The lymph vascular system has no intrinsic pumping mechanism.

The whole circulatory system has a common basic structure:

1. An inner lining comprising a single layer of extremely flattened epithelial cells called *endothelium* supported by a basement membrane and delicate connective tissue. This constitutes the *tunica intima*.
2. An intermediate muscular layer, the *tunica media*.
3. An outer connective tissue layer called the *tunica adventitia*.

The tissues of the walls of large vessels cannot be sustained by diffusion from their lumens. Thus they are supplied by small arteries called *vasa vasorum* (i.e. 'vessels of vessels') which are derived either from the main vessel itself or from adjacent arteries. The vasa vasorum give rise to a capillary network within the tunica adventitia which may extend into the tunica media.

The muscular layer exhibits the greatest variation throughout the system; for example, it is totally absent in capillaries but comprises almost the whole mass of the heart. Blood flow is predominantly influenced by variations in activity of the muscular layer.

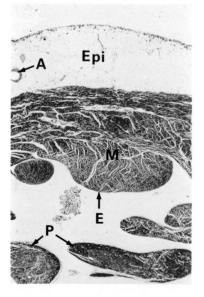

Fig. 8.1 Heart: wall of ventricle

(Masson's trichrome × 20)

This micrograph illustrates the three basic layers of the heart wall. The tunica intima of the heart is called the *endocardium* **E**, and is difficult to see at this magnification. The tunica media of the heart is called the *myocardium* **M** and is thickest in the ventricular walls. The myocardium is made up of cardiac muscle, the structure of which meets the unique functional requirements of the heart (see Ch. 6).

The tunica adventitia of the heart, the *epicardium* **Epi** (also called *visceral pericardium*), is surrounded by a space, the *pericardial cavity*, enclosed by a fibrous sac, the *pericardium* (the *parietal pericardium*) which is not shown in this micrograph. The parietal pericardium is loosely fixed to the surrounding mediastinal structures. The parietal and visceral layers of the pericardium move freely against one another thus permitting relatively unimpeded movement of the heart.

Note a branch **A** of the coronary arterial system; these arteries represent the vasa vasorum of the heart. Note also papillary muscles **P** of the ventricle, extensions of the myocardium which, via the chordae tendinae, stabilise the cusps of the mitral and tricuspid valves.

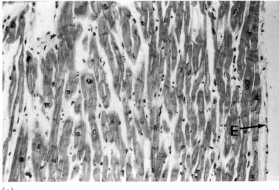

(a)

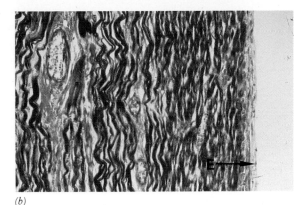

(b)

Fig. 8.2 Heart: myocardium and endocardium

(a) H & E × 128 (b) Masson's trichrome × 128

The endocardium, the innermost layer of the heart, consists of an endothelial lining and its supporting connective tissue. The endothelium E, is a single layer of flattened epithelial cells, which is continuous with the endothelium of the vessels entering and leaving the heart. The endothelium is supported by a delicate layer of fibro-elastic connective tissue which accommodates gross movements of the myocardium without damage to the endothelium.

The subendothelial connective tissue becomes continuous with the perimysium of the cardiac muscle; this is best demonstrated in micrograph (b) in which the collagen of the connective tissue is stained green. The endocardium contains blood vessels, nerves and branches of the conducting system of the heart.

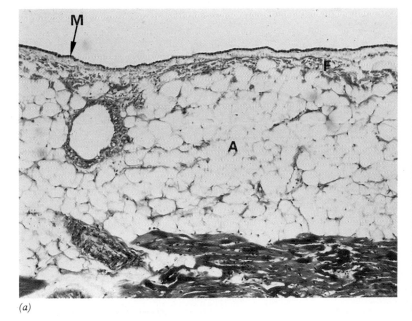

(a)

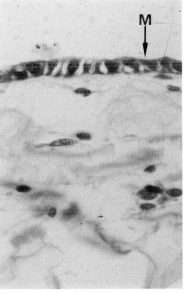

(b)

Fig. 8.3 Heart: epicardium

(H & E (a) × 200 (b) × 480)

The free surface of the epicardium is covered by a single layer of flattened epithelial cells, the mesothelium M; a similar mesothelial layer lines the opposing parietal pericardial surface. The mesothelial cells secrete a small amount of serous fluid which lubricates the movement of the epicardium on the parietal pericardium.

A thin layer of fibro-elastic connective tissue F supports the mesothelium; this layer is connected to the myocardium by a broad layer of adipose connective tissue A. Branches of the coronary vessels and autonomic nerves pass in the epicardium to supply the myocardium.

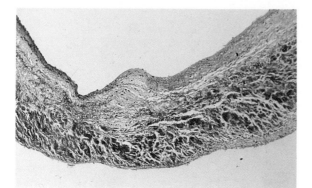

Fig. 8.4 Heart valve

(Elastic van Gieson × 64)

The valves of the heart consist of leaflets of connective tissue, the surfaces being invested with a thin endothelial layer continuous with that of the heart chambers and great vessels. The connective tissue of each leaflet forms a tough fibrous sheet, the *lamina fibrosa*; in this specimen, the collagen is stained red. The valve connective tissue also contains a significant amount of elastin, stained black in this preparation, best seen immediately beneath the surface endothelium.

At the attached margins of each valve, the collagenous tissue becomes condensed to form a fibrous ring (valve anulus) and the rings of the four valves together form a central fibrous 'skeleton' which is continuous with the connective tissue of the myocardium, endocardium and epicardium. The mitral and tricuspid leaflets are connected to the papillary muscles by collagenous strands, the *chordae tendinae*, which also merge with the fibrous lamina of the valve leaflet.

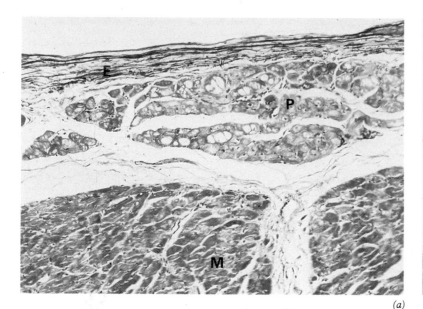

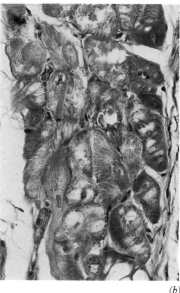

(a)   *(b)*

Fig. 8.5 Purkinje fibres

(H & E elastin (a) × 150 (b) × 400)

The coordinated contraction of the myocardium during each pumping cycle is mediated by a specialised conducting system of modified cardiac muscle fibres. With each cardiac cycle, a wave of excitation originates in the pacemaker region of the right atrium, the *sino-atrial node*, the excitatory stimuli arising spontaneously at regular intervals, the rate being modulated by the autonomic nervous system. The wave of excitation spreads throughout the atria causing them to contract thus forcing blood into the ventricles. The wave of excitation then spreads to the *atrioventricular node* from which an excitatory stimulus is passed rapidly throughout the whole ventricular myocardium via the *atrioventricular bundle* or *bundle of His*. This bundle divides within the interventricular septum to give rise to smaller branches called *Purkinje fibres* which cross in the subendocardial connective tissue before penetrating the ventricular myocardium. This system permits almost simultaneous

contraction of the entire ventricular myocardium.

The characteristics of the specialised muscle fibres of the conducting system are demonstrated in these micrographs. Note in micrograph (a), the subendocardial location of the bundle of Purkinje fibres **P** and the darkly staining endocardial elastin **E**. Note also the broad similarity of the Purkinje bundle to the adjacent myocardium **M**.

As seen in micrograph (b), the conducting cells are large, sometimes binucleate, with extensive pale cytoplasm containing relatively few myofibrils which are arranged in an irregular manner immediately beneath the plasma membrane of the cell. The cytoplasm is rich in glycogen and mitochondria but in contrast to cardiac muscle cells, there is no T tubule system. Connections between the Purkinje cells are via desmosomes and gap junctions rather than by intercalated discs as in the myocardium.

The arterial system

The function of the arterial system is to distribute blood from the heart to capillary beds throughout the body. The cyclic pumping action of the heart produces a pulsatile blood flow in the arterial system. With each stroke of the ventricles, blood is forced into the arterial system causing expansion of the arterial walls; subsequent recoil of the arterial walls assists in maintenance of arterial blood pressure between strokes of the ventricles. This expansion and recoil is facilitated by the presence of elastic tissue within the walls of the arterial system. The flow of blood to various organs and tissues may be regulated by varying the diameter of the distributing vessels. This function is performed by the smooth muscle component of vessel walls and is principally under the control of the sympathetic nervous system and adrenal medullary hormones.

Although the walls of the arterial vessels conform to the general structure of the circulatory system, they are characterised by the presence of variable amounts of elastic fibres and a smooth muscle wall which is thick relative to the diameter of the lumen. There are three main types of vessel in the arterial system:

1. Elastic arteries: these comprise the major distribution vessels and include the aorta, the innominate, common carotid and subclavian arteries and most of the pulmonary arterial vessels.

2. Muscular arteries: these are the main distributing branches of the arterial tree, for example the radial arteries.

3. Arterioles: these are the terminal branches of the arterial tree which supply the capillary beds.

There is a gradual transition in structure and function between the three types of arterial vessel. In general, the amount of elastic tissue decreases as the vessels become smaller and the smooth muscle component assumes greater prominence.

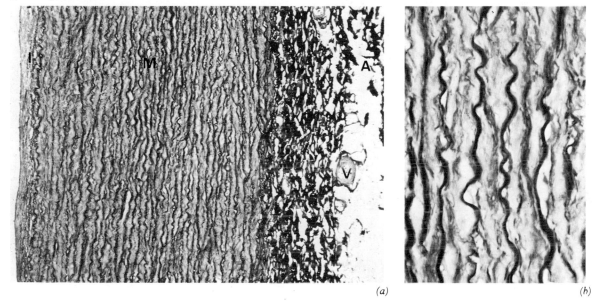

(a)   *(b)*

Fig. 8.6 Elastic artery: aorta

(Elastic van Gieson (a) × 33 (b) × 320)

The highly elastic nature of the aortic wall is demonstrated in these preparations in which the elastic fibres are specifically stained black. In micrograph (a) the three basic layers of the wall can be seen, the tunica intima **I**, the tunica media **M** and the tunica adventitia **A**.

The tunica intima consists of a single layer of flattened endothelial cells, which cannot be seen at this magnification, supported by a thin layer of collagenous connective tissue containing a few elastic fibres. The subendothelial connective tissue contains scattered fibroblasts and other cells with ultrastructural features akin to smooth muscle cells and known as *myointimal cells*. With increasing age, the myointimal cells accumulate lipid and the intima

progressively thickens; in a more extreme form this represents one of the early changes of atherosclerosis. The tunica media is particularly broad and extremely elastic; at high magnification it is seen to consist of fenestrated sheets of elastin separated by collagenous connective tissue and relatively few smooth muscle fibres which are stained yellow. The collagenous tunica adventitia, stained red in this preparation, contains small vasa vasorum **V**.

Blood flow within elastic arteries is highly pulsatile; with advancing age the arterial system becomes less elastic thereby increasing peripheral resistance and thus arterial blood pressure.

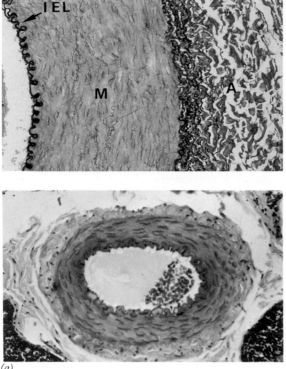

Fig. 8.7 Muscular artery
(TS: Elastic van Gieson × 64)

Muscular arteries have the same basic composition as elastic arteries but the elastic tissue is reduced to a well defined, fenestrated elastic sheet, the *internal elastic lamina* **IEL**, in the tunica intima, and a diffuse *external elastic lamina* in the tunica adventitia; elastin is stained black in this preparation. A few elastic fibres are scattered throughout the tunica media **M** which is mainly composed of a thick layer of smooth muscle, stained yellow in this preparation. Note the red-stained collagen fibres within each layer. The vasa vasorum are mainly confined to the adventitial layer **A**, although small branches may extend into the tunica media.

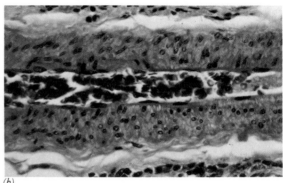

(a) *(b)*

Fig. 8.8 Large arterioles
(H & E (a) TS × 128 (b) LS × 320)

Arterioles may be defined as those vessels of the arterial system with a lumen less than 0.3 mm in diameter, although the distinction between small muscular arteries and large arterioles is somewhat artificial. Arterioles are characterised by the following features which are seen in these micrographs:

1. The tunica intima is very thin and comprises the endothelial lining, little collagenous connective tissue and a thin, but distinct, internal elastic lamina.
2. The tunica media is almost entirely composed of smooth muscle cells in six concentric layers or less.
3. The tunica adventitia may be almost as thick as the tunica media and merges with the surrounding connective tissues. There is no external elastic lamina.

The flow of blood through capillary beds is regulated mainly by the arterioles which supply them. Contraction of circularly arranged, smooth muscle fibres of the arteriolar wall reduces the diameter of the lumen and hence blood flow. Generalised constriction of arterioles throughout the body markedly increases peripheral resistance to blood flow and hence the arteriolar compartment of the circulatory system has an important role in the regulation of systemic blood pressure.

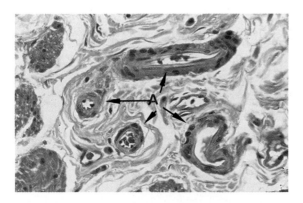

Fig. 8.9 Small arterioles
(H & E × 320)

This micrograph illustrates four small arterioles **A** in the loose connective tissue of the bowel wall. The smallest arterioles have only a single layer of smooth muscle cells and are almost devoid of elastin. The adventitial layer merges imperceptibly with the surrounding connective tissue.

The microcirculation

The microcirculation is that part of the circulatory system concerned with the exchange of gases, fluids, nutrients and metabolic waste products. Exchange occurs mainly within the capillaries. The arterioles, and muscular sphincters at the arteriolar-capillary junctions called *precapillary sphincters*, control blood flow within capillary networks. The capillary networks drain into a series of vessels of increasing diameter namely *post-capillary venules, collecting venules* and small *muscular venules* which comprise the venous component of the microcirculation.

In different tissues, the structure of the microcirculation varies to meet specific functional requirements. There are four main structural variables:

1. The diameter of the capillaries: capillary diameter varies between as little as 3 to 4 μm (i.e. half the diameter of a red blood cell) and 30 to 40 μm. Large diameter capillaries are called *sinusoids*.

2. The nature of the capillary endothelium: three types of capillary endothelium are found:

(a) *Continuous capillaries*: the endothelial cells form an uninterrupted capillary lining; this is the most common type of capillary.

(b) *Fenestrated capillaries*: the endothelial cells contain numerous large pores or fenestrations.

(c) *Discontinuous endothelium*: the endothelial cells do not form a continuous interface between the lumen and surrounding tissues; this arrangement is found only within the sinusoids of the liver (see Fig. 15.11).

3. The presence of arterio-venous shunts: direct connections between the arterial and venous systems.

4. The abundance of the capillary network: for example, dense connective tissue has a poor capillary network in contrast to cardiac muscle.

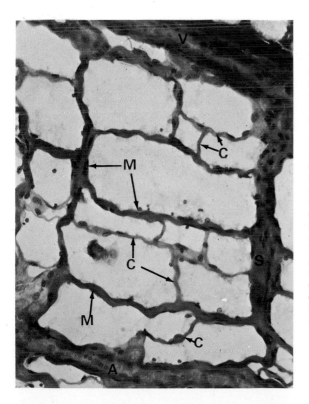

Fig. 8.10 The microcirculation

(Mesenteric spread, H & E × 120)

This micrograph demonstrates an anastomosing network of capillaries between an arteriole **A** and a venule **V**. The capillary network comprises small diameter capillaries **C** consisting only of a single layer of endothelial cells, and larger diameter capillaries with a discontinuous outer layer of smooth muscle cells, known as *metarterioles* **M**.

Note that small capillaries arise both from arterioles and metarterioles. At the origin of each capillary there is believed to be a sphincter mechanism which is involved in regulation of capillary blood flow. Note also a direct wide-diameter communication between the arteriole and venule, an arteriovenous shunt **S**. Metarterioles also form direct communications between arterioles and venules. Contraction of the smooth muscle of the shunts and metarterioles directs blood through the network of small capillaries. Thus, regulation of blood flow in the microcirculation is mediated by arterioles, metarterioles, precapillary sphincters and arteriovenous shunts. The smooth muscle activity of these vessels is modulated by the autonomic nervous system and circulating hormones. In addition, the concentration of oxygen and metabolites, such as lactic acid, regulate the local flow of blood within tissues; this process is called *autoregulation*.

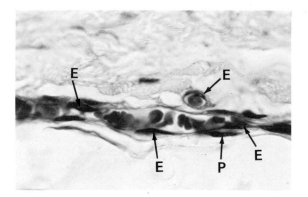

Fig. 8.11 Capillaries

(H & E × 800)

The vessels seen in longitudinal section and transverse section illustrate the characteristic features of capillaries:

1. A single layer of flattened endothelial cells **E**, the cytoplasm of which is difficult to resolve by light microscopy. The flattened endothelial cell nuclei bulge into the capillary lumen; in longitudinal section the nuclei appear elongated whereas in transverse section they appear more rounded in shape.

2. The absence of muscular and adventitial layers.

3. The presence of occasional flattened cells embracing the capillary endothelial cells; these cells are called *pericytes* **P** and may have a contractile function.

4. The diameter of capillaries is similar to that of the red blood cells contained within them.

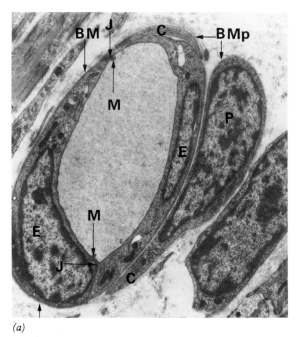

(a)

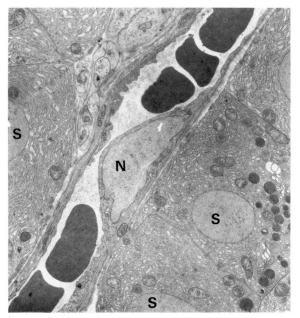

(b)

Fig. 8.12 Capillaries (continuous type)

(EM (a) TS × 7500 (b) LS × 4000)

These electron micrographs illustrate the ultrastructure of capillaries of the continuous endothelium type, the usual type found in most tissues.

In micrograph (a), two endothelial cells **E** are seen to encircle the capillary lumen; their plasma membranes approximate to one another very closely and in places form discrete junctional complexes **J**. Small cytoplasmic flaps called *marginal folds* **M** extend across the intercellular junctions at the luminal surface. The capillary endothelium is supported by a thin basement membrane **BM** containing a few reticular fibres. Note the pericyte **P** with its cytoplasmic extensions **C** which embrace the capillary. The pericyte is supported by its own basement membrane **BMp**.

In micrograph (b), an endothelial cell nucleus **N** is seen bulging into the capillary lumen. Note the diameter of the lumen relative to its contained erythrocytes and to the size

of the nuclei of the adjacent secretory cells **S**.

Exchange between the lumen of the continuous type capillary and the surrounding tissues is believed to occur in three ways:

1. Passive diffusion through the endothelial cell cytoplasm; exchange of gases, ions and small molecular weight metabolites occurs in this manner.

2. Transport by pinocytotic vesicles; proteins and some lipids may be transported in this manner.

3. Passage through the intercellular space between the endothelial cells; white blood cells are believed to migrate through the endothelial cell junctions by a process called *diapedesis*. Some workers maintain that the intercellular spaces also permit molecular transport. In capillaries of this type the basement membrane is thought to present little barrier to exchange between capillaries and the tissues.

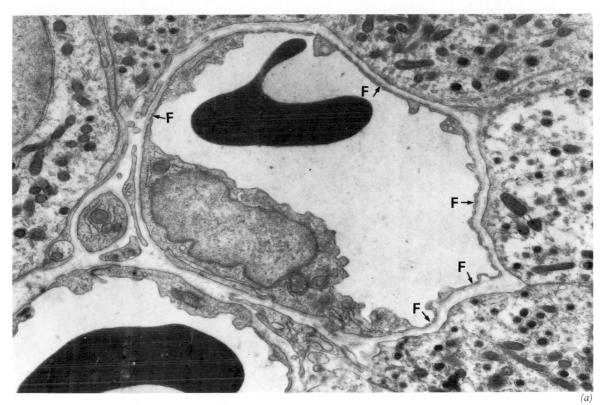

(a)

Fig. 8.13 Fenestrated capillary

(TS: EM (a) × 13 000 (b) × 54 000)

Fenestrated capillaries are found in some tissues where there is much molecular exchange with the blood; such tissues include the small intestine, endocrine glands and the kidney.

At low magnification, fenestrations **F** appear as pores through thin areas of the endothelial cytoplasm, however, only a small proportion of the thin areas are fenestrated. At high magnification, the fenestrations appear to be traversed by a thin electron-dense line which may constitute a diaphragm **D**, the biochemical and functional nature of which is in dispute. A diaphragm is not seen across the fenestrations of the glomerular capillaries of the kidney (see Fig. 16.14).

The permeability of fenestrated capillaries is much greater than that of continuous capillaries; molecular labelling techniques have demonstrated that fenestrations permit the rapid passage of macromolecules smaller than plasma proteins.

Like continuous capillaries, all fenestrated capillaries are supported by a basement membrane **BM** which is continuous across the fenestrations. Pericytes are rarely found in association with fenestrated capillaries.

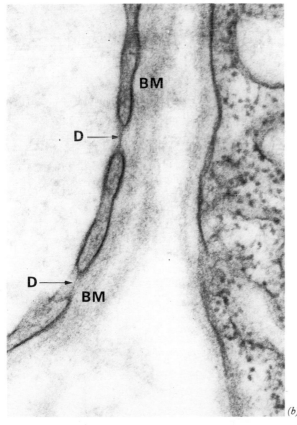

(b)

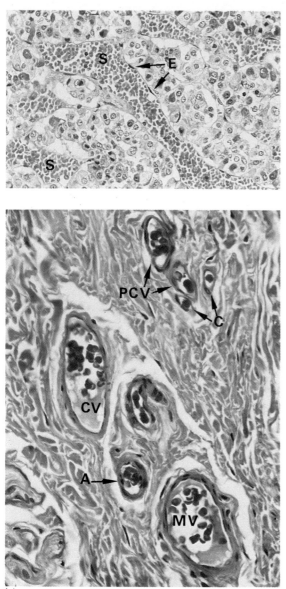

Fig. 8.14 Sinusoids

(H & E × 320)

Sinusoids are capillaries of wide diameter found in the liver, spleen, bone marrow and some endocrine glands. The endothelium of sinusoids may be continuous, fenestrated or discontinuous, the discontinuous type of endothelial lining being found only in the liver sinusoids (see Fig. 15.11). Sinusoids usually have an irregular outline which conforms to the cellular arrangement of the tissue in which they are found.

This micrograph illustrates sinusoids **S** between cords of secretory cells in the anterior pituitary. Several endothelial cell nuclei **E** can be distinguished by their flattened shape.

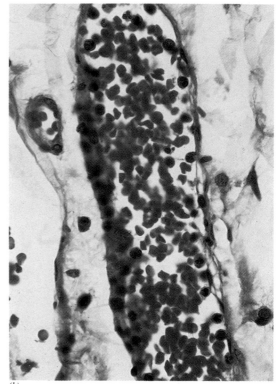

(a)

(b)

Fig. 8.15 Post-capillary and collecting venules

(H & E (a) × 480 (b) × 480)

The capillary beds are drained by a series of thin-walled vessels which form the first part of the venous system. Examples of each type of vessel are seen in micrograph (a).

Post-capillary venules **PCV** are the smallest of these vessels and are formed by the union of several capillaries **C** to produce a vessel similar in structure but of a wider diameter. Post-capillary venules perform metabolite exchange functions in a similar manner to that of capillaries but, in addition, they appear to be the main point at which white blood cells enter and leave the circulation. Post-capillary venules drain into collecting venules **CV** which are characterised by their larger diameter and a greater number of enveloping pericytes. Collecting venules drain into vessels of progressively greater diameter, the walls of which contain a recognisable layer of smooth muscle and which are

therefore known as muscular venules **MV**. This micrograph also shows a very small arteriole **A** with only a single layer of smooth muscle cells in its wall.

Micrograph (b) illustrates a post-capillary venule in the connective tissue of a mildly inflamed organ; the leucocytes are characteristically seen close to the endothelium at the margin of the erythrocyte stream, a phenomenon known as *margination*. Blood flow in post-capillary venules is extremely sluggish and this may facilitate the exit of leucocytes from the micro-circulation at this point. In contrast to capillaries, intercellular junctional complexes are relatively uncommon between the endothelial cells of post-capillary venules and this may also facilitate leucocyte emigration.

The venous system

With the exception of the venous components of the microcirculation, the venous system merely functions as a low-pressure collecting system for the return of blood from the capillary networks to the heart. Blood flow in veins occurs passively down a pressure gradient towards the heart. With each respiratory inspiration, a negative pressure is created within the thorax and hence within the right atrium of the heart. Venous return from the extremities is aided by the contraction of skeletal muscles which compress the veins contained within them. With each respiratory expiration, the pressure gradients are reversed and blood tends to flow in the opposite direction. This tendency is prevented by the presence of valves in veins of medium size.

The structure of the venous system conforms to the general structure of the whole circulatory system, but the elastic and muscular components are much less prominent features. A major part of the total blood volume is contained within the venous system. Variations in relative blood volume, for example, due to dilation of capillary beds or haemorrhage, may be compensated for by changes in the capacity of the venous system. These changes are mediated by smooth muscle in the tunica media which controls the luminal diameter of muscular venules and veins.

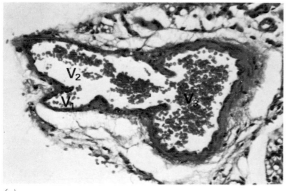

(a)

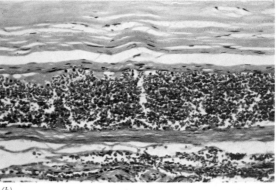

(b)

Fig. 8.16 Muscular venules and small veins

(H & E (a) × 128 (b) × 128)

Micrograph (a) illustrates the confluence of a small muscular venule V_1 with a larger muscular venule V_2 which then joins a small vein V_3 cut in transverse section. Note the valve at the junction of the large venule and vein. Muscular venules are characterised by a clearly defined intimal layer devoid of elastic fibres and a tunica media consisting of one or two layers of smooth muscle fibres. Veins are characterised by a thicker muscular wall and a poorly developed internal elastic lamina. Note that the tunica adventitia of these vessels is continuous with the surrounding connective tissue.

Micrograph (b) shows a small vein cut in longitudinal section and fixed whilst still distended with blood. The wall of the vein consists of two to three layers of smooth muscle fibres. Note the wide diameter of the lumen relative to the thickness of the wall.

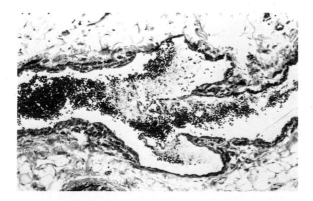

Fig. 8.17 Vein with valve

(LS: Masson's trichrome × 128)

This micrograph demonstrates a valve in a small vein. The valve consists of delicate semilunar projections of the tunica intima of the vein wall; the projections are composed of fibro-elastic connective tissue lined on both sides by endothelium. Each valve usually consists of two leaflets, the free edges of which project in the direction of blood flow. Valves only occur in veins of more than 2 mm in diameter, particularly those draining the extremities.

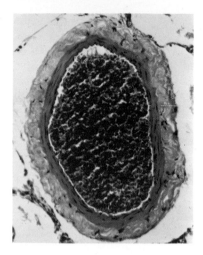

Fig. 8.18 Vein

(TS: H & E × 128)

Small and medium size veins are characterised by the following features demonstrated in this micrograph of a medium size vein:

1. The tunica intima consists of little more than the endothelial lining. In veins that are not distended with blood the endothelium may be thrown up into small folds.

2. The tunica media is thin compared with that of arteries and consists of two or more layers of circularly arranged smooth muscle fibres.

3. The tunica adventitia is the thickest layer of the vessel wall and is composed of longitudinally arranged thick collagen fibres which merge with the surrounding connective tissue.

Note that the wall of the vein is thin relative to the diameter of the lumen. In contrast, in most arteries, the thickness of the wall approaches the diameter of the lumen.

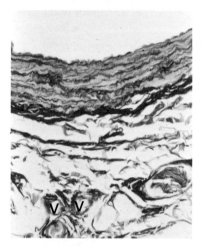

Fig. 8.19 Large muscular vein

(TS: Elastic van Gieson × 128)

Large veins such as the femoral and renal veins have a relatively thick muscular wall consisting of several layers of smooth muscle, stained yellow in this specimen, separated by layers of collagenous connective tissue, stained red. The tunica media and tunica intima also contain a few elastic fibres, stained black in this preparation, but there is no distinct elastic lamina as in arteries of comparable size.

The tunica adventitia is broad and contains numerous vasa vasorum **V** reflecting the need for arterial blood by the tissues of the vein wall.

The largest vessels of the venous system, the *venae cavae*, have a structure similar to that just described except that the smooth muscle is disposed longitudinally rather than in a circular fashion.

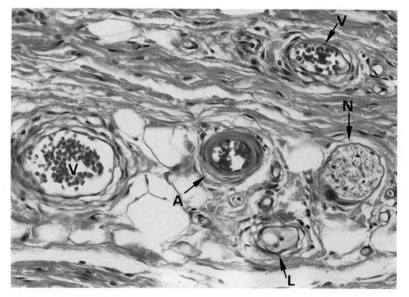

Fig. 8.20 Small neurovascular bundle

(H & E × 150)

The vessels supplying and draining a particular area of tissue tend to pass together, frequently accompanied by a peripheral nerve and invested by a condensation of the surrounding connective tissue which forms an ill-defined protective sheath. This micrograph shows such a small neurovascular bundle containing a small arteriole **A**, venules **V**, lymphatic **L** and nerve **N**. These structures lie in loose areolar connective tissue and are surrounded by a more condensed collagenous sheath.

The lymph vascular system

The lymph vascular system drains excess fluid called lymph from extracellular spaces and returns it to the blood vascular system. Lymph is formed in the following manner. At the arterial end of blood capillaries, the hydrostatic pressure of blood exceeds the colloidal osmotic pressure exerted by plasma proteins. Water and electrolytes therefore pass out of capillaries into the extracellular spaces; some plasma proteins also leak out through the endothelial wall. At the venous end of blood capillaries the pressure relationships are reversed and fluid tends to be drawn back into the blood vascular system. In this way, about two percent of plasma passing through the capillary bed is exchanged with the extracellular tissue fluid. The rate of tissue fluid formation at the arterial end of capillaries generally exceeds the re-uptake of fluid at the venous end. The excess fluid, lymph, is drained by a system of lymph capillaries which converge to form progressively larger diameter lymphatic vessels. Lymph enters the venous system by a single vessel on each side of the body, the thoracic duct and the right lymphatic duct. Movement of lymph in the lymph vascular system is similar to movement of blood in the venous system but valves are more numerous in lymphatic vessels.

Along the course of the larger lymphatic vessels are aggregations of lymphoid tissue called lymph nodes where cells of the immune system and antibodies join the general circulation (see Chapter 11). Lymphatic vessels are found in all tissues except the central nervous system, cartilage, bone, bone marrow, thymus, placenta and teeth. The structure of lymphatic vessels conforms closely to that of vessels of similar diameter in the venous system. Lymphatic vessels may be distinguished from venous vessels by the absence of erythrocytes and the presence of small numbers of leucocytes mainly lymphocytes. Lymphatic capillaries differ from blood capillaries in several respects which reflect the greater permeability of lymphatic capillaries: the endothelial cell cytoplasm is extremely thin and a basement membrane and pericytes are absent.

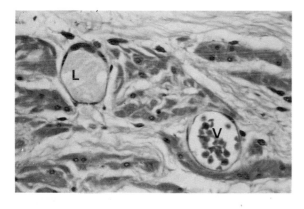

Fig. 8.21 Small lymphatic vessel
(H & E × 320)

This micrograph illustrates the characteristic histological differences between a small lymphatic **L** and a venule **V**. Lymphatics do not contain erythrocytes but often contain a few lymphocytes. The stained amorphous material seen in this lymphatic is the protein of lymph which becomes precipitated during tissue processing. The presence of such material is often a distinguishing feature of lymphatics in histological preparations.

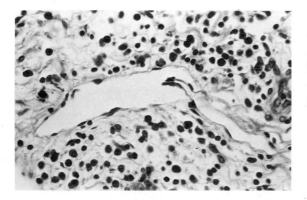

Fig. 8.22 Valve of a lymphatic vessel
(H & E × 320)

A characteristic feature of the lymphatic system is the numerous delicate valves in small and medium sized vessels. The structure of these valves is similar to that of valves in the venous system, but the connective tissue core consists merely of reticulin fibres and a little ground substance.

9. Skin

Introduction

The skin, or integument, forms the continuous external surface of the body and in different regions of the body varies in thickness, colour and the presence of hairs, glands and nails. Despite these variations, which reflect different functional demands, all types of skin have the same basic structure. The external surface of skin consists of a keratinised squamous epithelium called the *epidermis*. The epidermis is supported and nourished by a thick layer of dense, fibro-elastic connective tissue called the *dermis* which is highly vascular and contains many sensory receptors. The dermis is attached to underlying tissues by a layer of loose connective tissue called the *hypodermis* or *subcutaneous layer* which contains variable amounts of adipose tissue. Hair follicles, sweat glands, sebaceous glands and nails are epithelial structures termed *epidermal appendages* since they originate during embryological development from downgrowths of epidermal epithelium into the dermis and hypodermis.

The skin is the largest organ of the body, constituting almost one sixth of the total body weight; it has four major functions:

1. **Protection**: the skin provides protection against ultraviolet light and mechanical, chemical and thermal insults; its relatively impermeable surface prevents excessive dehydration and acts as a physical barrier to invasion by micro-organisms.

2. **Sensation**: the skin is the largest sensory organ in the body and contains a variety of receptors for touch, pressure, pain and temperature.

3. **Thermoregulation**: in man, skin is a major organ of thermoregulation. The body is insulated against heat loss by the presence of hairs and subcutaneous adipose tissue. Heat loss is facilitated by evaporation of sweat from the skin surface and increased blood flow through the rich vascular network of the dermis.

4. **Metabolic functions**: subcutaneous adipose tissue constitutes a major store of energy, mainly in the form of triglycerides. Vitamin D is synthesised in the epidermis and supplements that derived from dietary sources.

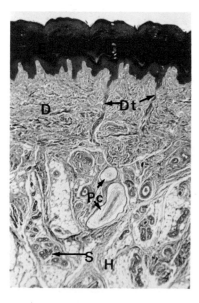

Fig. 9.1 Skin (fingertip)
(Masson's trichrome × 8)

The general structure of skin is illustrated in this preparation of thick skin from the fingertip. The epidermis **E** consists of a stratified squamous keratinising epithelium which, in this site, has an extremely thick keratinised surface layer. A prominent feature of the skin of the fingertips, palms and soles of the feet is a pattern of surface ridges formed by the epidermis; this pattern is unique to each individual.

The epidermis is supported by the dermis **D**, a layer of dense fibro-elastic tissue, the fibres of which are stained blue-green in this preparation. The dermis merges with the loose connective tissue of the hypodermis **H** which consists largely of adipose tissue; in this site, adipose tissue acts as a soft, shock-absorbing layer. Numerous sweat glands **S** are located in the dermis and hypodermis and discharge their secretions on to the skin surface via long excretory ducts **Dt**. Pressure receptors, Pacinian corpuscles **Pc** (see Fig. 7.28) are located deep in the dermis and are a prominent feature of fingertip skin.

The junction between the epidermis and dermis is characterised by downward folds of the epidermis called *epidermal ridges* which interdigitate with upward projections of the dermis called *dermal papillae*. This arrangement, which is shown diagrammatically in Figure 9.6, enhances the adhesion of the epidermis to the dermis and is accentuated in skin subject to considerable frictional forces.

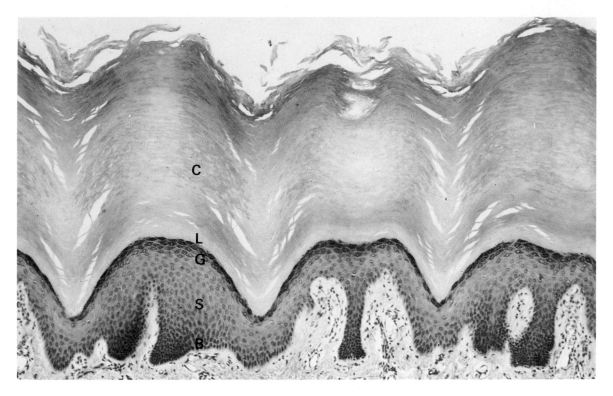

Fig. 9.2 Epidermis (fingertip)

(H & E × 104)

This section of thick skin, taken from the same specimen as Fig. 9.1, demonstrates the general features of the epidermis. Cells produced by mitosis in the germinal layer adjacent to the dermis undergo maturational changes concerned with the production of keratin. The outer keratinised layer is shed continuously and is replaced by the progressive movement and maturation of cells from the germinal layer. The rate of mitosis in the germinal layer generally equals the rate of desquamation of keratin from the outer surface and the process of maturation of a basal cell through to desquamation takes approximately 27 days in humans.

The phases of this dynamic process are represented in five morphological layers:

1. The stratum germinativum or stratum basale B is the germinal layer of the epidermis. This layer is also sometimes referred to as the *stratum malpighii*.

2. The stratum spinosum or prickle cell layer S, so named for the 'prickly' appearance of the cells at high magnification (see Fig. 9.4), contains cells which are in the process of growth and early keratin synthesis.

3. The stratum granulosum or granular layer G is characterised by the presence within the cells of granules which contribute to the process of keratinisation.

4. The stratum lucidum L is only present in extremely thick skin, and appears as a homogeneous layer between the stratum granulosum and the keratinised layer.

5. The stratum corneum or cornified layer C consists of flattened, fused cell remnants composed mainly of the fibrous protein, keratin.

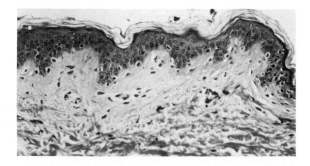

Fig. 9.3 Epidermis (abdomen)

(H & E × 128)

In this preparation of thin skin from the abdomen, the individual cellular layers are more difficult to discern and a stratum lucidum is not present.In comparison with thick skin, the stratum corneum is much reduced in thickness and the combined thickness of the other layers is reduced to a lesser extent.

Fig. 9.4 Epidermis

(a) Masson's trichrome × 600 (b) Thin section, toluidine blue × 1200

The cytological details of the layers of the epidermis are illustrated in micrograph (a) whilst micrograph (b) focuses on the prickle cell layer.

Stratum basale B: the cells of this layer are cuboidal and form a single layer separated from the dermis **D** by a basement membrane too thin to be resolved by light microscopy. The basal aspect of each germinal cell is highly irregular and bound to the basement membrane by numerous hemi-desmosomes (see Fig. 5.24). Like the cells of the adjacent stratum spinosum, small cytoplasmic projections extend across the intercellular spaces to abut upon those of adjacent cells; desmosomes bind these contact points. Mitotic figures are most frequently observed in this layer but cell division also occurs to a lesser extent in the stratum spinosum.

Stratum spinosum S: the so-called 'prickle cells' of this zone are relatively large and polyhedral in shape and have extremely numerous cytoplasmic 'prickles' bound by desmosomes to adjacent cells. Prominent nucleoli and cytoplasmic basophilia indicate active protein synthesis. A fibrillar protein, the predominant synthetic product of these cells, aggregates to form intracellular fibrils known as *tonofibrils* which converge upon the desmosomes of the cytoplasmic 'prickles'; tonofibrils are stained red in this preparation and become more prominent towards the stratum granulosum.

Stratum granulosum G: the cells of this layer are characterised by numerous, dense basophilic granules which crowd the cytoplasm and tend to obscure the tonofibrils. The chemical nature of these so-called *keratohyalin granules* is distinct from that of the fibrous protein of the tonofibrils. The process of keratinisation is thought to involve the combination of tonofibril and keratohyalin elements to form the mature keratin complex. In addition, the cells of the stratum granulosum also synthesise glycoprotein granules which are believed to form an intercellular cementing substance. In the outermost aspect of the stratum granulosum, cell death occurs due to rupture of lysosomal membranes; released lysosomal enzymes may play an important role in the final process of keratinisation.

Stratum lucidum: this layer is seen only in some specimens of thick skin and is not seen in this preparation. When present, it appears as a homogeneous layer between the stratum granulosum and stratum corneum; it may merely represent a compressed transitional zone between these layers.

Stratum corneum C: the morphology and staining characteristics of this layer are strikingly different from that of the underlying layers. The stratum corneum consists of layers of fused, flattened cells devoid of organelles and filled with mature keratin. In the deeper aspect of this layer the cornified cells retain their desmosomal junctions and the intracellular keratin has an ordered pattern. Towards the surface, the desmosomes and internal structure of the cells become disrupted, a process which precedes desquamation.

In addition to the keratinocytes, which form the bulk of the epidermis, three other cell types, all poorly stained, are found in the epidermis. The most common of these are the melanocytes responsible for skin pigmentation (see Fig. 9.5) which are usually confined to the basal layer.

The second of these cells, known as *Merkel cells*, are associated with free nerve endings and are presumed to serve

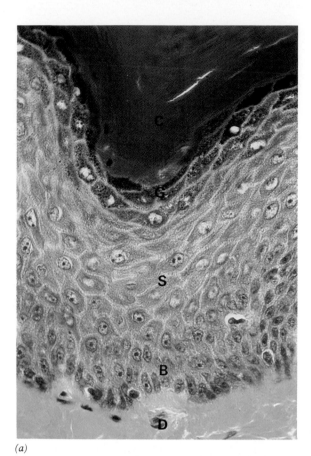

(a)

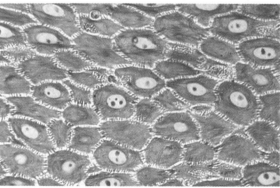

(b)

as sensory receptors. The ultrastructural features of Merkel cells suggest that they form part of the diffuse neuroendocrine system (see Ch. 17).

Langerhan's cells are the other cell type found in the epidermis. With electron microscopy, they have been shown to have cytoplasmic granules and other organelles distinct from those of keratinocytes and evidence is accumulating that they represent part of the immune system with a role in detecting foreign antigens. In micrograph (a), a poorly stained cell can be seen in the lower prickle cell layer representing either a Merkel or Langerhan's cell.

Fig. 9.5 Skin pigmentation

*(a) Caucasian abdominal skin: H & E × 320 (b) Negroid
abdominal skin: H & E × 320 (c) Caucasian forearm skin: thin
section, toluidine blue × 600*

The colour of human skin depends on three major factors.
Firstly, the skin has an inherent yellowish colour due partly
to the presence of various carotene pigments in the
subcutaneous fat. Secondly, the concentration and state of
oxygenation of haemoglobin, and the presence of other
pigments such as bile pigments in blood are reflected in skin
colour. Thirdly, skin colour is determined by the amount of
the pigment *melanin* present in the epidermis; this is the
most important variable between parts of the body, between
individuals of the same race and between members of
different races.

Melanin is synthesised by cells associated with the
epidermis called *melanocytes*. These cells are of neuroectodermal origin and migrate during development to the
epidermis where they become scattered in the basal layers.
Melanocytes have long, dendritic processes which ramify
between the epithelial cells but which do not establish cell
junctions with the epithelial cells. The cell bodies of the
melanocytes are usually located between the basal epithelial
cells and the basement membrane but may be seen between
the epithelial cells at higher levels.

The ratio of melanocytes to basal epithelial cells varies
from about one in five to one in ten in different regions of
the body, being highest in the skin of the face and external
genitalia. The number of melanocytes is relatively constant
between different individuals irrespective of race; differences
in skin colour are thus due to the amount of melanin
produced rather than the number of melanocytes present.

Melanin synthesis involves conversion of the amino-acid
tyrosine, via intermediates including dihydroxyphenylalanine
(DOPA), to melanin. Within melanocytes, melanin
accumulates in secretory vesicles known as *melanosomes*
which are then disseminated throughout the long,
cytoplasmic processes from which they are transferred to
surrounding epithelial cells. Hence, the pigmented cells of
skin are both the melanocytes which synthesise melanin and
the epithelial cells which have taken up melanin; commonly,
the epithelial cells contain much more melanin than the
melanocytes themselves. The size, shape, and rate of
production of melanosomes varies between individuals of
one race and between racial groups. In blond and red-haired
people there are biochemical differences in the form of
melanin produced. Sunlight promotes melanin synthesis and
causes darkening of previously synthesised melanin. In
addition, melanin synthesis is stimulated by the pituitary
hormone, melanocyte stimulating hormone (MSH) although
the physiological importance of this in humans is not well
understood (see Ch. 17).

Micrographs (a) and (b) permit comparison of caucasian
and negro skin. In the caucasian, there are merely traces of
melanin in the basal epithelial cells and the relatively
inactive melanocytes **M** are unstained. In contrast, the basal

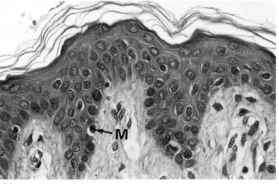

(a)

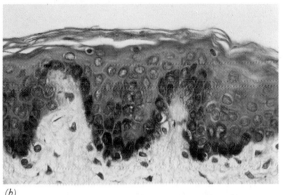

(b)

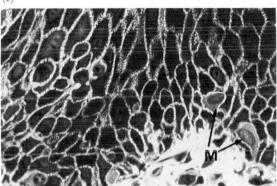

(c)

epithelial cells of negro skin are packed with melanin and
melanocytes themselves are difficult to identify. In thin
sections, as in micrograph (c), melanocytes **M** and their
major dendritic processes are readily distinguishable from
the surrounding epithelial cells.

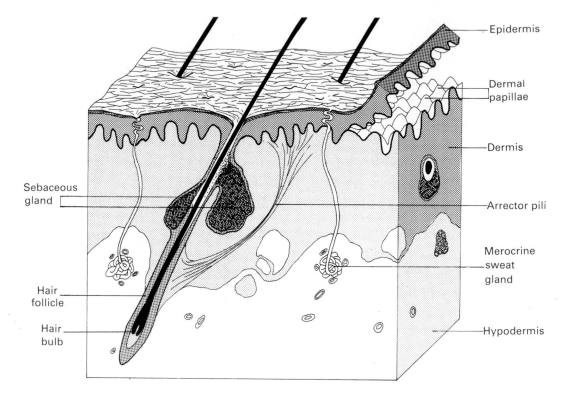

Fig. 9.6 Skin appendages

Skin has a variety of appendages, principally hairs, sebaceous glands and sweat glands, which are derived embryonically from the surface epithelium. The distribution, arrangement and detailed structure of the appendages varies from one part of the skin to another but nevertheless the general structure conforms to a basic pattern. The three-dimensional arrangement shown in this diagram has been deduced from studies of serial sections of skin; individual sections of skin rarely demonstrate all these features.

Hairs: hairs are highly modified keratinised structures produced by *hair follicles* which are essentially cylindrical downgrowths of the surface epithelium ensheathed by connective tissue. Hair growth takes place within a terminal expansion of the follicle, the *hair bulb*, which consists of actively dividing epithelial cells surrounding a papilla of connective tissue, the *dermal papilla*.

A bundle of smooth muscle, the *arrector pili* muscle, is attached to the connective tissue sheath of each follicle and is inserted into the dermal papillary zone. Contraction of the arrector pili erects the hair and pulls down its point of insertion, producing the effect known as 'goose-flesh'.

The arrector pili muscles are innervated by the sympathetic nervous system and pilo-erection is activated by cold or fear. In furry animals, hair erection traps a thicker layer of air over the skin surface thus increasing insulation against heat loss; hair erection also makes the animal appear larger and is thus a protective mechanism in aggressive circumstances. These functions are probably of little physiological significance in man.

Sebaceous glands: one or more sebaceous glands are associated with each hair follicle; these glands secrete an oily substance called *sebum* on to the hair surface in the upper part of the follicle. Sebum acts as a waterproofing agent on the hair and skin surface. In regions of transition from the skin to the body tracts such as the lips, eyelids, glans penis, labia minora and nipples, sebaceous glands are independent of hair follicles and secrete directly on to the skin surface.

Sweat glands: in most areas of the skin, sweat glands are simple, coiled tubular glands which secrete a watery fluid on to the skin surface by the process of merocrine secretion (see Ch. 5). The coiled, secretory portions of these glands are found in the dermis and hypodermis where they are surrounded by a rich plexus of capillaries. Sweat glands are an important component of the thermoregulatory mechanism in man. When the body requires to lose heat, skin blood flow and sweat production are increased; evaporation of sweat causes cooling of the skin surface and loss of heat from the underlying vascular bed. Merocrine sweat glands are innervated by cholinergic fibres of the sympathetic nervous system; sweating is stimulated not only by excessive body heat but also by fear-provoking stimuli.

A different type of sweat gland is found in the skin of the axilla and genital regions of humans. In contrast to the merocrine sweat glands, these glands are believed to secrete by the apocrine process (see Ch. 5) and are thus called *apocrine sweat glands*. They also differ in that they produce a viscid secretion which is discharged into hair follicles rather than directly on to the surface. Apocrine sweat glands are innervated by adrenergic fibres of the sympathetic nervous system.

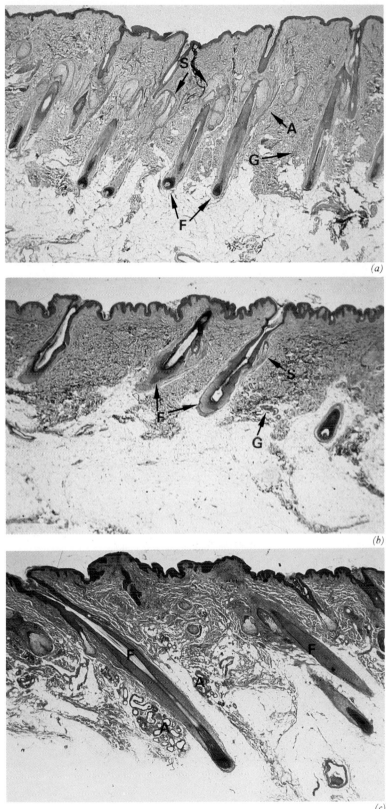

(a)

(b)

(c)

Fig. 9.7 Regional variations of skin structure

(a) Scalp skin: Masson's trichrome × 12
(b) Abdominal skin: Masson's trichrome × 12
(c) Pubic skin: H & E × 12

The structure of the skin differs considerably from one part of the body to another, the principal differences being in epidermal thickness, the size, density and state of activity of the hair follicles, and the nature and density of sweat glands and sensory receptors. These micrographs illustrate three extremes of structure in hairy skin.

As seen in micrograph (a), the skin of the scalp is robust due to a thick, densely collagenous dermis, stained blue-green in this preparation, and the hair follicles **F** are numerous and closely packed. In fair-haired people, the follicles are fewer in number and somewhat smaller in size producing finer hair. The follicles of the scalp are particularly long and have more numerous sebaceous glands **S** than those of other areas. Note the arrector pili muscles **A** extending from the base of the follicles towards the upper dermis. Merocrine sweat glands **G** are numerous though less prominent than in the skin of the trunk and limbs due to the profusion of other appendages.

Micrograph (b) illustrates the typical histological appearance of the skin which covers most of the body. The hair follicles **F** and associated sebaceous glands **S** are sparse and merocrine sweat glands **G** are relatively abundant. The hair follicles are shorter and the hairs produced are finer.

The skin of the axillae and pubic region, shown in micrograph (c), contains a moderate density of hair follicles **F** which, unlike those of the scalp, tend to be oriented obliquely to the skin surface and are often curved rather than straight causing the hairs to be curled. Apocrine sweat glands **A** are a common feature of this type of skin and are seen typically associated with hair follicles into which they discharge their secretions.

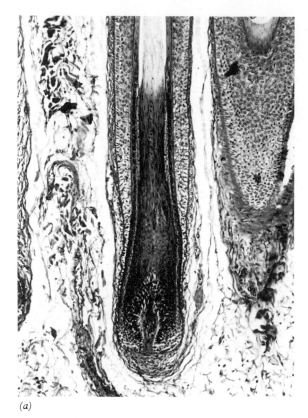

(a)

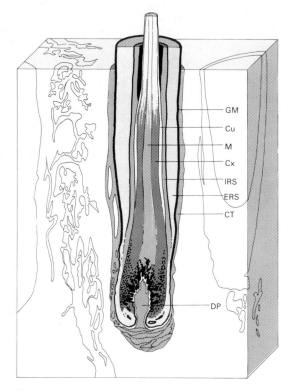

(b)

Fig. 9.8 Hair follicle

(a) LS: H & E × 120 (b) Explanatory diagram

The hair follicle is a tubular structure consisting of five concentric layers of epithelial cells. At the base, there is a bulbous expansion, the hair bulb, enclosing the dermal papilla **DP**. As they are pushed towards the skin surface from the hair bulb, the inner three epithelial layers undergo keratinisation to form the hair shaft whilst the outer two layers form an epithelial sheath. At the hair bulb, all the layers merge to become indistinguishable from one another.

During active hair growth, the epithelial cells surrounding the dermal papilla proliferate to form the innermost four layers of the follicle whilst the outermost layer merely represents a downward continuation of the stratum germinativum of the surface epithelium. The whole epithelial mass surrounding the dermal papilla constitutes the *hair root*.

The cells of the innermost layer of the follicle undergo moderate keratinisation to form the *medulla* **M** or core of the hair shaft; the medullary layer is often not distinguishable in fine hairs. The medulla is surrounded by a broad, highly keratinised layer, the *cortex* **Cx** which forms the bulk of the hair. The third cell layer of the follicle undergoes keratinisation to form a hard, thin *cuticle* **Cu** on the surface of the hair. The cuticle consists of overlapping keratin plates, an arrangement which is said to prevent matting of the hair.

The fourth layer of the follicle constitutes the *internal root sheath* **IRS**; the cells of this layer become only lightly keratinised and disintegrate at the level of the sebaceous gland ducts leaving a space into which sebum is secreted around the maturing hair. The outermost layer, the *external root sheath* **ERS**, does not take part in hair formation; this layer is separated from the sheath of connective tissue **CT** surrounding the follicle by a thick, specialised basement membrane known as the *glassy membrane* **GM**.

In the growing follicle, large active melanocytes (see Fig. 9.5) are scattered amongst the proliferating cells forming the cortex of the hair shaft thereby determining hair colour.

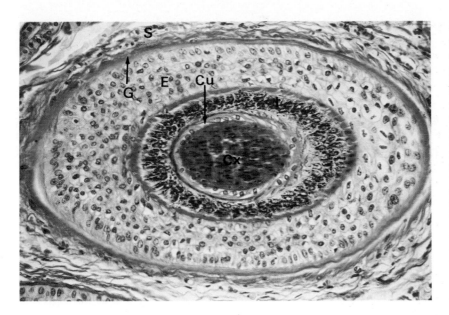

Fig. 9.9 Hair follicle

(H & E × 198)

This is a slightly oblique, transverse section through the lower part of a hair follicle. The broad external root sheath **E** is separated from the connective tissue sheath **S** by the glassy membrane **G**. Passing inwards, the internal root sheath **I** is recognised by its content of eosinophilic (keratohyaline) granules; the outermost cells of the internal root sheath have a more homogeneous appearance. Deep to the internal root sheath is the thin, pale-stained cuticle layer **Cu** which surrounds the strongly stained cortex **Cx**. A medulla is not present in this specimen.

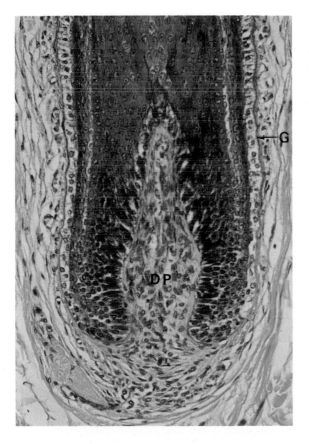

Fig. 9.10 Hair bulb

(Masson's trichrome × 198)

This staining method permits clear delineation of the epithelial and connective tissue elements of the hair follicle. The dermal papilla **DP** is highly vascular and is separated from the epithelial cells by a basement membrane which is continuous with the glassy membrane **G** surrounding the follicle externally. The connective tissue sheath of the follicle is also richly vascular and contains a delicate plexus of sensory nerve endings which are receptive to minute movements of the hair follicle and thus act as highly sensitive touch receptors.

Note the five cell layers of the hair follicle merging with the proliferating cells of the hair root. Note also the large amount of pigment in the basal layer extending up into the cortical layer and produced by melanocytes scattered along the basement membrane of the hair root.

Hair follicles undergo periods of growth and quiescence and this is reflected in changes in their structure. Actively growing follicles penetrate deeply into the hypodermis and the hair bulb is prominent, whereas quiescent follicles are shorter and the hair bulb is smaller and lacking in a dermal papilla; quiescent follicles are known as *club hairs*. In addition, the structure of hair follicles depends on the type of hair being produced. For example, the follicles of the scalp tend to be long and straight, whereas those of the trunk, which produce fine, downy hair, are relatively short and plump; curly hair may be produced by curved follicles or follicles in which the hair bulb lies at an angle to the hair shaft.

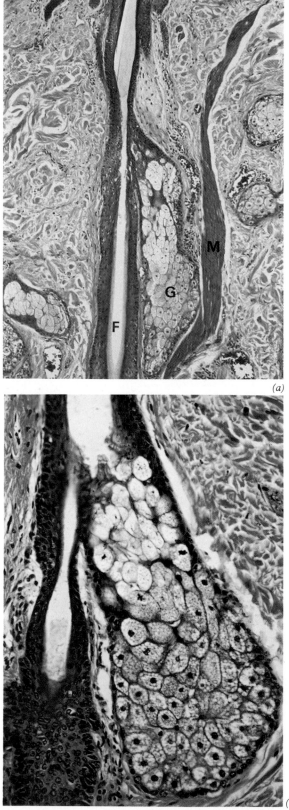

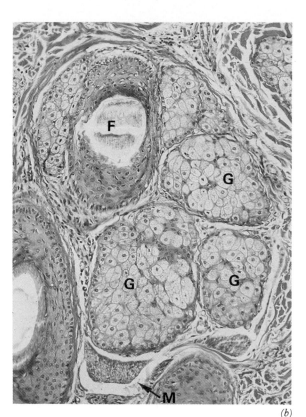

(a)

(b)

Fig. 9.11 Sebaceous glands

(H & E (a) × 33 (b) × 150 (c) × 198)

Micrograph (a) illustrates the relationship of a sebaceous
gland **G** and an arrector pili muscle **M** to a hair follicle **F**.
At a point about one-third of its length from the surface,
each hair follicle is surrounded by one or more sebaceous
glands which discharge their secretions on to the hair shaft
and thence on to the skin surface. As seen in micrograph
(b), sebaceous glands lie within the connective tissue sheath
surrounding the hair follicle and the glandular epithelium
represents an outgrowth of the external root sheath.

The arrector pili muscle of each follicle consists of a
bundle of smooth muscle fibres. The muscle inserts at one
end into the connective tissue sheath of the follicle, at a
point below the sebaceous glands, and at the other end into
the dermal papillary area beneath the epidermis. Each hair
follicle and its associated arrector pili muscle and sebaceous
glands is known as a *pilosebaceous unit*.

More detail of sebaceous gland structure can be seen in
micrograph (c). Each sebaceous gland has a branched acinar
form, the acini converging upon a short duct which empties
into the hair follicle beside the maturing hair. Each acinus
consists of a mass of rounded cells which are packed with
lipid-filled vacuoles; during tissue preparation the lipid is
largely removed, thus the cytoplasm of these cells is poorly
stained. Towards the duct, the lipid content of the acinar
cells increases greatly and the distended cells degenerate, so
releasing their contents, sebum, into the duct by the process
known as *holocrine secretion* (see Ch. 5). Cells lost by
holocrine secretion are replaced by mitosis in the basal layer
of the acinus.

(c)

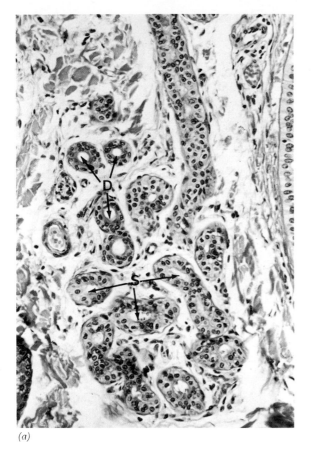

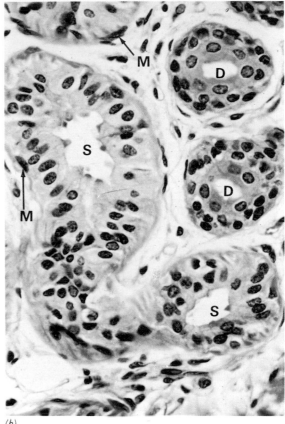

(a)

(b)

Fig. 9.12 Merocrine sweat glands

(H & E (a) × 198 (b) × 480)

Merocrine sweat glands are distributed in the skin of most parts of the body with the exception of areas such as the margins of the lip and the glans penis. Merocrine sweat glands secrete a watery fluid, hypotonic with respect to plasma, the evaporation of which plays an important role in thermoregulation. Sweat contains significant quantities of sodium and chloride ions, some other ions, urea and small molecular weight metabolites; thus sweating may be considered as a minor mode of excretion.

Merocrine sweat glands are unbranched, tubular glands, the secretory portion of which forms a compact coil deep in the dermis. In histological section, the glands appear as a mass of tubules cut in various planes; secretory portions are interspersed with sections of the first part of the excretory duct. The secretory portion **S** consists of a single layer of large cuboidal or columnar cells, whereas the excretory duct **D** is lined by two layers of smaller cuboidal cells. The surrounding dermal connective tissue contains a rich capillary plexus.

At higher magnification, the secretory portions **S** of merocrine sweat glands are seen to be mainly composed of pale-stained, pyramidal-shaped cells which rest on a prominent basement membrane. These cells are believed to pump sodium ions into the gland lumen; this is followed by passive diffusion of water. A second, darkly-stained cell type which is difficult to identify with light microscopy is described; this cell type has ultrastructural features typical of protein secreting cells. The dark cells are believed to secrete a glycoprotein, nevertheless the content of such in sweat is very low. Myoepithelial cells **M** form a discontinuous layer between the secretory cells and the basement membrane; contraction of these cells expels sweat into the excretory ducts.

Sections of the excretory duct **D** are readily distinguishable from sections of the secretory portion. The excretory duct has a narrower lumen, a double layer of small cuboidal cells, no underlying myoepithelial cells and a characteristically eosinophilic luminal aspect which may result from adsorption of the glycoprotein product of the dark secretory cells. The duct epithelium is thought to reabsorb sodium ions from the basic secretion thus making it hypotonic with respect to plasma.

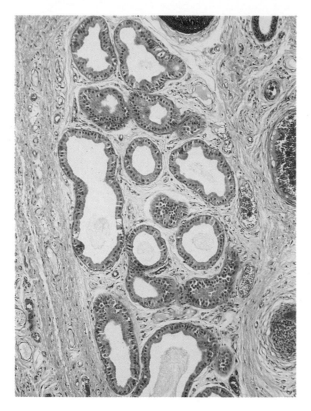

Fig. 9.13 Apocrine sweat glands

(H & E × 128)

Apocrine sweat glands are mainly confined to the axillae and genital regions where they produce a viscid, milky secretion which becomes odorous after the action of skin commensal bacteria.

Apocrine sweat glands are large glands which always secrete into an adjacent hair follicle via a duct which is histologically similar to that of merocrine sweat glands. The secretory portion of the gland is of the coiled, tubular type with a widely dilated lumen. The secretory cells are usually low cuboidal and have an eosinophilic cytoplasm. The budding appearance of the apical cytoplasm of some cells gave rise to the belief that the mode of secretion was of the apocrine type but recent evidence suggests that this appearance may be due to a fixation artefact and that the original interpretations were erroneous. Like merocrine sweat glands, apocrine glands have a discontinuous layer of myoepithelial cells between the base of the secretory cells and the prominent basement membrane.

Apocrine sweat glands do not become functional until puberty and in women undergo cyclical changes under the influence of the hormones of the menstrual cycle.

These glands are analogous to the odiferous glands of many mammals but their biological significance in humans is unknown.

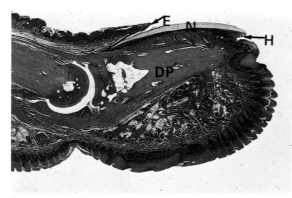

(a)

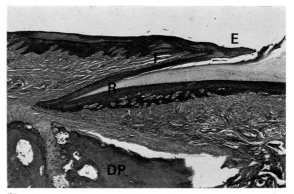

(b)

Fig. 9.14 Fingernail

(Monkey: H & E (a) × 5 (b) × 20)

The dorsal skin surface of the tip of each finger and toe forms a highly specialised appendage, the nail. Each nail **N** is a dense, keratinised plate which rests on a stratified squamous epithelium called the *nail bed*. The proximal end of the nail, the *nail root* **R**, and the underlying nail bed extend deeply into the dermis to lie in close apposition to the distal interphalangeal joint, and the dermis beneath the nail plate is firmly attached to the periosteum of the distal phalanx **DP**.

Nail growth occurs by proliferation and differentiation of the epithelium surrounding the nail root, and the nail plate slides distally over the rest of the nail bed which does not actively contribute to nail growth. Reflecting its proliferative activity, the epithelium beneath the nail root is thicker than that of the rest of the nail bed and exhibits pronounced epidermal ridges as seen in micrograph (b).

The skin overlying the root of the nail is known as the *nail fold* **F** and its highly keratinised free edge is known as the *eponychium* **E**. The skin beneath the free end of the nail is known as the *hyponychium* **H**.

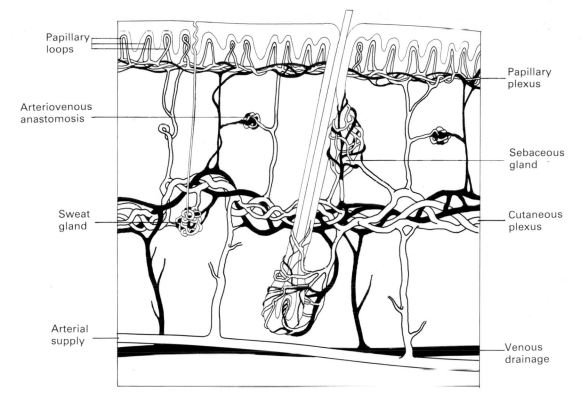

Papillary loops

Arteriovenous anastomosis

Sweat gland

Arterial supply

Papillary plexus

Sebaceous gland

Cutaneous plexus

Venous drainage

Fig. 9.15 The skin circulation

The circulation of the skin has an unusual arrangement which accommodates several different, sometimes conflicting, functional requirements: nutrition of the skin and appendages, increased blood flow to facilitate heat loss in hot conditions, and decreased blood flow to minimise heat loss in cold conditions whilst maintaining adequate nutritional flow.

The arteries supplying the skin are located deep in the hypodermis from which they give rise to branches passing upwards to form two plexuses of anastomosing vessels. The deeper plexus lies at the junction of the hypodermis and dermis and is known as the *cutaneous plexus*; the more superficial plexus lies just beneath the dermal papillae and is known as the *papillary plexus*. Branches of the cutaneous plexus supply the fatty tissue of the hypodermis, the connective tissues of the deeper aspect of the dermis and capillary networks which envelop the hair follicles and deep sebaceous glands and sweat glands. The papillary plexus supplies the upper aspect of the dermis and the capillary networks around the superficial appendages. The papillary plexus also gives rise to a capillary loop in each dermal papilla. The venous drainage of the skin is arranged into plexuses broadly corresponding to the arterial supply.

Numerous shunts provide direct arterio-venous communications which play an important role in thermoregulation by controlling blood flow to the appropriate part of the dermis.

The skin has a rich lymphatic drainage which forms plexuses corresponding to those of the blood vascular system.

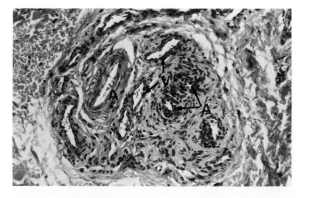

Fig. 9.16 Glomus body
(*H & E × 128*)

In the dermis of the finger tips, and other odd peripheral sites prone to excessive cold such as the external ear, the flow in arteriovenous shunts appears to be controlled by structures called *glomus bodies*. The glomus consists of a highly convoluted segment of an arteriovenous shunt enveloped by condensed connective tissue. In histological section, one or more convolutions of the arterial **A** and venous **V** elements of the shunt are usually seen. Just before the arteriovenous junction, the wall of the artery becomes greatly thickened and its smooth muscle cells assume an epithelial appearance.

10. Skeletal tissues

Introduction

The skeletal system is composed of a variety of specialised forms of connective tissue. Bone provides a rigid protective and supporting framework for most of the soft tissues of the body, whereas cartilage provides semi-rigid support in limited sites such as the respiratory tree and external ear. Joints are composite structures which unite the bones of the skeleton and, depending on their structure, permit varying degrees of movement of the skeleton. Ligaments are flexible bands which contribute to the stability of joints. Tendons provide strong, flexible connections between muscles and their points of insertion into bones.

The functional differences between the various tissues of the skeletal system relate principally to the different nature and proportion of the ground substance and fibrous elements of the extracellular matrix. The cells of all the skeletal tissues, like the cells of connective tissues in general, have close structural and functional relationships and a common origin from primitive mesenchymal cells (see Ch. 4).

Cartilage

Cartilage is a semi-rigid form of connective tissue, the characteristics of which mainly stem from the nature and predominance of ground substance in the extracellular matrix. Glycoproteins, containing a high proportion of sulphated polysaccharide units, make up the ground substance and account for the solid, yet flexible, property of cartilage.

Within the ground substance are embedded varying proportions of collagen and elastic fibres giving rise to three main types of cartilage: *hyaline cartilage, fibro-cartilage* and *elastic cartilage.*

Cartilage formation commences with the differentiation of stellate-shaped, primitive mesenchymal cells (see Fig. 4.2) to form rounded cartilage precursor cells called *chondroblasts*. Subsequent mitotic divisions give rise to aggregations of closely packed chondroblasts which grow and begin synthesis of ground substance and fibrous extracellular material. Secretion of extracellular material traps each chondroblast within the cartilagenous matrix thereby separating the chondroblasts from one another. Each chondroblast then undergoes one or two further mitotic divisions to form a small group of mature cells separated by a small amount of extracellular material. Mature cartilage cells, known as *chondrocytes*, maintain the integrity of the cartilage matrix. This differentiation and maturation sequence is most advanced in the centre of a mass of growing cartilage. Towards the periphery of the cartilage, chondroblasts at progressively earlier stages of differentiation merge with the surrounding loose connective tissue. On completion of growth, the cartilage mass consists of chondrocytes embedded in a large amount of extracellular matrix. At the periphery of mature cartilage is a zone of condensed connective tissue called *perichondrium*, containing chondroblasts with cartilage-forming potential. Growth of cartilage occurs by *interstitial growth* from within and *appositional growth* at the periphery.

Most cartilage is devoid of blood vessels and consequently the exchange of metabolites between chondrocytes and surrounding tissues depends on diffusion through the water of solvation of the ground substance. This limits the thickness to which cartilage may develop, whilst maintaining viability of the innermost cells; in sites where cartilage is particularly thick, e.g. intercostal cartilage, *cartilage canals* convey small vessels into the centre of the cartilage mass.

In mature mammals, cartilage has a limited distribution, whereas in immature mammals cartilage occurs more extensively since it forms a template for most of the developing bony skeleton.

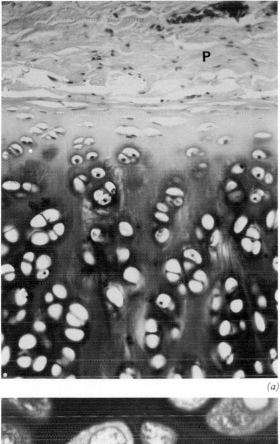

(a)

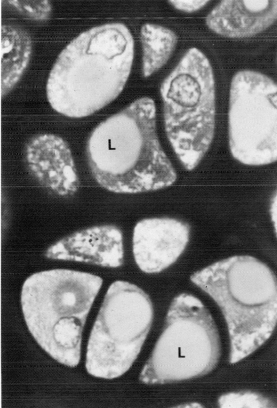

(b)

Fig. 10.1 Hyaline cartilage

(a) H & E × 78 (b) Thin section, toluidine blue × 1200

Hyaline cartilage is the most common type of cartilage and is found in the nasal septum, larynx, tracheal rings, most articular surfaces and the sternal ends of the ribs. Mature hyaline cartilage is characterised by small aggregations of chondrocytes embedded in an amorphous matrix of ground substance reinforced by collagen fibres.

In the preparation of mature hyaline cartilage shown in micrograph (a), two distinct zones are evident: an inner, strongly basophilic zone and an outer, pale-stained zone which merges with adjacent connective tissue. The chondrocytes of the inner zone are arranged in characteristic clusters usually consisting of two or four fully differentiated cells. The clusters are separated by a large mass of amorphous cartilage matrix whilst the cells of each cluster are separated by only a thin zone of extracellular matrix. In standard histological preparations, considerable shrinkage distorts the cellular detail of the chondrocytes and thus they appear not to fully occupy their spaces within the matrix.

Extending from the inner zone towards the outer surface of the cartilage, the chondrocytes are progressively less differentiated so that the cells of the outer surface in the *perichondrium* **P** resemble mature fibroblasts. Note that the cells of the outer zone have not divided to form clusters. The morphological gradation of cartilage cells from the perichondrium to the most mature chondrocytes of the inner zone represents the progressive changes that occur during the development of cartilage. In adult cartilage, cell differentiation in the perichondrium and outer zone is suspended unless growth is stimulated. When growth is stimulated, isolated chondrocytes divide to form clusters thereby promoting interstitial growth, and chondroblasts of the perichondrium differentiate into chondrocytes resulting in appositional growth.

The matrix of hyaline cartilage appears fairly amorphous since the ground substance and collagen have similar refractive indices. With the exception of articular cartilage, the collagen of hyaline cartilage, designated as collagen Type II (see Ch. 4) is not cross-banded and is arranged in an interlacing network of fine fibrils; this collagen cannot be demonstrated by light microscopy. The variable staining intensity of the cartilage matrix reflects the concentration of acidic, sulphated glycoproteins; this is greatest around the clusters of fully differentiated cells and least in the perichondrium.

With the technique employed in micrograph (b), the cellular detail of chondrocytes is preserved. Note that the chondrocytes fully occupy the spaces in the matrix each space containing a single chondrocyte. Mature chondrocytes are characterised by small nuclei with dispersed chromatin and basophilic, granular cytoplasm reflecting a well developed rough endoplasmic reticulum. Lipid droplets **L**, often larger than the nuclei, are a prominent feature of chondrocytes; the cytoplasm is also rich in glycogen. These characteristics reflect the active role of chondrocytes in synthesis of both the ground substance and fibrous elements of the cartilage matrix. In fully formed cartilage, the constituents of the extracellular matrix are continuously turned over; the integrity of the matrix is thus dependent on the viability of the chondrocytes.

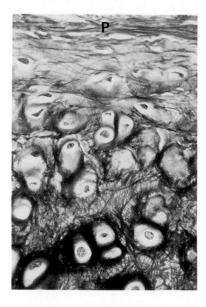

Fig. 10.2 Elastic cartilage

(Elastic van Gieson × 128)

Elastic cartilage occurs in the external ear and external auditory canal, the epiglottis, parts of the laryngeal cartilages and the walls of the Eustachian tubes.

The histological structure of elastic cartilage is similar to that of hyaline cartilage, its elasticity, however, being derived from the presence of numerous bundles of branching elastic fibres in the cartilage matrix; this network of elastic fibres, stained black in this preparation, is particularly dense in the immediate vicinity of the chondrocytes. Collagen, stained red in this preparation, is also a major constituent of cartilage matrix and makes up the bulk of the perichondrium **P** intermingled with a few elastic fibres.

Development and growth of elastic cartilage occurs by both interstitial and appositional growth in the same manner as for hyaline cartilage.

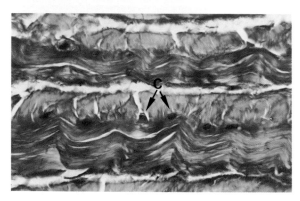

Fig. 10.3 Fibrocartilage

(H & E / Alcian blue × 320)

Fibrocartilage, which has features intermediate between cartilage and dense fibrous connective tissue, is found in the intervertebral discs, some articular cartilages, the pubic symphysis, and in association with dense connective tissue in joint capsules, ligaments and the connections of some tendons to bone.

Fibrocartilage consists of alternating layers of hyaline cartilage matrix and thick layers of dense collagen fibres oriented in the direction of the functional stresses. In this micrograph, pink-stained collagen characteristically permeates the blue-stained cartilage ground substance. Chondrocytes **C** are usually arranged in rows between the dense collagen layers within lacunae in the glycoprotein matrix.

Bone

Bone is a specialised form of connective tissue in which the extracellular components are mineralised, thus conferring the property of marked rigidity and strength whilst retaining some degree of elasticity. In addition to its supporting and protective function, bone constitutes a variable store of calcium and other inorganic ions, and actively participates in the maintenance of calcium homeostasis in the body as a whole. The structure of individual bones provides for the maximum resistance to mechanical stresses whilst maintaining the least bony mass. To accommodate changing mechanical stresses and the demands of calcium homeostasis, all bones in the body are in a dynamic state of growth and resorption throughout life.

Like other connective tissues, bone is composed of cells and an organic extracellular matrix containing glycoprotein ground substance and collagen fibres. Inorganic salts, predominantly *calcium hydroxyapatite* crystals, form the mineral component of bone matrix. Ground substance constitutes only a small proportion of the organic extracellular matrix of bone and contains glycoproteins similar to those found in cartilage except that the proportion of sulphated glycoproteins is much less than in cartilage. The fibrous component of the extracellular material is mainly Type I collagen which exhibits a similar banding pattern to that of common collagenous connective tissues (see Ch. 4).

The cells found in bone are of three types: *osteoblasts, osteocytes* and *osteoclasts,* the first two cell types being derived from mesenchymal-type cells called *osteoprogenitor cells.* Osteoblasts are immature bone cells responsible for the synthesis and secretion of the organic component of the extracellular matrix of bone, a substance known as *osteoid*; osteoid rapidly undergoes mineralisation to form bone. Osteoblasts become trapped within bone as osteocytes and are then responsible for maintenance of the bone matrix. Osteoclasts are multinucleate cells probably derived from cells of the macrophage-monocyte system (see Fig. 3.12) which are actively involved in resorptive processes associated with continuous remodelling of bone.

Bone exists in two main forms: *woven bone* and *lamellar bone*. Woven bone is an immature form and is characterised by a random (woven) organisation of its collagen, the fibres of which are much coarser than those of lamellar bone. During bone development, woven bone is the first form of bone to be produced; it is then remodelled to form lamellar bone, the form which constitutes most of the mature skeleton. Lamellar bone is composed of successive layers each of which has a highly organised infrastructure. Lamellar bone may be formed as a solid mass, when it is described as *compact bone*, or may be formed as a spongy mass, described as *cancellous bone*.

The mineralised component of bone makes it too brittle to be cut into histological sections to say nothing of the unsuitability of traditional microtome knives for this task. Consequently, for routine histological purposes, bone is first decalcified in acid solutions prior to sectioning and staining. With this method, cellular detail and the organic component of the matrix is preserved though the stains are taken up less readily as a result of the initial decalcification process. Recently, acrylics have become available for embedding bone without prior decalcification, and using diamond-edged knives, sections can be cut and then stained preserving detail in both the cells and the calcified matrix. Such methods are used in the study of the mineralisation process and its disorders, and examples are shown in Figures 10.13 (b) and 10.14 (b).

Finally, for the study of the morphology of the mineralised matrix, *ground sections* are made. This involves sawing undecalcified bone into relatively thick sections and the surfaces are then ground thin and smooth with grinding stones. All cellular detail is lost in such preparations.

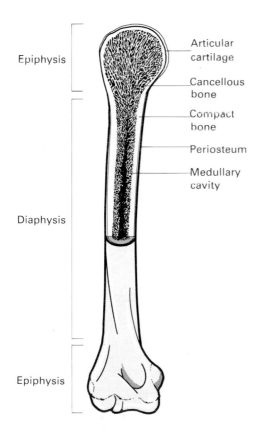

Epiphysis

Diaphysis

Epiphysis

Articular cartilage

Cancellous bone

Compact bone

Periosteum

Medullary cavity

Fig. 10.4 Long bone

This diagram illustrates the general structure of long bones and the gross morphological appearance of the two types of lamellar bone found in the mature skeleton: compact bone and (cancellous) spongy bone.

Compact bone forms the dense walls of the shaft or *diaphysis* while spongy bone occupies part of the large central *medullary cavity*. Spongy bone consists of a network of fine, irregular plates called *trabeculae* separated by intercommunicating spaces. In immature animals, the medullary cavities of most bones contain active (red) marrow which is responsible for the production of the cellular elements of blood. In the adult, active marrow is restricted to a few sites (see Ch. 3); the medullary cavities of other bones are filled with inactive (yellow) marrow which is largely composed of adipose tissue.

The articular (joint) surfaces of the expanded ends, or *epiphyses*, of long bones are protected by a layer of specialised hyaline cartilage called *articular cartilage*. The external surface of the bone is invested in a dense fibrous connective tissue layer called the *periosteum* into which are inserted muscles, tendons and ligaments. The inner surface of the bone, including the trabeculae of spongy bone, is invested by a delicate connective tissue layer called the *endosteum*. The endosteum and periosteum contain cells of the osteogenic series which are responsible for growth, continuous remodelling and repair of bone fractures.

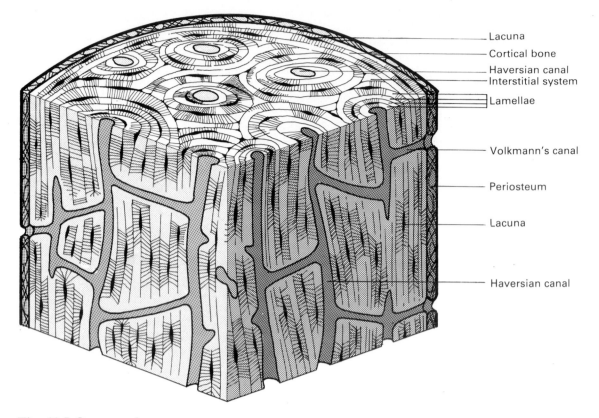

Lacuna
Cortical bone
Haversian canal
Interstitial system
Lamellae
Volkmann's canal
Periosteum
Lacuna
Haversian canal

Fig. 10.5 Compact bone

Compact bone is made up of parallel bony columns which, in long bones, are disposed parallel to the long axis i.e. in the line of stress exerted on the bone. Each column is made up of concentric bony layers or *lamellae* disposed around central channels containing blood and lymphatic vessels, and nerves. The neurovascular channels are known as *canals of Havers* or *Haversian canals,* and with their concentric lamellae form *Haversian systems.* The neurovascular bundles interconnect with one another, and with the endosteum and periosteum, via *Volkmann's canals* which pierce the columns at right angles, or obliquely, to the Haversian canals.

Each Haversian system begins as a broad channel, at the periphery of which osteoblasts lay down lamellae of bone. With the deposition of successive lamellae, the diameter of the Haversian canal decreases and osteoblasts are trapped as osteocytes in spaces called *lacunae* in the matrix. The

osteocytes are thus arranged in concentric rings within the lamellae. Between adjacent lacunae and the central canal are numerous minute interconnecting canals called *canaliculi* which contain fine cytoplasmic extensions of the osteocytes.

As a result of the continuous resorption and redeposition of bone, complete, newly formed Haversian systems are disposed between partly resorbed systems formed earlier. The remnants of lamellae no longer surrounding Haversian canals form irregular *interstitial systems* between intact Haversian systems.

At the outermost aspect of compact bone, Haversian systems give way to concentric lamellae of dense *cortical bone* laid down at the bone surface by osteoblasts of the periosteum. At the inner medullary aspect, similar but irregular circumferential lamellae merge with trabeculae of spongy bone.

Fig. 10.6 Compact bone

(TS: Ground section, unstained × 80)

In this ground section, the bone has been cut transversely thereby demonstrating newly formed Haversian systems **H₁** and older, partly resorbed Haversian systems **H₂** amongst irregular interstitial systems **I**.

Concentric rings of flattened lacunae surround the Haversian canals and numerous fine canaliculi, barely visible at this magnification, interconnect lacunae with Haversian canals.

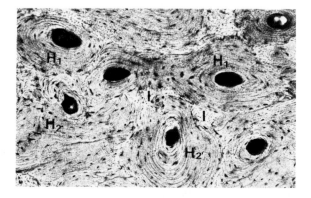

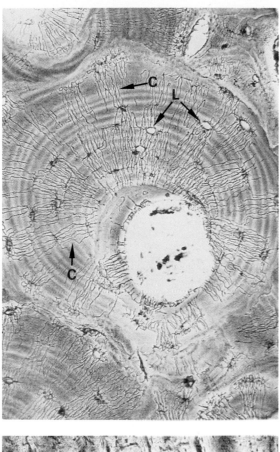

Fig. 10.7 Haversian system

(TS: Ground section, unstained × 600)

This micrograph focuses on a single Haversian system, the central canal being surrounded by concentric lamellae of bone matrix containing empty lacunae **L**. Fine canaliculi **C** radiate from each lacuna to anastomose with those of adjacent lacunae. In life, the oesteocytes do not completely fill the lacunae, the remaining narrow space being filled with unmineralised matrix. Fine cytoplasmic processes of the osteocytes pass in the canaliculi to communicate via gap junctions with the processes of osteocytes in adjacent lamellae. The canaliculi provide passages for circulation of tissue fluid and diffusion of metabolites between the lacunae and vessels of the Haversian canals.

Osteocytes are believed to maintain the dynamic state of the mineralised matrix and to mediate short-term release or deposition of calcium for the process of calcium homeostasis. The activity of osteocytes in calcium regulation is controlled directly by plasma calcium concentration and indirectly by the hormones parathyroid hormone and calcitonin secreted by the parathyroid and thyroid glands respectively (see Ch. 17).

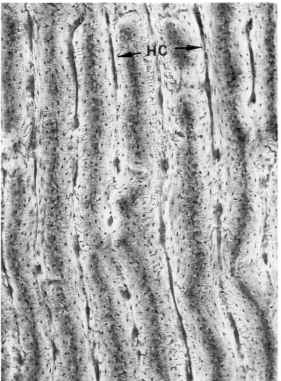

Fig. 10.8 Compact bone

(LS: Ground section, unstained × 150)

This micrograph shows compact bone cut in longitudinal section, the plane of section including some Haversian canals **HC**. In ground sections, these appear dark in colour since air is contained within them, all cellular material being destroyed during processing. Likewise, the tiny osteocyte lacunae also appear as brown specks elongated in shape and arranged in concentric layers around the Haversian canals.

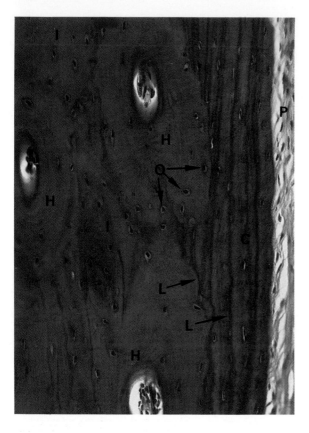

Fig. 10.9 Compact bone
(TS: H & E × 198)

The morphology of the cells and organic components of bone may be studied in standard decalcified preparations, as in this micrograph which illustrates several Haversian systems **H** in transverse section separated by irregular interstitial systems **I**. The matrix of decalcified mature bone is strongly eosinophilic because of its high content of collagen. The collagen of the lamellae is disposed in a helical manner around the long axes of the Haversian systems.

At its outer aspect, the Haversian bone gives way to lamellae of cortical bone **C** which provides a more dense, protective outer surface to most bones. Where the Haversian systems and cortical lamellae abut one another, fine basophilic cement lines **L** rich in glycoprotein ground substance, are seen. Note the fibrous periosteum **P** investing the surface of the cortical bone.

Osteocytes **O** have densely stained, irregular nuclei and pale, basophilic cytoplasm which undergoes considerable shrinkage in routine preparations such as this. Unlike the chondrocytes of cartilage, osteocytes do not usually completely occupy their lacunae in bone matrix. Canaliculi, containing the fine cytoplasmic processes of osteocytes, are not usually visible in this type of preparation. Within the Haversian canals, note the presence of small blood vessels and nuclei representing endosteal osteoblasts.

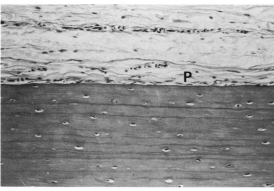

(a)

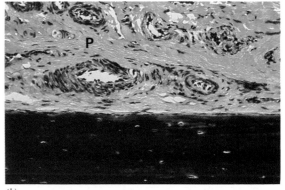

(b)

Fig. 10.10 Mature periosteum
(a) H & E × 128 (b) Masson's trichrome × 200

The outer surface of most bone is invested by a layer of condensed fibrous tissue, the periosteum **P**, which contains numerous osteoprogenitor cells which are practically indistinguishable from fibroblasts. During bone growth or repair, the osteoprogenitor cells differentiate into osteoblasts which are responsible for the deposition of concentric lamellae of cortical bone by appositional growth. The periosteum is bound to the underlying bone by bundles of collagen fibres called *Sharpey's fibres* which may penetrate the whole thickness of the cortical bone; collagen is stained green in micrograph (b). The periosteum is richly supplied with blood vessels from adjacent connective tissues.

Periosteum is not present on the articular surfaces of bone, the sites of insertion of tendons and ligaments, and at several other discrete sites such as the subcapsular area of the neck of the femur. The periosteum plays an important role in the repair of bone fractures and its absence may lead to delay or failure of healing particularly of subcapsular fractures of the femoral neck.

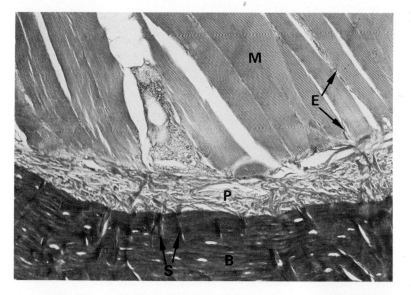

Fig. 10.11 Muscular insertion into bone

(Phosphotungstic acid / Haematoxylin × 480)

Muscle may be attached directly to bone, in which case the area of attachment is relatively extensive, or alternatively, the muscle may be inserted into a tendon which is attached to bone over a more localised area.

This micrograph shows the direct attachment of skeletal muscle **M** to bone **B**. The end of the muscle fibres abut onto the periosteum **P**, the collagenous fibres of which extend between the muscle fibres to mingle with the collagen of the endomysium **E**; collagen stains red with this staining method. In areas of muscle attachment, the surface of the cortical bone tends to be roughened and the periosteal Sharpey's fibres **S** are robust and extend deeply into the bony cortex.

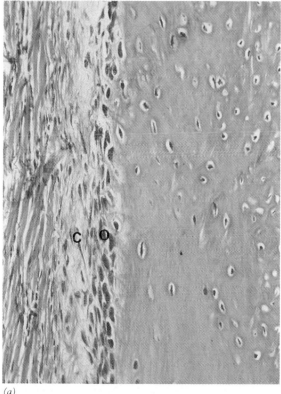

(a)

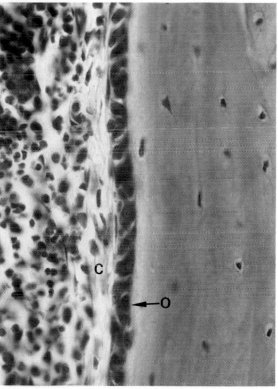

(b)

Fig. 10.12 Active periosteum

(H & E (a) × 200 (b) × 480)

These micrographs illustrate highly active periosteum from a developing fetal long bone. The periosteum consists of plump, basophilic osteoblasts **O** two to three cells deep on the surface of the developing bone, and a thin layer of immature, loose connective tissue **C**. The cytoplasmic basophilia of active osteoblasts is due to the large content of rough endoplasmic reticulum involved in synthesising the fibres and ground substance of bone matrix. When appositional bone growth at the periosteal surface is complete, osteoblasts revert to quiescent, osteoprogenitor cells which closely resemble fibroblasts. Note that the bone of the developing shaft is of the woven type; the process of remodelling, to form lamellar bone, occurs at a later stage (see Fig. 10.25).

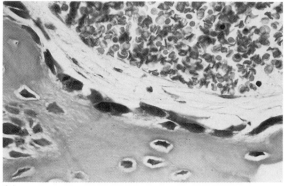

(a)

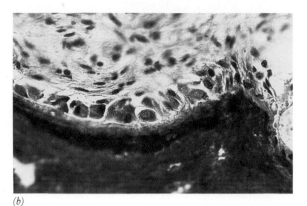

(b)

Fig. 10.13 Osteoblasts and osteoid

(a) H & E × 320 (b) Undecalcified section, Goldner's trichrome × 320

These micrographs illustrate active osteoblasts in the process of laying down the organic components of bone matrix; before mineralisation occurs the organic matrix is known as osteoid. In comparison with mature osteocytes, osteoblasts are large cells with abundant basophilic cytoplasm, a large Golgi apparatus and a pale stained nucleus with a prominent nucleolus. These features reflect a high rate of protein and proteoglycan synthesis.

In normally developing bone, as seen in (a), osteoid becomes calcified almost immediately after deposition. Under conditions in which adequate calcium and phosphate ions are not available, for example in rickets or chronic renal failure, there is a lag in mineralisation of osteoid; under such circumstances osteoid tissue accumulates. Osteoid is readily demonstrated in undecalcified sections as shown in (b), a biopsy specimen from an individual with chronic renal failure. With this staining method, osteoid appears as a red-stained zone between a layer of active osteoblasts and the mineralised bone (stained blue).

Little is known about the process of mineralisation but it has been suggested that calcium and phosphate ions form hydroxyapatite crystals under the influence of collagen and associated ground substance; the organic components may act as nucleation centres for crystallisation.

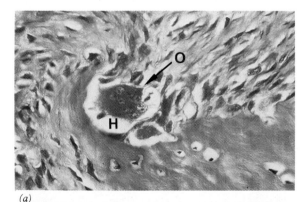

(a)

(b)

Fig. 10.14 Osteoclasts

(a) H & E × 320 (b) Undecalcified section, Goldner's trichrome × 320

Resorption of bone is performed by large multinucleate cells called osteoclasts **O** which are often seen lying in depressions resorbed from the bone surface called *Howship's lacunae* **H**.

In decalcified preparations as in micrograph (a), osteoclasts tend to shrink and become detached from the bone surface; the intimate relationship of osteoclasts with bone is seen better in micrograph (b).

Osteoclastic resorption contributes to bone remodelling in response to growth or changing mechanical stresses upon the skeleton. Osteoclasts also participate in the long-term maintenance of blood calcium homeostasis by their response to parathyroid hormone and calcitonin (see Ch. 17). Parathyroid hormone stimulates osteoclastic resorption and the release of calcium ions from bone, whereas calcitonin inhibits osteoclastic activity.

The specimen shown in micrograph (b) is from an individual with a low serum calcium level. This condition stimulates release of parathyroid hormone which promotes excessive osteoclastic resorption in an attempt to restore serum calcium levels. In addition, under these circumstances there is a lag in mineralisation of newly deposited bone matrix which is manifest by the presence of osteoid **Os**.

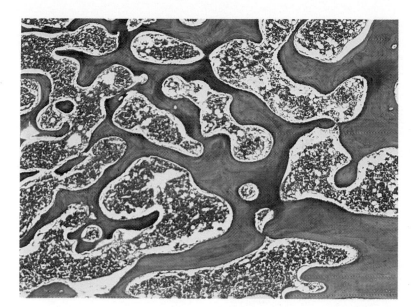

Fig. 10.15 Cancellous bone
(H & E × 50)

Cancellous (spongy) bone is composed of a network of bony trabeculae separated by a labyrinth of interconnecting spaces containing bone marrow. The trabeculae are thin and composed of irregular lamellae of bone with lacunae containing osteocytes. Spongy bone does not usually contain Haversian systems and the osteocytes exchange metabolites via canaliculi with blood sinusoids in the marrow. The trabeculae are lined by a delicate layer of connective tissue called endosteum which contains osteoprogenitor cells, osteoblasts and osteoclasts.

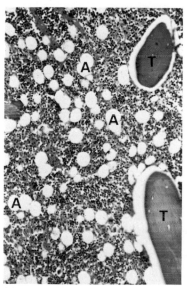

(a)

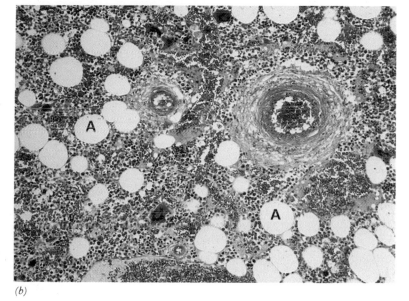

(b)

Fig. 10.16 Bone marrow
(H & E (a) × 128 (b) × 480)

The intertrabecular spaces of all bones are filled with bone marrow containing the primitive stem cells from which all the cellular elements of blood are derived (see Ch. 3). Active bone marrow is crammed with dividing stem cells and the precursors of mature blood cells and the predominance of maturing erythrocytes confers a deep red colour on active marrow and hence the name *red marrow*. In the newborn, all bone marrow is involved in haemopoiesis; however, with increasing age, the marrow of peripheral long bones becomes less active and is progressively dominated by adipocytes. In mature mammals, therefore, much of the marrow is inactive and yellow in colour; *yellow marrow* may, however, be reactivated if the need arises for increased haemopoiesis.

These preparations from a 7-year-old child contain much active haemopoietic tissue and scattered adipocytes **A**. Note two thin trabeculae **T** of cancellous bone in micrograph (a). Micrograph (b) shows a moderate sized artery and one of its branches passing through the marrow. The arteries of the marrow are derived from the nutrient artery of the bone and supply the extensive sinusoidal network between the cords of haemopoietic tissue. The sinusoids then drain to a vein which passes out of the marrow in company with the nutrient artery.

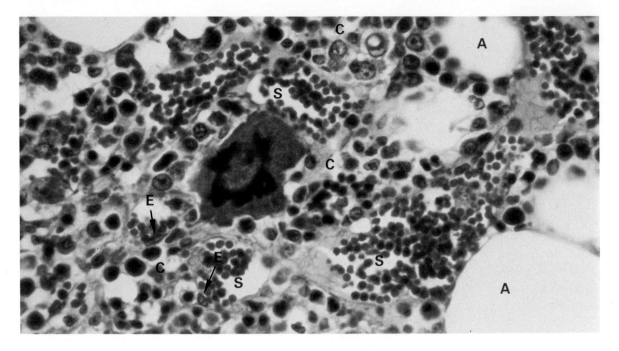

Fig. 10.17 Bone marrow

(H & E × 800)

This micrograph shows a small area of bone marrow at very high magnification. Active bone marrow consists of two main components, a reticulin framework which supports developing blood cells and a system of interconnected blood sinusoids which drain towards the central vein.

Haemopoiesis occurs within the reticulin framework, thus forming cords of cells which contain a mixture of developing blood cell lines. Draped on the supporting reticulin framework among the haemopoietic cells are macrophages which engulf the cell debris resulting from the haemopoietic process; they are probably also responsible for elaboration and maintenance of the supporting reticulin framework. When development is complete or almost complete, blood cells pass from the cords through the delicate sinusoidal endothelium to enter the general circulation.

The endothelium lining the sinusoids is of the continuous type with the endothelial cells overlapping each other at their margins in such a way as to allow passage of blood cells between them. The endothelial cells also exhibit phagocytic activity and are also probably involved in clearing haemopoietic cellular debris. The efflux of blood cells from the bone marrow depends on the functional demands of the body but the mechanism which controls the entry of specific blood cell types into the sinusoids is unknown.

This micrograph of active bone marrow illustrates haemopoietic cords **C** separated by broad sinusoids **S** which are filled with erythrocytes and occasional leucocytes. Note two flattened endothelial cell nuclei **E**. Of the haemopoietic cells, only one can be reliably identified, namely a huge megakaryocyte near the centre of the field. Note also a few scattered adipocytes **A**.

The functional relationship between bone and bone marrow is obscure; bone may merely provide protection and support for the delicate bone marrow tissue or there may be some specific metabolic relationship between the two tissues. In support of the latter, it has been observed that transplanted bone marrow is unable to survive in sites other than the medullary cavities of bone marrow.

Bone development and growth

The fetal development of bone occurs in two ways, both of which involve replacement of connective tissues by bone. The resulting woven bone is then extensively remodelled by resorption and appositional growth to form the mature adult skeleton which is made up of lamellar bone. Thereafter, resorption and deposition of bone occur at a much reduced rate to accommodate changing functional stresses and to effect calcium homeostasis. The bones of the vault of the skull, the maxilla and most of the mandible are formed by the deposition of bone within primitive mesenchymal tissue; this process of direct replacement of mesenchyme by bone is known as *intramembranous ossification* and the bones so formed are called *membrane bones*. In contrast, the long bones, vertebrae, pelvis and bones of the base of the skull are preceded by the formation of a continuously growing cartilage model which is progressively replaced by bone; this process is called *endochondral ossification* and the bones so formed are called *cartilage bones*. Bone development is controlled by growth hormone, thyroid hormone and the sex hormones.

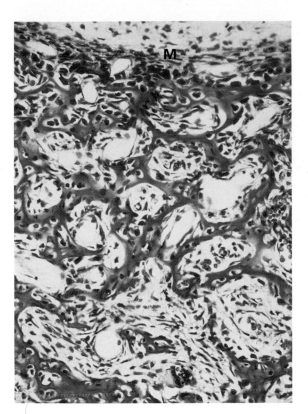

Fig. 10.18 Intramembranous ossification

(H & E × 75)

Intramembranous bone formation occurs within 'membranes' of condensed, primitive mesenchymal tissue. Mesenchymal cells differentiate into osteoblasts which begin synthesis and secretion of osteoid at so-called *centres of ossification*; mineralisation of osteoid follows closely. As osteoid is laid down, osteoblasts are trapped in lacunae to become osteocytes and their cytoplasmic extensions shrink to form the fine processes contained within canaliculi. Osteoprogenitor cells at the surface of the centres of ossification divide mitotically to produce further osteoblasts which lay down more bone. Progressive bone formation results in the fusion of adjacent bony centres to form bone which is spongy in gross appearance.

The collagen fibres of developing bone are randomly arranged in interlacing bundles giving rise to the term woven bone. The woven bone then undergoes progressive remodelling by osteoclastic resorption and osteoblastic deposition to form mature compact or spongy bone. The primitive mesenchyme remaining in the network of developing bone differentiates into bone marrow.

This preparation from the developing skull vault of a cat fetus illustrates spicules of woven bone, separated by primitive mesenchymal tissue. Note the condensed primitive mesenchyme **M** which delineates the outer margin of the developing bone.

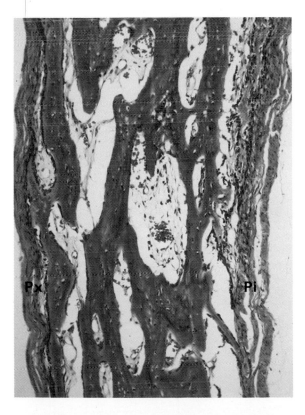

Fig. 10.19 Skull

(Cat: TS, H & E × 30)

This micrograph shows a full thickness view of the skull vault of a mature cat which, like that of the human, is formed by the process of intramembranous ossification. The skull vault consists of cancellous bone which is condensed at its internal and external aspects to form continuous, relatively smooth surfaces. The external surface of the skull is invested by periosteum **Px** which merges with the deep layers of the overlying skin. The internal surface of the skull is also lined by periosteum **Pi**; this layer also constitutes the outermost membranous covering of the brain, the dura mater.

During skeletal growth, the skull vault expands in response to the pressure of the growing brain within. The developing skull bones, which are bound together by sutures of periosteum, are pushed outwards and new membrane bone is laid down at the sutural margins. At the same time, periosteal deposition of new bone on the outer surfaces, and corresponding osteoclastic resorption at the inner surfaces, provides for the necessary recontouring of the skull bones which become progressively flatter. At skeletal maturity the sutures between the skull bones become almost closed and filled with dense fibrous tissue which represents the periosteal layers of opposing bones. With advancing age the sutures tend to ossify.

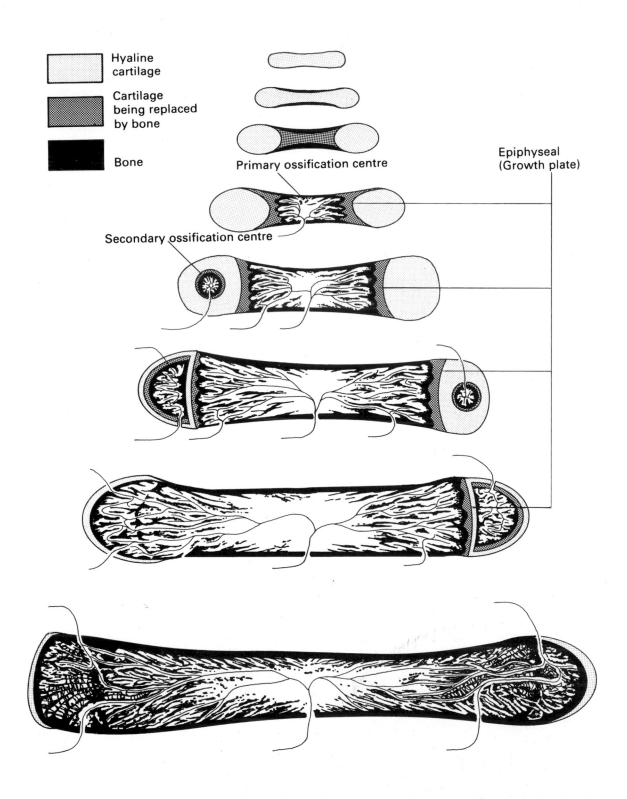

Hyaline cartilage

Cartilage being replaced by bone

Bone

Primary ossification centre

Secondary ossification centre

Epiphyseal (Growth plate)

Fig. 10.20 Endochondral ossification *(Illustration opposite)*

Endochondral ossification is a method of bone formation which permits functional stresses to be sustained during skeletal growth and is well demonstrated in the development of the long bones.

A small model of the long bone is first formed in solid hyaline cartilage which undergoes mainly appositional growth to form an elongated, dumb-bell shaped mass of cartilage consisting of a shaft (diaphysis) and future articular portions (epiphyses) surrounded by perichondrium.

Within the shaft of the cartilage model the chondrocytes enlarge greatly, resorbing the surrounding cartilage so as to leave only slender perforated trabeculae of cartilage matrix. This cartilage matrix then calcifies and the chondrocytes degenerate leaving large, interconnecting spaces. During this period the perichondrium of the shaft develops osteogenic potential and assumes the role of periosteum. The periosteum then lays down a thin layer of bone around the surface of the shaft and primitive mesenchymal cells and blood vessels invade the spaces left within the shaft after degeneration of the chondrocytes. The primitive mesenchymal cells differentiate into osteoblasts and blood-forming cells of the bone marrow. Osteoblasts form a layer of cells on the surface of the calcified remnants of the cartilage matrix and commence the formation of irregular, woven bone.

The ends of the original cartilage model have by now become separated by a large site of *primary ossification* in the shaft. The cartilaginous ends of the model, however, continue to grow in diameter. Meanwhile, the cartilage at the ends of the shaft continues to undergo regressive changes followed by ossification so that the developing bone now consists of an elongated, bony diaphyseal shaft with a semilunar cartilage epiphysis at each end. The interface between the shaft and each epiphysis constitutes a *growth* or *epiphyseal plate.* Within the growth plate, the cartilage proliferates continuously, resulting in progressive elongation of the bone. At the diaphyseal aspect of each growth plate, the chondrocytes mature and then die, the degenerating zone of cartilage being replaced by bone. Thus the bony diaphysis lengthens and the growth plates are pushed further and further apart. On reaching maturity, hormonal changes inhibit further cartilage proliferation and the growth plates are replaced by bone causing fusion of the diaphysis and epiphyses.

In the meantime, in the centre of the mass of cartilage of each developing epiphysis, regressive changes and bone formation similar to that in the diaphyseal cartilage occur along with appositional growth of cartilage over the whole external surface of the epiphysis. This conversion of central epiphyseal cartilage to bone is known as *secondary ossification.* A thin zone of hyaline cartilage always remains at the surface as the articular cartilage.

Under the influence of functional stresses the calcified cartilage remnants and the surrounding irregular woven bone are completely remodelled so that the bone ultimately consists of a compact outer layer with a medulla of cancellous bone. By maturity, the medullary bone is almost completely resorbed to leave a large medullary space filled with bone marrow.

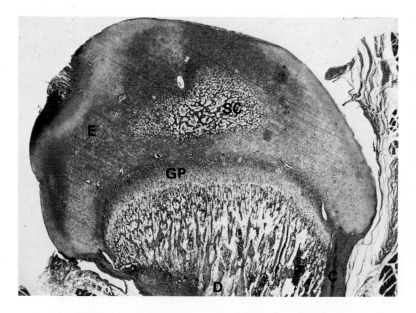

Fig. 10.21 Epiphysis
(H & E/Alcian blue × 12)

This micrograph illustrates the head of a kitten femur at an advanced stage of development.

The cartilaginous epiphysis **E** is separated from the diaphysis **D** by the epiphyseal growth plate **GP.** Note the thickening compact bone **C** at the outer aspect of the diaphysis and the trabeculae of bone in the medulla. Note also the centre of secondary ossification **SC** in the epiphyseal cartilage.

Epiphyseal growth plates provide for growth in length of long bones whilst accommodating functional stresses in the growing skeleton. The following three micrographs focus, at higher magnification, on particular regions of this field.

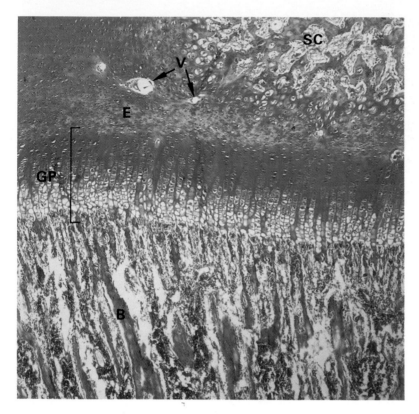

Fig. 10.22 Epiphyseal growth plate

(H & E/Alcian blue × 40)

At higher magnification, the epiphyseal growth plate **GP** shows a progression of morphological changes between the epiphyseal cartilage **E** and the newly forming bone **B** of the diaphysis. Similar, but less organised, morphological changes are seen between the epiphyseal cartilage and the centre of secondary ossification **SC** within the epiphysis although this does not represent a growth plate. Note blood vessels **V**, cut in transverse section, passing into the secondary ossification centre in cartilage canals.

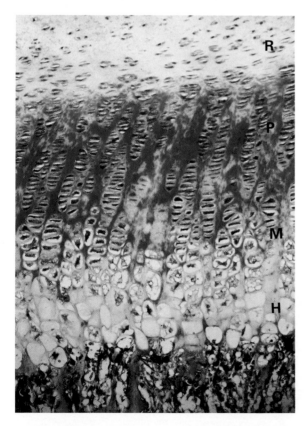

Fig. 10.23 Epiphyseal growth plate

(H & E/Alcian blue × 120)

The dynamic process of endochondral ossification is summarised in this micrograph of the epiphyseal growth plate at high magnification. The transition between epiphyseal cartilage and new bone occurs in six functional and morphological stages:

1. Zone of reserve cartilage R: this consists of typical hyaline cartilage (see Fig. 10.1) with the chondrocytes arranged in small clusters surrounded by a large amount of moderately stained matrix.

2. Zone of proliferation P: the clusters of cartilage cells undergo successive mitotic divisions to form columns of chondrocytes separated by strongly stained, glycoprotein-rich matrix.

3. Zone of maturation M: cell division has ceased and the chondrocytes increase in size.

4. Zone of hypertrophy and calcification H: the chondrocytes become greatly enlarged and vacuolated and the matrix becomes calcified.

5. Zone of cartilage degeneration D: the chondrocytes degenerate and the lacunae of the calcified matrix are invaded by osteogenic cells and capillaries from the marrow cavity of the diaphysis.

6. Osteogenic zone O: the osteogenic cells differentiate into osteoblasts which congregate on the surface of the spicules of calcified cartilage matrix where they commence bone formation. This transitional zone is known as the *metaphysis*.

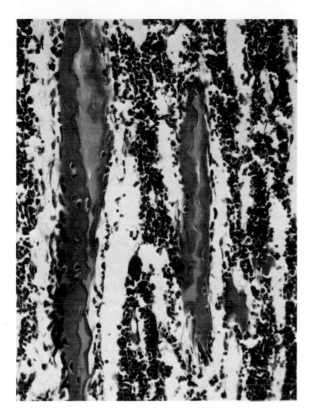

Fig. 10.24 Endochondral ossification: metaphysis
(H & E/Alcian blue × 198)

In the metaphysis seen in this preparation, the blue-stained spicules of calcified cartilage matrix are surrounded by osteoblasts and newly formed woven bone which is stained pink. Further growth of metaphysial woven bone is followed by extensive remodelling to produce mature compact and spongy bone.

At physical maturity the process of endochondral ossification ceases. This stage is recognised by the fusion of the diaphysis with the epiphysis, resulting in the obliteration of the growth plates. From this point onwards no further endochondral ossification is possible. Although endochondral ossification is the means of growth in length of a long bone, growth in diameter of the shaft occurs by appositional growth at the periosteal surface and complementary osteoclastic resorption at the endosteal surface.

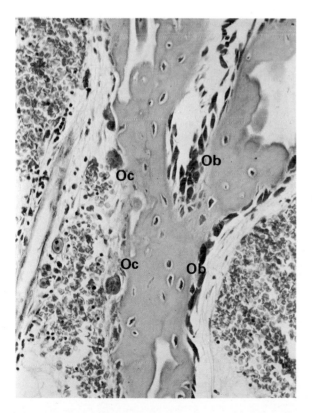

Fig. 10.25 Bone remodelling and repair
(H & E × 480)

This micrograph illustrates an irregular spicule of woven bone from a fetus. Some of the surfaces of the spicule exhibit osteoblastic deposition **Ob** whereas other surfaces are in the process of being resorbed by osteoclasts **Oc**.

Woven bone is not only the first type of bone to be formed during skeletal development but is also the first bone to be laid down during the repair of a fracture. At the fracture site, a blood clot initially forms, later being replaced by highly vascular connective tissue which becomes progressively more dense and infiltrated by cartilage. This firm but still flexible bridge is known as the *provisional callus*. The provisional callus is then strengthened by deposition of calcium salts within the cartilage matrix. Meanwhile, osteoprogenitor cells in the endosteum and periosteum are activated and lay down a meshwork of woven bone within and around the provisional callus; the provisional callus thus becomes transformed into the so-called *bony callus*. *Bony union* is achieved when the fracture site is completely bridged by woven bone. Under the influence of functional stresses, the bony callus is then slowly remodelled to form mature lamellar bone.

Joints

Joints may be classified into two main functional groups both of which have wide morphological variations:

1. Synovial joints: in this type of joint there is extensive movement of bones upon one another at articular surfaces. The articular surfaces are maintained in apposition by a fibrous capsule and ligaments, and the surfaces are lubricated by *synovial fluid*. Synovial joints are known as *diarthroses*. In some diarthroses such as the temporomandibular and knee joints, plates of fibrocartilage may be completely or partially interposed between the articular surfaces but remain unattached to the articular surfaces.

2. Non-synovial joints: these joints have limited movement; the articulating bones have no free articular surfaces but are joined by dense connective tissue which may be of three types:

(a) *Dense fibrous connective tissue:* this forms the sutures between the bones of the skull, and permits moulding of the fetal skull during its passage through the birth canal. The sutures are progressively replaced by bone with advancing age. Such fibrous connective tissue joints are called *syndesmoses*, and when replaced by bone are called *synostoses*.

(b) *Hyaline cartilage:* this type of joint, called a *synchondrosis* or *primary cartilaginous joint*, unites the first rib with the sternum and is the only synchondrosis found in the human adult.

(c) *Fibrocartilage:* the opposing surfaces of some bones are covered by hyaline cartilage but are directly connected to each other by a plate of fibrocartilage. Such fibrocartilaginous joints are called *symphyses* or *secondary cartilaginous joints* and occur in the pubic symphysis and at the intervertebral discs. The fibrocartilage disc of the pubic symphysis develops a hollow central cavity and the intervertebral discs have a fluid-filled central cavity.

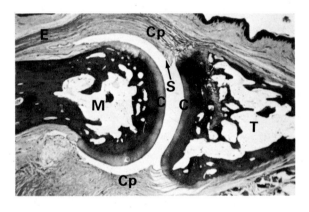

Fig. 10.26 Synovial joint

(Monkey: H & E × 12)

This micrograph illustrates a typical synovial joint, the distal interphalangeal joint of the finger. The articular surfaces of the terminal phalanx **T** and the middle phalanx **M** are covered by hyaline cartilage **C**. The joint cavity is artefactually enlarged. In vivo the articular surfaces are maintained in close contact by a fibrous capsule **Cp** which is inserted into the articulating bones at some distance from the articular cartilages. The *synovium* **S** is a specialised connective tissue layer on the inner aspect of the capsule. Note the extensor tendon **E** which inserts into the terminal phalanx.

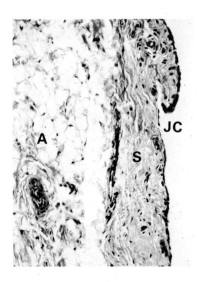

Fig. 10.27 Synovium

(H & E × 128)

The inner surface of the capsule of synovial joints is lined by a specialised connective tissue layer of variable thickness and density called the synovium **S**. The surface of the synovium is thrown up into folds which may extend for some distance into the joint cavity **JC**. The synovial connective tissue contains numerous blood and lymphatic vessels, nerves, and variable numbers of adipocytes **A**.

The free surface of the synovium is lined by a discontinuous layer of cells which are of two morphological types: fibroblast-like cells and macrophage-like cells. These cells are not connected by junctional complexes and do not rest on a basement membrane; the synovial surface, therefore, does not constitute an epithelium.

The synthesis of synovial fluid is poorly understood but it is thought to be formed by a transudate from synovial capillaries into which hyaluronic acid is secreted by the surface cells.

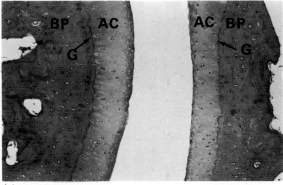

(a)

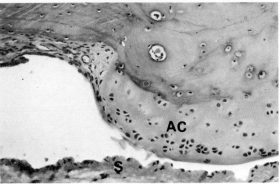

(b)

Fig. 10.28 Articular cartilage

(H & E (a) × 20 (b) × 128)

Micrograph (a) focuses on the opposing articular cartilages **AC** of the synovial joint shown in Fig. 10.26 and micrograph (b) shows the lower rim of the articular cartilage of the middle phalanx of the same specimen.

Each articular cartilage is bonded to its long bone at a region called the *bony end plate* **BP**; this region is composed of an unusual type of bone which lacks Haversian systems and canaliculi and in which osteocytes occupy particularly large lacunae. The articular cartilage is sharply demarcated from the underlying bony end plate by a thick layer of glycoprotein-rich substance **G** which resembles the cement lines of Haversian bone.

Articular cartilage differs from other hyaline cartilage in two respects. Firstly, the articular surface is not covered by perichondrium. Secondly, the collagen fibres of the cartilage matrix exhibit the characteristic cross-banding of the collagen fibres of loose connective tissue and bone whereas the collagen fibres of other hyaline cartilage are not cross-banded (see Ch. 4).

Articular cartilage, like other hyaline cartilage, is avascular; it is nourished by diffusion from the synovial fluid of the joint cavity. In micrograph (b), note part of the synovial layer **S** of the joint capsule.

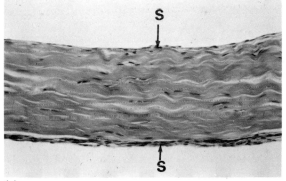

(a)

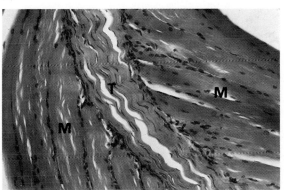

(b)

Fig. 10.29 Tendon

(H & E (a) × 128 (b) × 128)

Tendons are tough inextensible but flexible straps which connect certain muscles to various skeletal structures allowing the muscular forces to be exerted at some distance from the body of the muscle itself and, in some cases, in a different direction.

Tendon is the densest form of fibrous connective tissue, consisting of bundles of coarse collagen fibres among which are scattered rows of fibroblasts with elongated nuclei. Each tendon is composed of small bundles of such dense tissue bound together by a small amount of looser connective tissue which contains the scanty blood supply and tiny nerve fibres from the tendon stretch receptors. The connective tissue of the tendon surface is smooth and condensed with minimal connections with the surrounding tissue so as to allow relatively unimpeded movement of the tendon. In some sites, as shown in micrograph (a), tendons are invested in a connective tissue sheath lined by synovium **S**, movement of the tendon within the sheath being lubricated by synovial fluid.

Micrograph (b) shows the insertion of two masses of skeletal muscle **M** into a common tendon **T**; in this case, the tendon will exert the muscular force in a direction different from the direction of pull of the individual skeletal muscles attached to it.

Ligaments are dense bands of fibrous connective tissue which reinforce joint capsules and maintain bones in the correct anatomical arrangement. Ligaments are histologically similar to tendons but have a less ordered arrangement of the collagen fibres and a variable amount of elastic fibres.

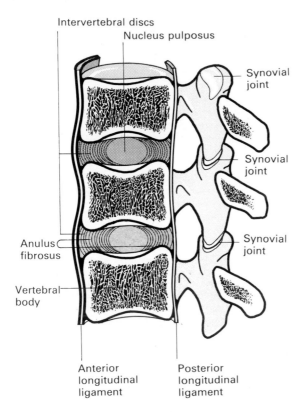

Intervertebral discs

Nucleus pulposus

Synovial joint

Synovial joint

Synovial joint

Anulus fibrosus

Vertebral body

Anterior longitudinal ligament

Posterior longitudinal ligament

Fig. 10.30 The intervertebral joints

The vertebrae articulate by means of two different types of joints:

1. The vertebral bodies are united by symphyseal joints, the *intervertebral discs*, which permit movement between the vertebral bodies whilst maintaining a union of great strength. The fibrocartilage of each intervertebral disc is arranged in concentric rings forming the *anulus fibrosus*. Within the disc, there is a cavity containing a viscous fluid, called the *nucleus pulposus*, which acts as a shock absorber. The anulus fibrosus is reinforced peripherally by circumferential ligaments. A thick ligament extending down the anterior aspect of the spinal column further reinforces the anulus fibrosus and a similar, but thinner, ligament reinforces the posterior aspect.

2. The vertebral arches articulate with each other by pairs of synovial joints. Strong elastic ligaments connecting the bony processes of the vertebral arches contribute to the stability of the spinal column.

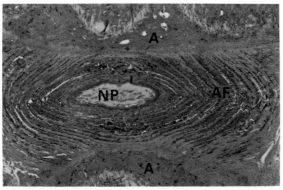

(a)

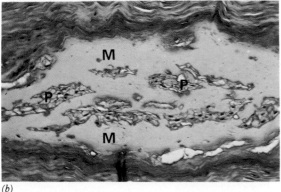

(b)

Fig. 10.31 Intervertebral disc
(Rat: H & E/Alcian blue (a) × 20 (b) × 128)

An intervertebral disc is shown in these micrographs of the tail of an immature rat. The intervertebral disc lies between the articular surfaces **A** of adjacent vertebral bodies. The disc consists of concentric layers of fibrocartilage, constituting the anulus fibrosus **AF**, which surrounds the central nucleus pulposus **NP**. This staining method distinguishes the collagen component of the fibrocartilage, which is stained pink, from the ground substance component, which is stained blue.

At high magnification, the nucleus pulposus is seen to consist of an unusual fluid form of connective tissue; this is the only remnant of the embryonic notochord persisting in adult mammals. The cells of the nucleus pulposus, called *physaliphorous cells* **P**, are scattered in irregular clumps throughout an extracellular matrix **M** which consist of ground substance only.

The intervertebral disc functions in the manner of a hydraulic shock absorber, the nucleus pulposus acting as hydraulic fluid. With advancing age, the fibrocartilage of the anulus fibrosus becomes thinned and weakened and the nucleus pulposus tends to be extruded, particularly at the posterior aspect where the disc is least reinforced by surrounding ligaments. This gives rise to the inappropriately named condition, 'slipped disc'.

11. Immune system

Introduction

All living tissues are subject to the constant threat of invasion by disease-producing organisms or *pathogens* such as bacteria, viruses, fungi and multicellular parasites. Mammals have three main lines of defence against invading pathogens: protective surface phenomena, non-specific cellular responses and specific immune responses.

1. Protective surface phenomena: in man, these provide a first line of defence. The skin constitutes a relatively impenetrable surface to most micro-organisms, unless breached by injury such as abrasion or burning. The sero-mucous surfaces of the body, such as the conjunctiva and oral cavity, are protected by a variety of antibacterial substances including the enzyme lysozyme, secreted in tears and saliva. The respiratory tract is protected by a layer of surface mucus which is continuously disposed of by ciliary action and replaced by goblet cell activity. The maintenance of an acidic environment in the stomach, vagina and to a lesser extent the skin, inhibits the growth of bacteria in these sites. When such defences fail to prevent access of pathogens to the tissues, the two other main types of defence mechanisms are activated.

2. Non-specific cellular responses: many types of pathogenic bacteria are spontaneously destroyed by the phagocytic cells of loose connective tissue after breaching an epithelial surface. Macrophages and neutrophils are the principal cells which carry out this function. Viral infections induce many cell types in the body to secrete an anti-viral substance called *interferon*, which disrupts viral multiplication within cells. Many pathogens evoke a multifactorial tissue response called *acute inflammation*; this process involves local changes in blood flow and attraction of blood-borne phagocytes to the site of pathogenic insult. When both protective surface phenomena and non-specific responses fail to check the invasion of pathogenic organisms, specific responses are activated, collectively known as the *immune response*.

3. Specific immune responses: many pathogens activate immune responses at the time of initial invasion, although these specific responses may not be effective until a later stage, non-specific responses being operative in the interim period. The primary function of the *immune system* is the production of specific responses directed against specific pathogens. Thus, activation of the immune system involves recognition of characteristics peculiar to a particular pathogen; such characteristics, usually specific surface macromolecules, are termed *antigens* since they generate responses directed at their own destruction which at the same time also destroy the pathogenic organism as a whole.

Lymphocytes are the functional units of the immune system; they express their specific activity in two main ways. Firstly, certain types of lymphocyte produce *antibodies* in response to the recognition of a particular antigen. Antibodies bind to antigens to promote destruction of antigen by a variety of mechanisms; the defence mechanism mediated by antibody is called the *humoral immune response*. Secondly, some lymphocytes are stimulated by antigens to produce a response in which circulating antibodies are not formed but in which lymphocytes and macrophages co-operate in the direct destruction of pathogenic organisms. This defence mechanism is called the *cellular immune response*. Although the humoral and cellular immune responses may occur separately, a single pathogen often evokes both responses concurrently.

The cells of the immune system, principally lymphocytes, are disseminated throughout the body either as isolated cells, diffuse aggregations particularly in the gastrointestinal and respiratory tracts, or within the *lymphoid organs*. The principal lymphoid organs are the *thymus*, *lymph nodes* and the *spleen*.

Many of the detailed mechanisms constituting the immune response are still poorly understood despite rapid advances in research; however, most of the histological features of lymphoid tissue can be interpreted in terms of known immunological defence phenomena.

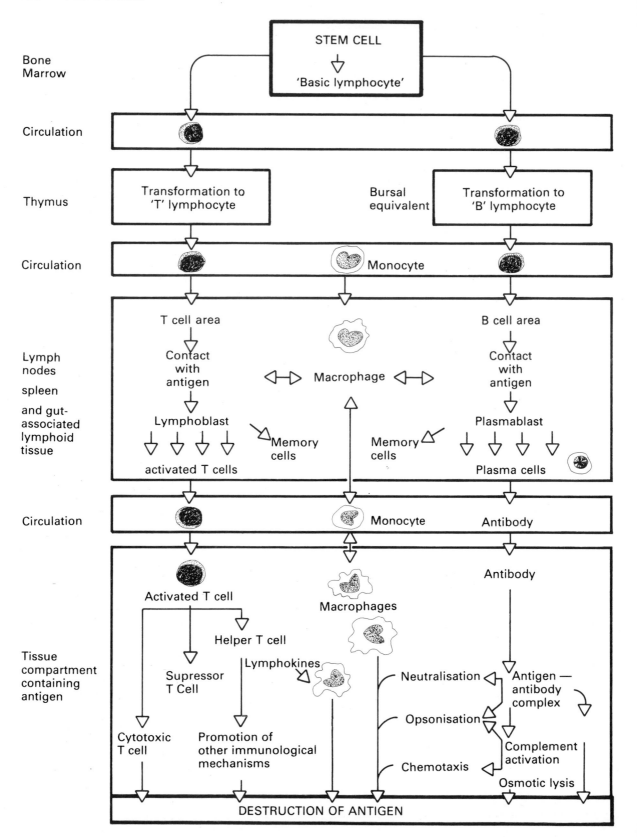

Fig. 11.1 The immune system *(illustration opposite)*

This diagram summarises the principal mechanisms of the immune system. Lymphocytes are a heterogeneous population of cells which can be divided into a number of subpopulations, each with a different role in immunological defence.

Lymphocytes, like all other blood cells, are derived from a common stem cell in bone marrow (see Ch. 3). At some unknown point during development within the bone marrow, each lymphocyte acquires the potential to recognise one specific antigen. These 'basic lymphocytes' are then released from bone marrow into the circulation and undergo either of two main maturation processes which determines the manner in which they will express their activity, that is via the cellular or humoral mechanism.

1. The cellular immune response: basic lymphocytes destined to be involved in this type of response enter the thymus and undergo a series of changes before being released into the circulation; lymphocytes which mature in the thymus are called *thymus dependent* or *T lymphocytes*. From the circulation, T lymphocytes localise in particular lymphoid tissues throughout the body, from which they then circulate continuously via the blood and lymphatic systems. This constant circulation of T lymphocytes has been interpreted as a 'quest for antigens'.

When a specific antigen is encountered in the tissues, the T lymphocytes which are programmed to recognise that particular antigen return to the specific T lymphocyte domains of the lymphoid tissues where they transform into *lymphoblasts*. Lymphoblasts then divide by mitosis to produce activated T lymphocytes which enter the circulation and migrate to the site of antigenic stimulation.

There are at least three subpopulations of activated T lymphocytes employing different means of dealing with antigen:

(a) *Cytotoxic T cells* cause direct destruction of antigen-containing cells by some as yet unknown mechanism; cytotoxic destruction is particularly important in dealing with viruses which are otherwise relatively inaccessible within the host cells.

(b) *Helper T cells* are so named for their ability to promote the activity of other immunologically competent cells including cytotoxic T cells and the cells responsible for the humoral response; indeed helper T cells are essential in initiating most immunological responses, exerting their influence by a variety of highly specific regulatory factors. Helper T cells also produce a variety of relatively non-specific substances, collectively called *lymphokines* or *interleukins*, which enhance the phagocytic effectiveness of local and blood-borne macrophages; mechanisms of *macrophage activation* include enhanced lysosomal activity, attraction of macrophages to antigen, and inhibition of macrophage migration from antigen-exposed sites. Macrophage activation is particularly important in dealing with organisms such as Mycobacterium tuberculosis which is otherwise relatively resistant to phagocytic destruction.

(c) *Suppressor T cells* inhibit the activity of certain immunologically activated cells being responsible for the phenomenon of *immunological tolerance* towards certain antigens.

A small proportion of activated T lymphocytes remain in lymphoid tissues where they act as 'memory cells'; these are capable of mounting a more effective *secondary immune response* on subsequent exposure to that particular antigen.

2. The humoral immune response: in mammals, those basic lymphocytes which will ultimately respond to antigens by producing antibodies, develop immunological competence in some as yet unknown organ. In birds, however, such lymphocytes mature in the *Bursa of Fabricius*, a lymphoid organ associated with the gastrointestinal tract. Thus, these lymphocytes are called *Bursa dependent* or *B lymphocytes*. Several 'bursal equivalents' have been suggested in mammals, including the tonsils, Peyer's patches and appendix, but recent evidence suggests that the bone marrow itself may function as the mammalian bursal equivalent. By convention, the mammalian lymphocytes involved in the humoral response are called B lymphocytes.

Immunocompetent B lymphocytes, each programmed to recognise one particular antigen only, are released into the general circulation from which they seed the lymphoid tissues, mainly lymph nodes and spleen. In contrast to T lymphocytes, it is thought that most B lymphocytes do not continuously recirculate throughout the body but rather make contact with antigens taken up and processed by macrophages. Once activated, a process usually involving helper T cells, B lymphocytes transform into *plasmablasts* which then divide to form antibody-producing cells called *plasma cells*. A proportion of plasma cells is thought to revert to B lymphocytes and remain in lymphoid tissue as 'memory cells'.

The secretion of antibody molecules by plasma cells takes place either within lymphoid tissue or at the site of antigenic stimulation. In the first case, antibodies are carried to the appropriate site by both the lymph and blood vascular systems.

The combination of antibody and antigen produces a complex which induces antigen destruction in four main ways:

(a) Simple neutralisation of soluble antigen: the complex is destroyed by phagocytosis.
(b) Opsonisation: some antigens are made more amenable to phagocytosis by combination with antibody. Antibodies which enhance phagocytosis are called *opsonins* (see also Fig. 4.17).
(c) Complement activation: the combination of antibody and antigen may activate a system of plasma factors comprising the *complement system*. Activation of complement has three main effects. Firstly, some components of complement may act as opsonins; secondly, other components of complement attract neutrophils, thus acting as *chemotaxins*; thirdly, all nine components of complement act together to create holes in the plasma membranes of pathogenic cells resulting in cell death by osmotic lysis.
(d) Killer cells: a population of cells described as *K (killer) cells* have been discovered which have a direct cytotoxic effect on cells coated with antibody. These cells are morphologically similar to lymphocytes but do not appear to be either T or B lymphocytes.

Antigens often initiate co-operative responses of both the cellular and humoral type. Furthermore, the co-operation of non-specific phagocytes is often necessary to produce the final destruction of antigen. Thus the response of lymphoid tissue to any particular antigen often shows histological features of cellular, humoral and non-specific responses.

Thymus

The thymus is a large lymphoid organ located in the anterior aspect of the thoracic cavity and lower part of the neck. The major activity of the thymus takes place during childhood after which it gradually involutes such that, in human adults, the thymus is often difficult to differentiate macroscopically from surrounding connective tissue. During embryological development, the thymus is the first lymphoid organ to appear, being derived from epithelial outgrowths of the third branchial pouches which merge in the midline; subsequently, the primitive thymus becomes infiltrated by lymphocytes derived from haemopoietic tissue elsewhere in the developing embryo.

The principal function of the thymus is the production of immunocompetent T lymphocytes by proliferation and modification of 'basic lymphocytes' produced by bone marrow lymphopoiesis. It has been postulated that the thymus also controls lymphopoiesis and the development of lymph nodes and spleen during infancy by the production of a hormone called *thymosine*.

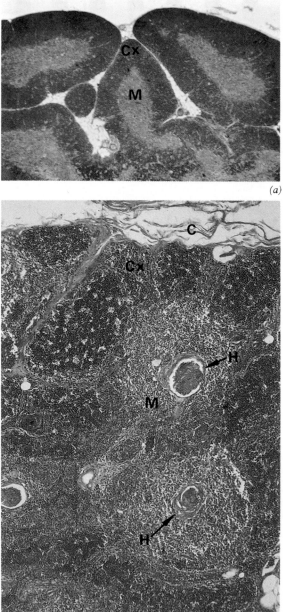

(a)

(b)

Fig. 11.2 Thymus

(H & E (a) Guinea pig × 20 (b) Human × 40)

The thymus is a highly lobulated organ invested by a loose connective tissue capsule from which short septa containing blood vessels radiate into the substance of the organ.

As seen in micrograph (a), the thymic tissue is divided into two distinct zones, a dense outer cortex **Cx** and an inner, pale-stained medulla **M**.

From birth to puberty, the thymus grows approximately three-fold but thereafter, the gland involutes, being progressively replaced by adipose tissue.

Micrograph (b) shows part of a human thymus at higher magnification. The cortex **Cx** is highly cellular whereas the medulla **M** is more loosely packed and contains fewer lymphocytes. Note that the demarcation between cortex and medulla is much less regular in humans than in the guinea pig.

The thymus is unique among the lymphoid organs in being of epithelial origin, the epithelial element forming a sponge-like framework radiating in irregular, interconnected sheets from the medulla into the cortex. The epithelial cells form a continuous sheet beneath the capsule **C** and also ensheath the blood vessels penetrating the thymus from the outer capsule. Between the epithelium and connective tissue elements, i.e. capsule and blood vessels, there is a prominent basement membrane which is thought to limit access of blood products including antigens to the thymus, particularly the cortex, and which has been described as a *blood-thymus barrier*.

The epithelial framework of the medulla is relative coarse and bulky, the interstices being much smaller than those of the cortex and therefore accommodating fewer lymphocytes. The eosinophilia of the epithelial framework, and the relative paucity of lymphocytes, explains the pale pink staining characteristics of the medulla.

The epithelial framework of the cortex is more delicate and finely branched than that of the medulla, the much larger interstices being packed with lymphocytes. The word 'reticular' is often used to describe the sponge-like epithelial framework of the thymus but there is no evidence that the cells are phagocytic or represent part of the so-called reticuloendothelial system (see Ch. 4). At an ultrastructural level, the epithelial cells are found to have typical desmosomes at their points of contact and contain electron-dense granules which are thought to represent an endocrine secretory product, probably the hormone thymosine.

In the centre of the medulla are eosinophilic lamellated structures known as *Hassal's corpuscles* **H** representing degenerate epithelial cells (see Fig. 11.4).

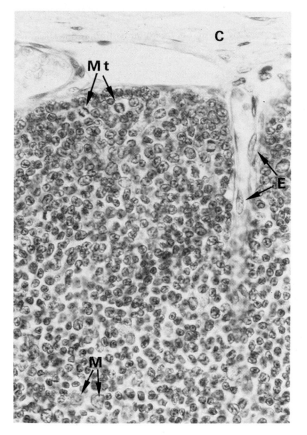

Fig. 11.3 Thymic cortex
(H & E × 480)

The thymic cortex is predominantly populated by lymphocytes and, as seen in this micrograph, those of the outer cortex are larger than those deeper in the cortex. The large lymphocytes of the outer cortex represent lymphoblasts which divide by mitosis to produce large numbers of smaller lymphocytes which are pushed into the deeper layers; several mitotic figures **Mt** can be seen in the outer cortex in this micrograph.

The thymic lymphoblasts are derived from 'basic lymphocytes' produced by bone marrow haemopoiesis. Of the vast number of lymphocytes produced in the thymic cortex, the majority die before ever leaving the cortex, and the remainder leave the thymus via post-capillary venules to enter the circulation as immunocompetent T lymphocytes (*thymocytes*). This extraordinary wastage of thymus-produced lymphocytes is not understood but may be the means by which lymphocytes, programmed to recognise the body's own indigenous constituents, are eliminated, retaining only those programmed to recognise foreign antigens.

The thymic cortex also contains numerous pale-stained, vacuolated macrophages **M** responsible for engulfing dead lymphocytes but which also may be involved in 'processing' antigens before presentation to the lymphocytes.

Note also in this micrograph, a small capillary, lined by flattened endothelial cells **E**, entering the cortex from the capsule **C**. Around the capillary can be seen a distinct basement membrane constituting the blood-thymus barrier. Note that cells of the delicate cortical epithelial framework cannot be readily distinguished, being obscured by the mass of lymphocytes.

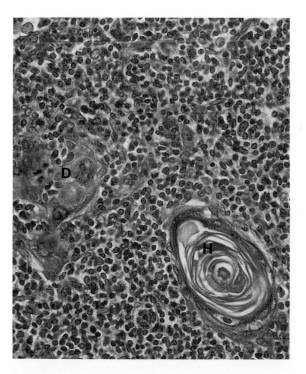

Fig. 11.4 Thymic medulla
(H & E × 480)

In the thymic medulla, cells of the epithelial framework can be more readily identified by their relatively large, pale-stained nuclei, eosoinophilic cytoplasm and prominent basement membranes.

A feature of the thymic medulla are the concentrically lamellated Hassal's corpuscles **H** which first appear in fetal life and increase in number throughout life. Initially, the corpuscles begin as a single medullary epithelial cell which enlarges and then degenerates to form a vacuolated eosinophilic (pink-stained) mass. Further epithelial cells become similarly involved to form a lamellated hyaline mass surrounded by flattened degenerating epithelial cells as seen in this example. Nearby is a small mass of large atypical degenerate epithelial cells **D** which may represent an early Hassal's corpuscle.

Some authorities maintain that macrophages, laden with debris from degenerate cortical lymphocytes, become incorporated in the Hassal's corpuscles.

Lymph nodes

Lymphocytes are distributed throughout the body where they are arranged in aggregations which exhibit various degrees of structural organisation. Isolated lymphocytes are found in most loose connective tissues and amongst epithelial cells, particularly the epithelium of the gastrointestinal and respiratory tracts; in addition, large diffuse aggregations of lymphocytes are found in the walls of these tracts. The vast majority of lymphocytes are, however, located in encapsulated, highly organised structures called lymph nodes, which are interposed along the larger regional vessels of the lymph vascular system. Lymph nodes tend to occur in groups, particularly in areas where the lymphatics converge to form larger trunks as in the axilla, groin and hilum of the lung.

Three principal, interrelated functions occur within lymph nodes:

1. Non-specific 'filtration' of particulate matter and bacteria from lymph by the phagocytic activity of macrophages;
2. Storage and proliferation of B lymphocytes and antibody production;
3. Storage and proliferation of T lymphocytes.

T and B lymphocytes occupy different areas within lymph nodes; each undergoes characteristic histological changes when stimulated by the presence of appropriate antigens. Even in the absence of overt disease, individuals are exposed to a wide range of antigenic stimulation from both within and without, thus the histological appearance of a lymph node at any particular time will reflect not only the response to local antigenic stimulation but also the immunological status of the individual as a whole.

Fig. 11. 5 Lymph node *(illustrations opposite)*

(a) Structure and vascular organisation (b) H & E × 8

Lymph nodes are small kidney-shaped organs situated in the course of the regional lymphatic vessels such that lymph draining back to the bloodstream passes through one or more lymph nodes.

The lymph node is encapsulated by dense connective tissue from which *trabeculae* extend for variable distances into the substance of the node. *Afferent lymphatic vessels* divide into several branches outside the lymph node, then pierce the capsule to drain into a narrow space called the subcapsular sinus. Lymph from the subcapsular sinus drains via a series of interconnected channels, *the medullary sinuses*, into the hilum of the node from which arises one or more *efferent lymphatic vessels*.

The body of the lymph node consists of an open meshwork of fine reticular fibres which provides a loose support for the ever changing populations of lymphocytes. The *cortex* consists of densely-packed lymphocytes and forms extensions called *medullary cords* which project into the medulla between the medullary sinuses.

Within the cortex, lymphocytes form into a variable number of densely packed *lymphoid follicles*, many of which

show less dense *germinal centres*.

The blood supply of the lymph node is derived from arteries which enter at the hilum and branch in the medulla, giving rise to extensive capillary networks in the cortex and medullary cords. Lymphocytes enter lymph nodes mainly via the arterial system, gaining access by migrating across the walls of post-capillary venules, which have an unusual structure well adapted for this purpose (see Fig. 11.10).

The micrograph illustrates the main geographical features of a lymph node; note that the plane of section passes through the hilum **H**.

Several trabeculae **T** extend from the capsule **C** into the substance of the node. The densely packed cellular mass of the cortex **Cx** contains several lymphoid follicles **F**, many of which have pale-stained germinal centres. Note that these follicles are located in the outer part of the cortex. The irregular medullary cords **MC** are continuous with the cortical cell mass. The narrow subcapsular sinus becomes continuous with the broad interconnected medullary sinuses. Blood vessels are seen in trabeculae within the medulla.

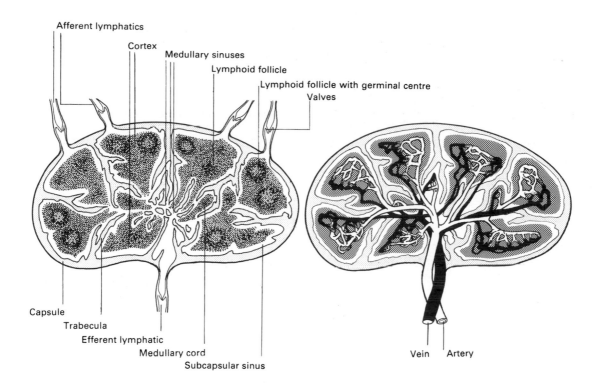

Afferent lymphatics
Cortex
Medullary sinuses
Lymphoid follicle
Lymphoid follicle with germinal centre
Valves

Capsule
Trabecula
Efferent lymphatic
Medullary cord
Subcapsular sinus

Vein   Artery

(a)

(b)

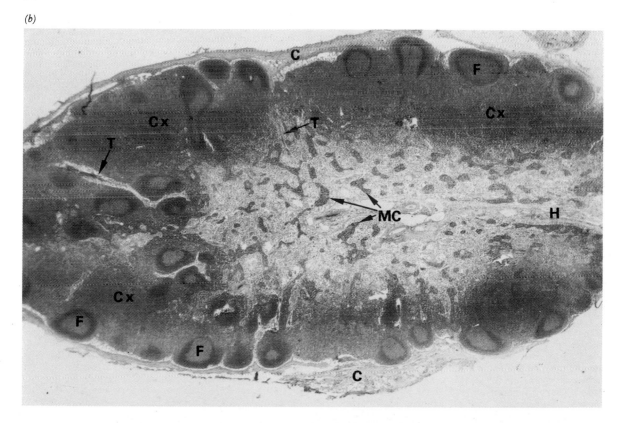

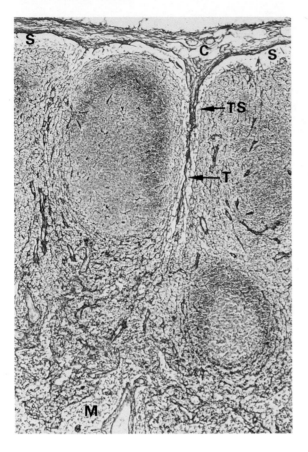

Fig. 11.6 Lymph node

(Reticulin method × 30)

This technique shows the fine reticular architecture of the lymph node; reticulin fibres are stained black and lymphocyte nuclei appear brown.

The main structural support for the lymph node is derived from the collagenous capsule **C** and trabecular extensions **T** into the body of the node. From these, a fine meshwork of reticulin fibres extends throughout the node providing a loose, supporting framework for the huge mass of lymphocytes within the cortex and medullary cords. The reticular network is particularly dense in the cortex except for the follicular areas where it is relatively sparse. The subcapsular sinus **S**, trabecular sinus **TS** and medullary sinuses **M** are also kept patent by this fine skeleton of reticulin fibres. All the lymph channels of the node are continuous, allowing afferent lymph to flow throughout the node; this arrangement reduces the rate of lymph flow and increases the contact of afferent lymph with the macrophages of the node.

The reticulin framework and collagen of the capsule and trabeculae are laid down by fibroblasts as in other connective tissues and a few fibroblast-like cells are found on the reticulin network. The spaces of the reticular network are lined by a discontinuous layer of endothelial cells continuous with those lining the afferent and efferent lymphatics. In addition, numerous macrophages are draped over the whole reticular meshwork, their long dendritic cytoplasmic processes providing a large surface area for the clearance of particles, organisms and soluble antigens from the afferent lymph.

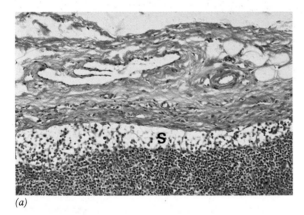

(a)

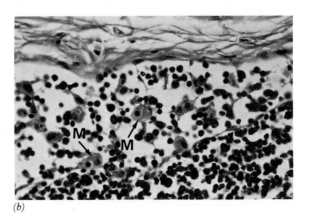

(b)

Fig. 11.7 Capsule and subcapsular sinus

(H & E (a) × 128 (b) × 320)

The fibrous capsule of the lymph node is pierced by branches of afferent lymphatic vessels, one such vessel seen in micrograph (a), containing a valve. Beneath the capsule, is the subcapsular sinus **S** which becomes continuous with trabecular sinuses which pass on either side of the trabeculae towards the medulla. The lymph node sinuses are traversed by fine reticular strands which, as seen in micrograph (b), provide support for large eosinophilic macrophages **M**. These macrophages, and those on the rest of the reticulin

skeleton of the node, engulf particles, soluble antigens and other debris from afferent lymph. In addition, macrophages are thought to be necessary for processing of many antigens before contact with the lymphocytes of the cortex. Antigens may also be sampled in peripheral tissues by macrophages and returned to regional lymph nodes via afferent lymph where activation of appropriate immune responses follows. Cortical lymphocytes may also sample antigen directly as it percolates through the node.

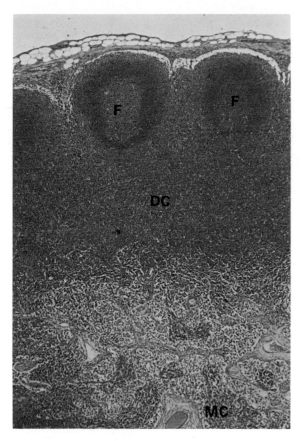

Fig. 11.8 Lymph node cortex
(H & E × 30)

Lymphocytes constitute the vast majority of the cells of the lymph node cortex within which T and B lymphocytes each have their own particular domains.

The lymphocytes of the outer cortex are mainly arranged in spheroidal lymphoid follicles F and these are the major sites in which B lymphocytes localise and proliferate. Traditionally, lymphoid follicles have been classified as 'primary follicles' if a central pale area is absent and 'secondary follicles' if such an area is present; however, the exact relationship between 'primary' and 'secondary' follicles is unclear. The pale central areas are known to be the site of B lymphocyte proliferation and are termed germinal centres and the 'primary' follicles probably merely represent quiescent 'secondary' follicles.

The deep cortical zone DC, or *paracortex*, consists mainly of T lymphocytes which are never arranged as follicles; discrete B lymphocyte follicles may however be seen in the deep cortical zone, particularly within immunologically active lymph nodes. The medullary cords MC mainly contain B lymphocytes and their derivatives.

The number of cortical lymphoid follicles and the depth of the paracortex vary greatly according to the immunological state of the particular lymph node and the individual as a whole. A purely cellular immunological response is associated with paracortical thickening whereas a humoral response is evidenced by the appearance of many cortical follicles with pale germinal centres.

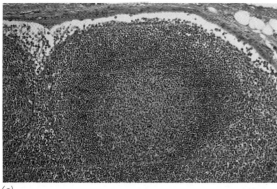

(a)

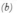

(b)

Fig. 11.9 Lymphoid follicle and germinal centre
(H & E (a) × 64 (b) × 480)

Lymphoid follicles are the principal sites of storage and proliferation of B lymphocytes including both memory cells and cells which have had no previous contact with the antigen which they were programmed to recognise; both types of B lymphocyte proliferate within germinal centres when stimulated by the appropriate antigen B lymphocytes transform into large cells called *plasmablasts* which then undergo mitosis to produce plasma cell precursors called *proplasmacytes*. Proplasmacytes pass to the follicle periphery and thence into the medullary cords where they mature into plasma cells and secrete antibodies into the efferent lymph. At some unknown stage during the process of B lymphocyte

activation, an expanded population of memory cells is formed which is capable of mounting a more rapid and intense humoral response on subsequent contact with the same antigen.

Micrograph (b) focuses on the cells of a germinal centre; these cells are a mixed population of B lymphocytes and the plasma cell precursors, plasmablasts and proplasmacytes. The latter cells have a more extensive cytoplasm than the surrounding lymphocytes; this results in a lower density of nuclei which accounts for the paler staining characteristics of germinal centres when viewed at lower magnification. Note several plasma cell precursors undergoing mitosis M.

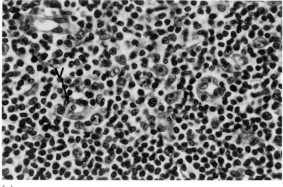

(a)

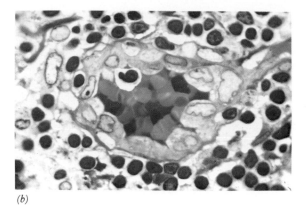

(b)

Fig. 11.10 Paracortical zone

(a) H & E × 320 (b) Thin section, toluidine blue × 800

T lymphocytes are the main cell type in the deep cortical area, also called the paracortex or paracortical zone.

Circulating T lymphocytes enter the lymph node in arterial blood then migrate through the walls of post-capillary venules **V** into the paracortical zone; to rejoin the circulation later, they pass out of the lymph node in efferent lymph.

When a cell-mediated immune response is stimulated, T lymphocytes in the paracortex transform into large cells called *lymphoblasts* which divide by mitosis to produce activated T lymphocytes. In contrast to plasma cells, T lymphocytes must migrate to the site of antigenic stimulation in order to exert their locally destructive effects. When an intense cellular response is evoked within a lymph node, the paracortex expands greatly, often obliterating the entire medulla; this process is called the *paracortical reaction*.

Post-capillary venules of the paracortex have an unusual structure which facilitates the passage of T lymphocytes from the blood circulation into the lymph node. As seen in micrograph (b) the endothelial lining is tall cuboidal rather than the usual squamous arrangement; this may allow lymphocytes to pass through the wall, between the endothelial cells, without causing leakage of blood into the lymph node. There is evidence that the endothelial cells have surface properties which enable T lymphocytes to recognise post-capillary venules as sites of exit into lymph nodes. Note in this micrograph, three lymphocytes in various stages of progress through the wall of the post-capillary venule.

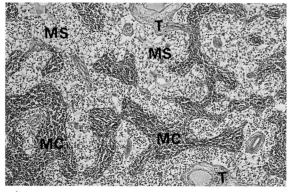

(a)

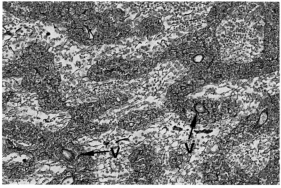

(b)

Fig. 11.11 Medullary cords and sinuses

(a) H & E × 20 (b) Reticulin method/neutral red × 20

Micrograph (a) illustrates the structure of the lymph node medulla with branching medullary cords **MC** separated by irregular medullary sinuses **MS**. Throughout the medulla are trabeculae **T** extending from the connective tissue of the capsule and hilum and conveying afferent and efferent blood vessels.

The medullary cords largely contain B lymphocytes, proplasmacytes and plasma cells although a few macrophages and T lymphocytes may also be present. As in the cortex, the cells of the medullary cords are supported on a reticulin framework as seen in micrograph (b), the black-staining reticulin being condensed around trabecular blood vessels **V**. As in the subcapsular and trabecular sinuses, fine reticular strands traverse the medullary sinuses providing support for macrophages, B lymphocytes and plasma cells.

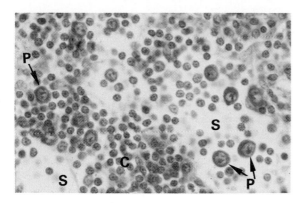

Fig. 11.12 Medullary cords and sinuses
(Methyl green/Pyronin × 480)

This preparation, taken from a lymph node undergoing an intense humoral response, has been stained by a technique to demonstrate plasma cells. The plasma cells **P** appear as large cells with an extensive, red-stained cytoplasm and a pale-stained nucleus with a prominent nucleolus. The red dye pyronin has a strong affinity for ribosomal RNA and hence stains the plasma cell cytoplasm strongly since it is packed with ribosomes involved in antibody synthesis. Note the presence of numerous plasma cells in both the medullary cords **C** and sinuses **S**.

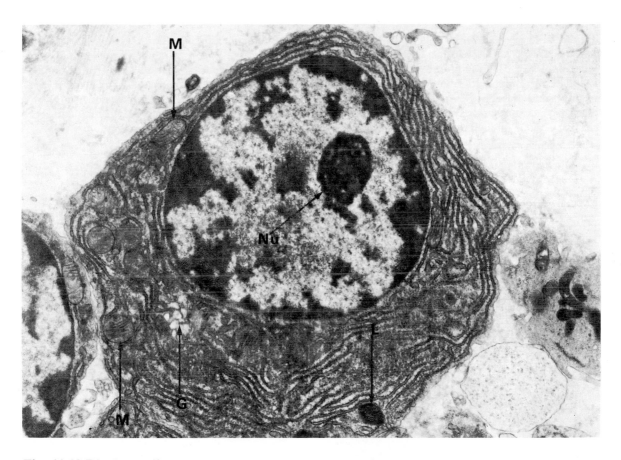

Fig. 11.13 Plasma cell
(EM × 13 860)

The mature plasma cell is a large, amoeboid cell with an eccentrically placed spherical or oval nucleus. Reflecting its intense activity in protein (antibody) synthesis, the nucleus contains much dispersed chromatin; the remaining heterochromatin tends to be distributed around the nuclear envelope. A large nucleolus **Nu** is a highly characteristic feature. The cytoplasm is packed with lamellae of rough endoplasmic reticulum which, during periods of active protein synthesis, become dilated and filled with amorphous

material. The Golgi apparatus **G** is usually well developed. Paradoxically, antibodies do not appear to be secreted by exocytosis of Golgi-derived vesicles; the mode of antibody secretion is not known.

The cytoplasm also contains a few rounded mitochondria **M** and occasional lysosomes **L**. The plasma membrane is usually regular in outline and exhibits few microvilli or pseudopodia.

Gut-associated lymphoid tissue

Lymphoid tissue is distributed throughout the gastrointestinal tract either as a diffuse lymphocytic infiltrate, especially in the lamina propria (see Fig. 11.15), or as large discrete though non-encapsulated aggregations such as in the tonsils (see Fig. 11.14), intestinal Peyer's patches (see Fig. 14.17) and the appendix (see Fig. 14.30) where they may form follicles with germinal centres similar to those of lymph nodes. Smaller follicular aggregations and diffuse lymphocytic infiltrates are also seen in the tracheo-bronchial tree (see Fig. 12.9).

The total mass of lymphoid tissue in the gastrointestinal and respiratory tracts is enormous but until recently its function was unknown and largely discounted. Recent studies have shown that these lymphoid tissues function in a manner analogous to lymph nodes, sampling antigenic material entering the tracts and mounting both cell-mediated and humoral immune responses where appropriate. In particular, the humoral response involves the production of antibodies of the IgA class which are secreted into the lumen where antigens can be dealt with before entering the tissues. Consequently, this mass of lymphoid tissue is now considered to be a lymphoid organ in its own right and is collectively known as *gut-associated lymphoid tissue (GALT)*.

The epithelium overlying all GALT aggregations is specialised for the sampling of luminal contents for antigen and acts as the equivalent of the afferent lymphatics of the lymph node. The lymphatics associated with GALT are all efferent, passing to regional, e.g. tonsillar and mesenteric lymph nodes, along with the lymphatics of the surrounding gut.

GALT is formed during fetal life but germinal centres do not develop until after exposure to antigen at birth. The amount of GALT is maximal during childhood undergoing progressive atrophy in adulthood.

The whole GALT organ probably acts as an integrated unit. When antigen is encountered, it is carried to local GALT tissue or regional lymph nodes where it evokes the relevant immunological response. Lymphocytes, antibodies and probably even plasma cells, then pass via the general circulation to the gastrointestinal and respiratory mucosae where lymphocytes and plasma cells await antigenic challenge. IgA is secreted either by diffusing directly through the lining epithelium or in specific secretions such as saliva, tears, and in the milk during lactation.

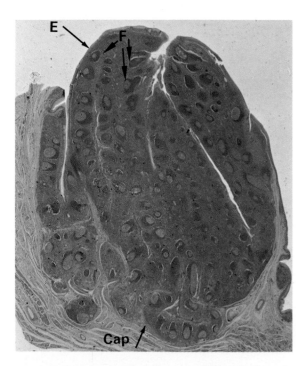

Fig. 11.14 Palatine tonsil

(H & E × 6)

The palatine tonsils are large masses of lymphoid tissue lying in the fossae created by the palatoglossal and palatopharyngeal muscles on either side of the oropharynx.

The luminal surface is covered by stratified squamous epithelium **E** which deeply invaginates the tonsil, forming blind-ended crypts. Note that the tonsil is separated at its base from underlying muscle by a dense hemi-capsule **Cap**. The crypts are lined by lymphoid tissue containing lymphoid follicles **F** with germinal centres similar to those found in lymph nodes. Lymphocytes, macrophages and plasma cells pass towards the crypt lumen through narrow passages between the epithelial lining cells presumably in the process of antigen sampling. Tracer studies have demonstrated that particulate matter entering the crypts from the oropharynx is passed to the follicles, a process that appears to involve phagocytosis by the epithelial cells of the crypt lining. Likewise, bacteria applied to the tonsils of germ-free animals have been shown to enter the follicle in a similar manner inducing the formation of germinal centres.

Antigen uptake occurs in a similar manner in the lingual tonsils and adenoids, the latter being covered with respiratory type epithelium rather than stratified squamous epithelium.

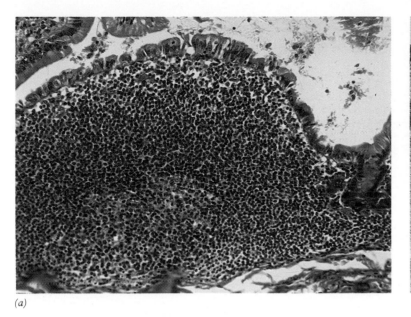

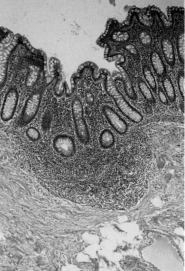

(a)   (b)

Fig. 11.15 Intestinal lymphoid aggregations
(H & E (a) Peyer's patch × 150 (b) Patch in colonic mucosa × 64)

Micrograph (a) illustrates a small ileal Peyer's patch with early germinal centre formation. Peyer's patches are largely confined to the lamina propria, bulging into the intestinal lumen but deeper tissues may become involved when hypertrophy occurs. The normal villous mucosal form is replaced by a single layer of columnar enterocytes similar to those of the surrounding villi; goblet cells are almost completely absent.

Ultra-structural studies have shown the presence within the covering epithelium of scattered cells specialised for the uptake of antigen. These cells, which are too thin to be seen with the light microscope, have a surface irregular with small folds, villi and pits, and contain numerous phagocytic vesicles which transport particles from the lumen to the underlying lymphoid cells.

Similar antigen transporting cells are present in the appendix and in the epithelium overlying lymphoid patches of the large intestine as shown in micrograph (b).

Spleen

The spleen is a large lymphoid organ situated in the left upper part of the abdomen; it receives a rich blood supply via a single artery, the *splenic artery*, and is drained by the *splenic vein* into the hepatic portal system.

In humans, the spleen has three main functions:

1. Removal of debris and other particulate matter from circulating blood;
2. Production of immunological responses against blood-borne antigens;
3. Removal of aged or defective blood cells, particularly erythrocytes, from the circulation.

In dogs and horses, the spleen also acts as a reservoir of blood which can be mobilised by contraction of the organ. In the human fetus, the spleen is an important site of haemopoiesis and this function may be resumed in adulthood in certain disease states.

Despite its large size and important functions, removal of the spleen appears to have few deleterious effects on the body as a whole and its functions are assumed to be taken over by the liver and bone marrow.

The manner in which the spleen performs its function, and many ultra-structural details, are still widely disputed; in many respects, however, the spleen may be considered analogous to a lymph node in which the lymphatic circulation is replaced by a blood circulation. The structure of the spleen provides for intimate contacts to be made between blood and immunologically active cells, just as the structure of lymph nodes facilitates the interaction of afferent lymph and lymphoid cells. Although it is well established that the spleen is involved in removal of aged or defective blood cells from the circulation, it is still not clear whether this is a purely mechanical process or whether immunological recognition plays an important role.

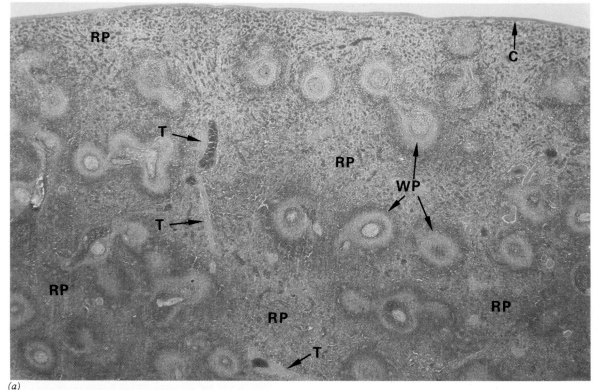

(a)

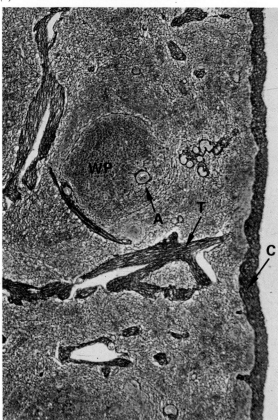

(b)

Fig. 11.16 Spleen

(a) H & E × 12 (b) Reticulin method/Neutral red × 42

On macroscopic examination of the cut surface, the spleen appears to consist of discrete white nodules, the so-called *white pulp*, embedded in a red matrix called the *red pulp*. Microscopically, as seen in micrograph (a), the white pulp **WP** is seen to consist of lymphoid aggregations and the red pulp **RP** making up the bulk of the organ, to be a highly vascular tissue.

Like lymph nodes, the spleen has a dense, fibro-elastic outer capsule **C** which is thickened at the hilum and gives rise to supporting connective tissue trabeculae **T** which conduct larger blood vessels throughout the spleen. In some mammals, the capsule and trabeculae contain smooth muscle which exerts a rhythmic pumping action, clearing the spleen of blood and allowing the spleen to act as a reservoir. In humans only a few smooth muscle cells persist.

The splenic artery divides into several major branches which enter the splenic hilum and pass into the spleen in the trabeculae. These trabecular arteries then give off arterioles which pass into the substance of the spleen where they become surrounded by sheaths of lymphoid tissue, the *peri-arteriolar lymphoid sheaths (PALS)*, which correspond to the white pulp 'nodules' seen in section.

The staining technique employed in micrograph (b) demonstrates the reticular architecture of the spleen. The capsule **C** and the trabeculae **T** provide a robust framework which supports a fine reticulin meshwork ramifying throughout the organ in the red pulp. The reticular skeleton is almost absent in the centre of the white pulp **WP** but is well developed at the white pulp margins and around the central arteriole **A**.

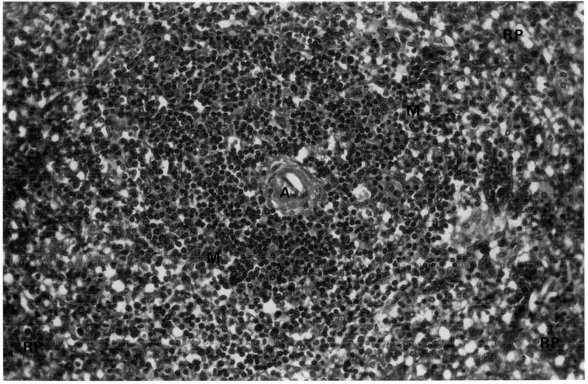

(a)

Fig. 11.17 Peri-arteriolar lymphoid sheaths

(H & E (a) × 160 (b) × 120)

The peri-arteriolar lymphoid sheaths bear a superficial resemblance to the follicles of lymph nodes when seen in transverse section; however, they are readily distinguished by the presence of the central arteriole.

The white pulp or peri-arteriolar lymphoid sheaths contain populations of both T and B lymphocytes, the central region containing predominantly B lymphocytes, which may form germinal centres if a humoral response is stimulated in the spleen by blood-borne antigen. The outer marginal zone consists mainly of closely packed T lymphocytes.

Micrograph (a) shows a classical peri-arteriolar lymphoid sheath with the arteriole **A** located centrally. In this situation there is no distinction between the central B lymphocyte area and the T lymphocyte containing *marginal zone* **M**. Note the highly vascular structure of the surrounding red pulp **RP**.

Micrograph (b) shows a more typical peri-arteriolar lymphoid sheath with a germinal centre **C** in which case the arteriole **A** is displaced into the marginal zone **M**. As in lymph nodes, germinal centre formation in the spleen is indicative of a humoral immune response with B lymphocyte proliferation and transformation into plasma cells.

The central arteriole gives off small side-branches which pass at right angles to supply a capillary network in the marginal zone. Thus the marginal zone, populated by T lymphocytes, is the first point of contact in the spleen between blood and immunologically active cells. This may well reflect the role of T lymphocytes in regulating immunological activity as helper or suppressor cells.

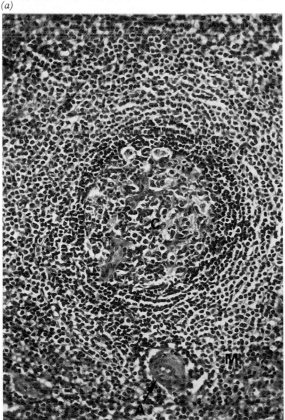

(b)

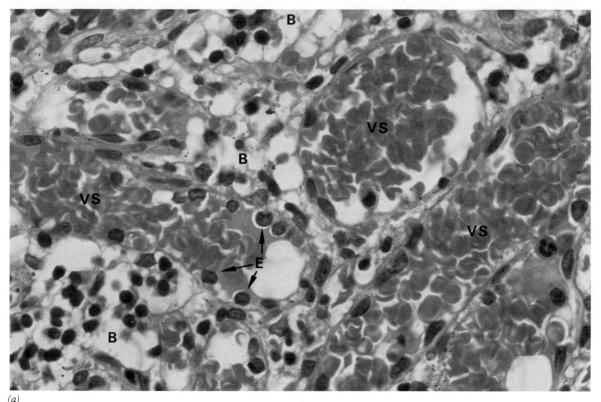

(a)

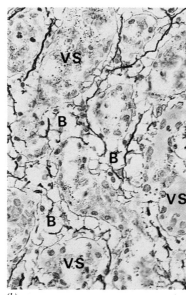

(b)

Fig. 11.18 Red pulp

(a) H & E × 800 (b) Reticulin method/Neutral red × 400

As seen in micrograph (a), the red pulp consists of irregular anastomosing plates, the *cords of Bilroth* **B**, separated by broad interconnected venous sinuses **VS**.

The pulp cords are supported by a delicate reticulin skeleton which supports a large population of highly phagocytic macrophages and the fibroblasts responsible for reticulin formation. The spaces between this meshwork in the pulp cords contain variable numbers of both erythrocytes and leucocytes, mainly lymphocytes. The phagocytic cells of the cords are known to effect the final destruction of aged or damaged blood cells; the mechanics of this process is, however, the subject of much controversy.

Reticulin is demonstrated specifically in micrograph (b) as strands which are stained black. All nuclei are counter-stained red and the plump nuclei of the sinusoid lining cells are particularly well demonstrated. Note that the sinusoid lumina appear almost empty in this preparation since they are occupied by erythrocytes (anucleate).

The venous sinuses are lined by unusual, highly elongated, spindle-shaped endothelial cells which lie parallel to the long axes of the sinuses. The venous sinuses have thus been likened to tall wooden barrels with both ends open, the epithelial cells being represented by the wooden staves and hence being described as *stave cells*. In micrograph (a), note the nuclei of endothelial stave cells **E** bulging into the sinus lumens. The stave cells are known to be moderately phagocytic and to contain numerous pinocytotic vesicles but the significance of these findings is not understood. Externally, the sinuses are encircled by reticulin fibres lying in the endothelial basement membrane in a manner reminiscent of the steel bands holding together a wooden barrel.

Spaces or pores occur between the endothelial cells, the endothelial basement membrane being discontinuous over the spaces or pores. Blood cells, particularly erythrocytes, are able to squeeze between the stave cells allowing passage to and from the pulp cords and venous sinuses.

The venous sinuses drain into progressively larger vessels, the trabecular veins, which converge to form the splenic vein which passes out of the spleen at the hilum.

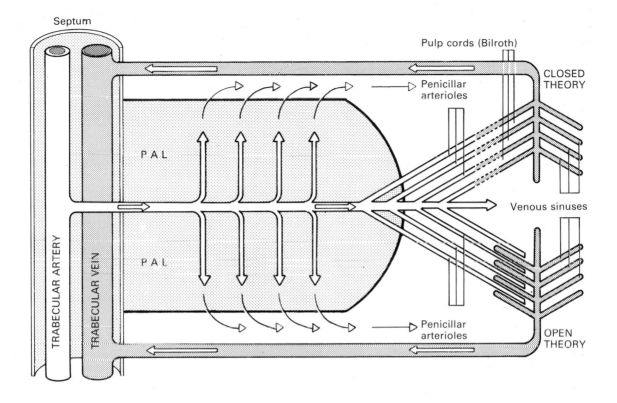

Fig. 11.19 Theories of the splenic circulation

Two main theories have been advanced to explain the passage of blood from the arterioles and marginal zones of peri-arteriolar lymphoid sheaths to the venous sinuses of the red pulp. As previously described, the main branches of the splenic arteries pass in the trabeculae, giving off arterioles which pass into the red pulp invested by peri-arteriolar lymphoid sheaths. After losing their sheaths, these arterioles appear to branch forming small straight arterioles known as *penicillar arterioles*. The fine side branches supplying the marginal zone capillaries of the peri-arteriolar lymphoid sheaths may also terminate in a similar fashion. At the origin of these vessels, the lumen is constricted by a thickening of the wall due to an aggregation of macrophages; these structures are known as *elipsoids*.

1. The *closed circulation theory* proposes that blood passes directly from the penicillar arterioles and marginal zone capillaries into the venous sinuses of the red pulp (i.e. the vascular system is continuous or closed). Blood then passes into the pulp cords where effete blood cells are destroyed by phagocytosis with normal blood cells being able to return to the circulation. The pores between endothelial stave cells of the venous sinuses would provide a route for passage in and out of the cords of Bilroth.

2. The *open circulation theory* proposes that blood passes from penicillar arterioles and marginal zone capillaries directly into the cords of Bilroth. Normal cells are then able to squeeze between the stave cells of the venous sinuses leaving effete cells in the pulp cords to be engulfed by macrophages.

Present evidence partly supports both theories and it seems likely that both circulatory routes co-exist; most of the splenic blood flow probably passes through the closed system since this is the path of least resistance, only a small proportion passing through the open circulation. It has been estimated that if only 3% of the splenic blood flow is diverted through the open circulation then the entire blood volume of the body would pass through the pulp cords at least once each day.

Whichever route is taken to gain entry into the pulp cords, the presence of a reticulin skeleton and the partial barrier of the venous sinus wall ensures a sluggish flow of blood within the cords. A slow rate of flow is likely to enhance the efficiency of phagocytosis by increasing the duration of contact between the macrophages of the cords and effete blood cells.

In order to pass through the pores in the walls of the venous sinuses, blood cells must be capable of considerable deformation. There is evidence that, with increasing age, erythrocytes become less deformable and are therefore more likely to be retained and engulfed by the phagocytes of the pulp cords. A second theory to explain the destruction of effete blood cells in the spleen proposes that effete cells assume antigenic characteristics which are recognised by the immune system. Such cells are then opsonised (see Fig. 11.1) in the general circulation, and actively destroyed by the macrophages of the pulp cords. Both mechanisms may contribute to the destruction of aged or damaged cells in the spleen.

Not shown in this diagram are the splenic lymphatics, a purely efferent drainage system, which pass with the blood vessels in the trabeculae and provide an important route for the emigration of leucocytes from the spleen into the general circulation.

12. Respiratory system

Introduction

Respiration is a term used to describe two different but interrelated processes: cellular respiration and mechanical respiration. Cellular respiration is the process in which cells derive energy by degradation of organic molecules (see Ch. I). Mechanical respiration is the process by which oxygen required for cellular respiration is absorbed from the atmosphere into the blood vascular system and the process by which carbon dioxide is excreted into the atmosphere. Mechanical respiration occurs within the respiratory system.

The respiratory system has two functional components: a conducting system for transport of inspired and expired gases between the atmosphere and the circulatory system, and an interface for passive exchange of gases between the atmosphere and blood. The conducting system begins essentially as a single tube which divides repeatedly to form airways of ever decreasing diameter. The terminal branches of the conducting system open into blind-ended sacs called *alveoli*, which are the sites of gaseous exchange. The alveoli, which constitute the bulk of the lung tissue, are thin-walled structures enveloped by a rich network of capillaries, the *pulmonary capillaries*. This arrangement provides a vast interface of minimal thickness for gaseous exchange between the atmosphere and blood. The continuous process of gaseous diffusion requires appropriate gaseous pressure gradients to be maintained across the alveolar wall. This is achieved by rapid and continuous perfusion of the pulmonary·capillaries by venous blood and regular replacement of alveolar gases by the process of breathing.

The respiratory system is divided anatomically into two parts, the *upper* and *lower respiratory tracts*, which are separated by the *pharynx*. The pharynx is best considered functionally and histologically as part of the gastrointestinal tract despite its important role as an airway.

1. Upper respiratory tract: the upper respiratory tract comprises a system of interconnected cavities, the *nose, paranasal sinuses* and the *nasopharynx,* and is principally involved in filtering, humidifying and adjusting the temperature of inspired air. In addition, the nose contains receptors for the sense of smell and the paranasal sinuses act as resonance chambers for speech, as well as reducing the bony mass of the facial skeleton. The nasopharynx is connected via the *auditory (Eustachian) tubes* to the middle ear cavities, an arrangement which permits equilibration of air pressure in the middle ear with that of the external environment.

The upper respiratory tract is lined by respiratory epithelium (see Figs. 5.10 and 5.11) which is supported by a connective tissue layer called the *lamina propria* containing numerous glands. Collectively, the epithelium and lamina propria are known as *respiratory mucous membrane* or *respiratory mucosa*. The terms *mucous membrane* and *mucosa* also have a common general use in describing the moist linings of other tracts such as the gastrointestinal tract and always refer to both the epithelium and its supporting lamina propria. A further connective tissue layer called the *submucosa* usually connects the mucosa to underlying structures.

2. Lower respiratory tract: the lower respiratory tract begins at the *larynx* then continues into the thorax as the *trachea* before dividing into numerous orders of smaller airways to reach the alveoli; there are about twenty orders of branches in man. The vocal cords of the larynx protect the lower respiratory tract against the entry of foreign bodies, in addition to performing a vital function in speech. The vocal cords are the only part of the lower respiratory tract which is not lined by respiratory epithelium; they are lined by stratified squamous epithelium which is better adapted to withstand frictional stress. The trachea first divides into left and right *primary* or *main bronchi* which supply the lungs. Each primary bronchus gives rise to *secondary bronchi* supplying the lobes of the lungs before dividing again to form *tertiary bronchi* which supply the segments of each lobe. The tertiary bronchi then ramify into numerous orders of progressively smaller airways called *bronchioles*, the smallest of which are called *terminal bronchioles* and mark the end of the purely conducting portion of the tract. The terminal bronchioles branch further into a series of transitional airways, the *respiratory bronchioles* and *alveolar ducts*, which become increasingly involved in gaseous exchange. These passages finally terminate in dilated spaces called *alveolar sacs* which open into the alveoli.

Each type of airway has its own characteristic structural features but there is a gradual, rather than abrupt, transition from one type of airway to the next along the whole length of the tract. In general terms, the airways are pliable tubes lined by respiratory mucosa and containing variable amounts of muscle and/or cartilage. The principal structural features of the lower respiratory tract are as follows:

1. The respiratory epithelium undergoes progressive transition from a tall, pseudostratified columnar, ciliated form in the larynx and trachea to a simple, cuboidal, non-ciliated form in the smallest airways. Goblet cells are numerous in the trachea but decrease in number and are absent in the terminal bronchioles. Throughout the respiratory tract are scattered cells which, with the electron microscope, have been shown to contain electron-dense, secretory granules and which are part of the diffuse neuroendocrine system (see Ch. 17).

2. The lamina propria consists of fibro-elastic connective tissue which contains lymphoid aggregations of variable size and density; these form part of the gut-associated lymphoid tissue (see Ch. 11). One of the functions of this immunological tissue is the production of antibodies of the IgA class which are secreted into the lumen as a defence against invading microorganisms.

3. A layer of smooth muscle lies deep to the mucosa (except in the trachea) and becomes increasingly prominent as the airway diameter decreases; it reaches its greatest prominence in the terminal bronchioles. Smooth muscle tone controls the diameter of the conducting passages and thus controls resistance to air flow within the respiratory tree. Smooth muscle tone is modulated by the autonomic nervous system, adrenal medullary hormones and local factors. Sympathetic activity causes smooth muscle relaxation and thus dilatation of the airways which is an obviously appropriate response in the 'fight or flight' situation. Parasympathetic activity, on the other hand, causes airway constriction; the functional significance of this may be to reduce 'dead space' on expiration.

4. Submucosal connective tissue underlies the smooth muscle layer and contains serous and mucous glands which become progressively less numerous in the narrower airways and are not present beyond the tertiary bronchi.

5. Cartilage provides a supporting skeleton for the larynx, trachea and bronchi and prevents the collapse of these airways during respiration. This layer lies outside the submucosa and diminishes in prominence as the calibre of the airway decreases being completely absent beyond the tertiary bronchi.

6. The outermost layer of cartilage or smooth muscle is surrounded by fibro-elastic connective tissue called the *adventitia* which merges with surrounding tissues.

Blood supply of the lungs

The lungs have a dual blood supply, the *pulmonary system* and the *bronchial system*. The pulmonary supply is the predominant system and conducts deoxygenated blood from the right side of the heart via a large pulmonary artery to each lung.

The pulmonary arteries enter the roots or *hila* of the lungs with the main bronchi and then divide and course in parallel with the branching airways to supply the pulmonary capillaries surrounding the alveoli. The pulmonary arterial system is structurally unusual in two respects. Firstly, the pulmonary arterial vessels are relatively thin-walled and of large calibre, their diameter approximating that of the accompanying airway. Secondly, the pulmonary arteries have the histological characteristics of elastic arteries rather than of muscular arteries. Elastic expansion and recoil of the vessels maintains the pulmonary arterial pressure at a relatively constant level throughout the cardiac cycle.

The bronchial arterial system constitutes the systemic circulation of the lower respiratory tract. It arises as small branches of the aorta and supplies oxygenated blood to the tissues of the airway walls and to the *pleura*, the layer which invests the outer surface of each lung. The bronchial vessels are of the usual type found in the rest of the systemic circulation.

A common venous system returns most of the blood to the left side of the heart via the pulmonary veins which are extremely thin-walled vessels. A small proportion of blood from the bronchial system drains to the right side of the heart via the azygos venous system.

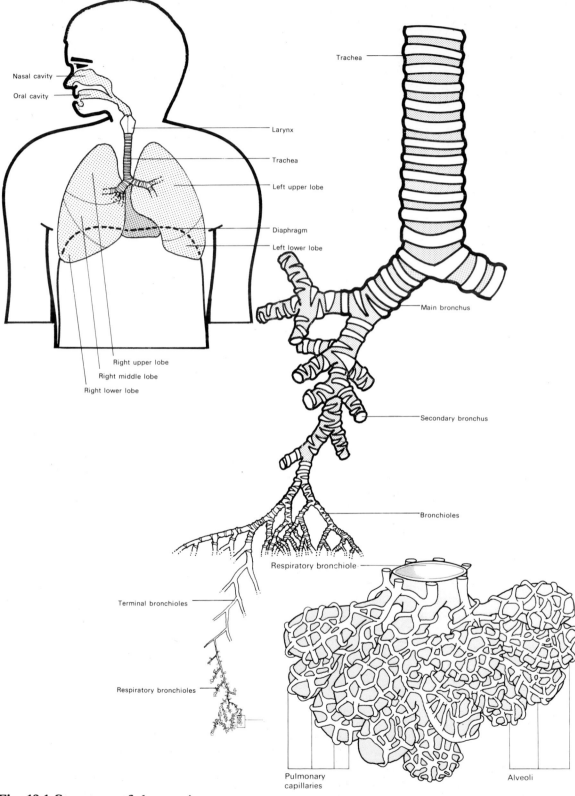

Fig. 12.1 Structure of the respiratory system

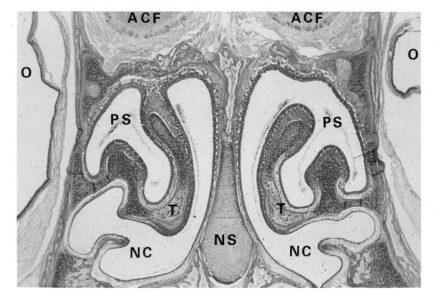

Fig. 12.2 Nasal cavity

(Kitten: coronal section, H & E Alcian blue × 12)

The first part of the upper respiratory tract, the nose, is subdivided into two nasal cavities **NC** by the cartilaginous nasal septum **NS**; cartilage is stained blue in this preparation.

The nasal cavities and paranasal sinuses **PS** are lined by respiratory mucosa, the major function of which is to filter particulate matter and to adjust the temperature and humidity of inspired air. These functions are enhanced by a large surface area provided by the turbinate system of bones **T** which project into the nasal cavities.

Part of the nasal mucosa, the *olfactory mucosa*, contains receptors for the sense of smell (see Fig. 21.2). Although the olfactory mucosa is extensive in lower mammals, in man it is confined to a relatively small area in the roof of the nasal cavities.

Note the close proximity of the nasal cavities to the orbital cavities **O** and the anterior cranial fossa **ACF**.

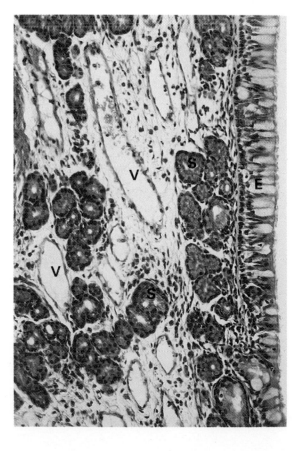

Fig. 12.3 Nasal mucosa

(H & E × 200)

The nasal mucosa consists of a pseudostratified, columnar, ciliated epithelium **E** with numerous goblet cells supported by a richly vascular lamina propria containing serous and mucous glands. These features reflect the protective functions of the nasal mucosa, processes which begin in the nasal cavities and continue throughout the respiratory tract.

Particulate matter in inspired air is trapped in a thin layer of surface mucus secreted by the goblet cells of the surface epithelium and the mucous glands of the lamina propria. Co-ordinated, wave-like beating of cilia propels mucus with trapped particles towards the pharynx where it is swallowed and inactivated in the stomach.

The entrance to each nasal cavity, the *nasal vestibule*, is lined by skin which has short, coarse hairs called *vibrissae* which trap the largest particles before they reach the nasal mucosa.

The temperature of inspired air is adjusted to that of the body by heat exchange between the air and blood flowing in a rich plexus of thin-walled venules **V** in the lamina propria. Inspired air is humidified by the watery secretions of serous glands **S** also located in the lamina propria.

A mucosa similar to that of the nasal cavities also lines the nasopharynx, paranasal sinuses and auditory tubes.

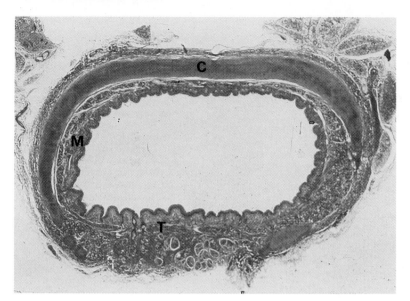

Fig. 12.4 Trachea

(TS: H & E/Alcian blue × 9)

This specimen from a newborn child shows the general structure of the trachea. The trachea is a flexible tube of fibro-elastic connective tissue and cartilage which permits expansion in diameter and extension in length during inspiration, and passive recoil during expiration.

A series of C-shaped rings of hyaline cartilage **C**, stained blue in this preparation, support the tracheal mucosa **M** and prevent its collapse during inspiration.

Bands of smooth muscle, called the *trachealis muscle* **T**, join the free ends of the rings posteriorly; contraction of the trachealis reduces tracheal diameter and thereby assists in raising intrathoracic pressure during coughing. A few strands of longitudinal muscle are disposed behind the trachealis muscle.

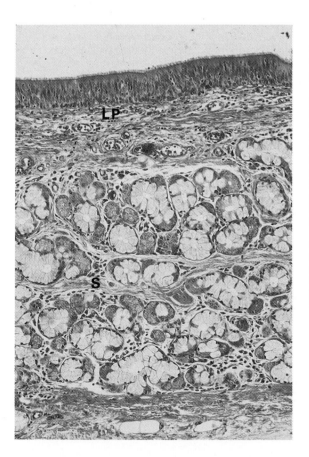

Fig. 12.5 Trachea

(LS: H & E × 198)

The layers of the tracheal wall are shown in this specimen from a young man.

The respiratory epithelium of the trachea is tall, pseudostratified and ciliated and contains goblet cells. In response to the irritation of tobacco smoke, the epithelium commonly undergoes morphological change (metaplasia) to a stratified squamous form with consequent loss of ciliary action; ciliary activity is essential for continuous movement of glandular secretions towards the pharynx. The tracheal epithelium is supported by a thick basement membrane. Beneath the basement membrane, the lamina propria **LP** consists of loose, highly vascular, connective tissue which becomes more condensed at its deeper aspect to form a band of fibro-elastic tissue.

Underlying the lamina propria is the loose submucosa **S** containing numerous mixed sero-mucous glands which decrease in number in the lower parts of the trachea; the serous cells stain strongly with H & E whilst the mucous cells remain poorly stained. The submucosa merges with the perichondrium of the underlying hyaline cartilage rings or with the external adventitial layer between the rings.

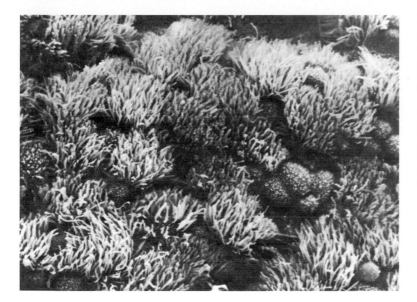

Fig. 12.6 Tracheal epithelium

(Scanning EM × 2000)

This micrograph illustrates the tracheal surface at high magnification; the film of surface mucus has been removed before fixation and processing.

The ciliated epithelial cells have an appearance reminiscent of clumps of seaweed, the cilia being several micrometres in length. Goblet cells are scattered amongst the ciliated cells being recognisable by their lack of cilia and the presence of a few small microvilli.

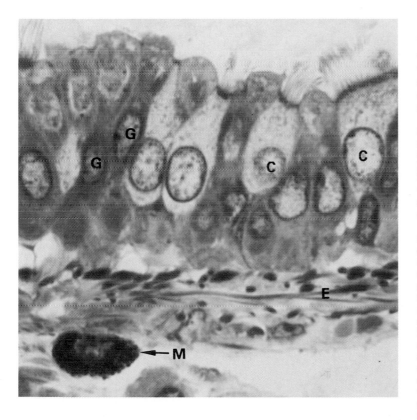

Fig. 12.7 Respiratory epithelium

(Rat: Thin section, toluidine blue × 800)

This micrograph illustrates the structure of the respiratory epithelium at the limit of resolution of the light microscope.

The epithelium is pseudostratified, the bases of all the cells extending down to the basement membrane, although not all the cells reach the luminal surface. The ciliated cells **C** have large nuclei and stain very poorly with this method. The goblet cells **G** stain most strongly due to their content of mucus, a mucopolysaccharide.

The underlying lamina propria contains a considerable amount of elastin **E** and mast cells **M** containing numerous darkly stained granules which contain histamine and heparin, a glycoprotein and thus responsible for the intense staining with this method (see also Fig. 4.15). The role of mast cells in normal function is unclear; however, when antigen-antibody complexes are formed on their cell membranes, they release large quantities of histamine. Histamine causes smooth muscle constriction and vasodilatation leading to mucosal swelling, these phenomena being responsible for the clinical condition of *asthma*.

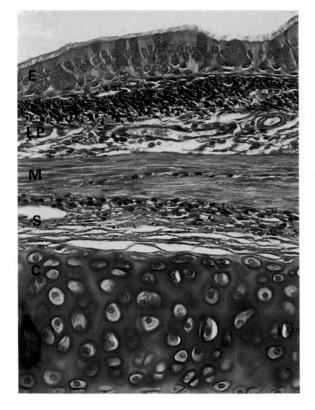

Fig. 12.8 Primary bronchus
(TS: Elastic van Gieson/Alcian blue × 150)

The basic structure of the primary bronchi is similar to that of the trachea, but it differs in several details. Firstly, the respiratory epithelium **E** is less tall and contains fewer goblet cells; the goblet cells have darkly stained, granular cytoplasm in this preparation. Secondly, the lamina propria **LP** is more dense with a large quantity of elastin in its more superficial aspect; elastic fibres are stained black in this preparation. Thirdly, the lamina propria is separated from the submucosa **S** by a discontinuous layer of smooth muscle **M** which becomes progressively more prominent further down the tract. Fourthly, the submucosal layer contains fewer sero-mucous glands; none are seen in this micrograph. Finally the cartilage framework **C** is arranged into flattened, interconnected plates rather than discrete C-shaped rings as in the trachea.

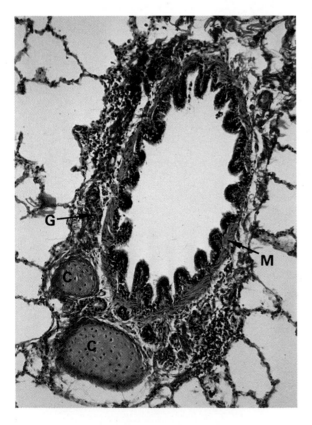

Fig. 12.9 Tertiary bronchus
(TS: Elastic van Gieson × 75)

As the bronchi diminish in diameter the structure progressively changes to more closely resemble that of large bronchioles. The respiratory epithelium, which cannot be seen at this magnification, is now tall columnar but not pseudostratified, and goblet cells have diminished in number.

The lamina propria is thin, elastic and completely encircled by smooth muscle **M** which is disposed in a spiral manner. This arrangement of smooth muscle permits contraction of the bronchi in both length and diameter during expiration. Sero-mucous glands **G** are sparse in the submucosa and are rarely found in smaller airways.

The cartilage framework **C** is reduced to a few irregular plates; cartilage also does not usually extend beyond the tertiary bronchi. Note that the submucosa merges with the surrounding adventitia and thence with the lung parenchyma. A small lymphoid aggregation is seen in the adventitia.

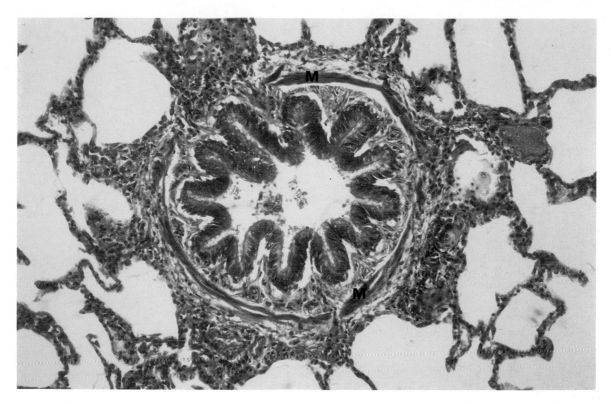

Fig. 12.10 Bronchiole

(TS: H & E × 160)

Bronchioles are airways of less than one millimetre in diameter and have no cartilaginous support. The respiratory epithelium is simple, columnar and ciliated and contains few goblet cells, these being completely absent beyond the terminal bronchioles.

The smooth muscle layer **M** is the most prominent feature of the bronchiole and is disposed in a spiral manner like that of the bronchi. The total cross-sectional area of all bronchioles combined is far greater than that of the rest of the conducting passages combined, thus the tone of the bronchiolar smooth muscle effectively controls resistance to air flow within the lungs.

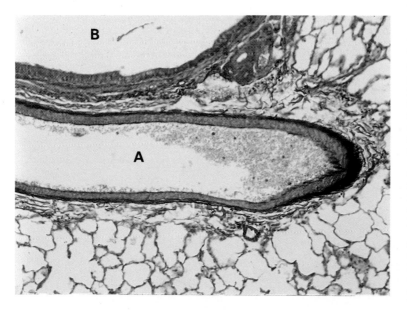

Fig. 12.11 Pulmonary artery

(Elastic van Gieson/Alcian blue × 75)

This micrograph shows a fairly major segmental branch of the pulmonary artery **A** traversing the lung parenchyma in close association with a tertiary bronchus **B**. The airway can be identified as such by the absence of cartilage, relatively thin muscular layer and presence of occasional submucosal glands.

The pulmonary arterial vessels are described as elastic arteries (see Fig. 8.6) and contain relatively little smooth muscle; elastin is stained black, and smooth muscle yellow, in this preparation.

The walls of the pulmonary arteries are relatively thin in relation to their diameter, the pressures being much lower than that in the systemic circulation. Note the red-stained collagen in the supporting connective tissue of the vessel and airway.

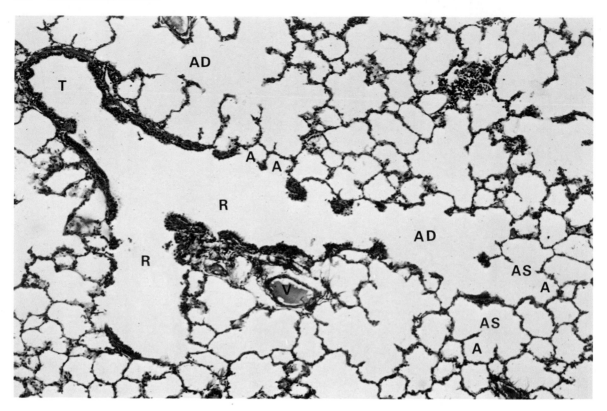

Fig. 12.12 Terminal portion of the respiratory tree

(Elastic van Gieson × 40)

Terminal bronchioles **T** are the smallest diameter passages of the purely conducting portion of the respiratory tree and beyond this, further branches become increasingly involved in gaseous exchange.

Each terminal bronchiole divides to form short, thinner-walled branches called respiratory bronchioles **R**, so named because their walls contain a small number of single alveoli **A**. The epithelium of the respiratory bronchioles is devoid of goblet cells and largely consists of ciliated, cuboidal cells and smaller numbers of non-ciliated cells called *Clara cells*. The epithelium of respiratory bronchioles undergoes further transition from that of the terminal bronchioles, and Clara cells become the predominant cell type in the most distal part of the respiratory bronchioles. Clara cells have the ultrastructural features of secretory cells, but the nature and function of their secretory product is not understood.

Each respiratory bronchiole divides further into several long, winding passages called alveolar ducts **AD** which open along their length into numerous alveolar sacs **AS** and alveoli **A**. In histological sections, all that can be seen of the walls of the alveolar ducts are minute aggregations of smooth muscle cells and associated collagen and elastic fibres which form rings surrounding the alveolar ducts and the openings of the alveolar sacs and alveoli. The smooth muscle of the respiratory bronchioles and alveolar ducts regulates alveolar air movements.

The alveolar ducts lead into alveolar sacs, distended spaces, each of which gives rise to several alveoli. Each alveolus consists of a pocket, open at one side and lined by extremely flattened epithelial cells. Surrounding each alveolus is a rich network of pulmonary capillaries supplied by pulmonary vessels **V** which follow the general course of the airways. Between adjacent alveoli, the wall or *alveolar septum* consists of the flattened epithelial lining cells of each alveolus separated by capillaries and extremely delicate reticular and elastic supporting elements. Fibres condense around the opening of each alveolus and merge with those around the openings of adjacent alveoli to form a fine, supporting system for the whole lung parenchyma.

The alveolar septa contain small openings called *alveolar pores* which are thought to enable equalisation of pressure between alveoli, and to provide a collateral air circulation when a bronchiole is obstructed.

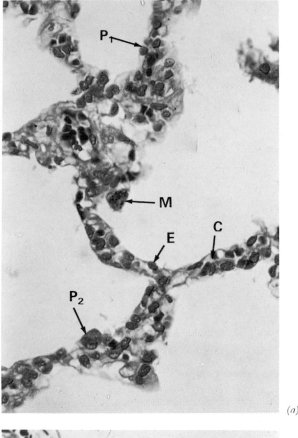

(a)

Fig. 12.13 Alveoli

(a) H & E × 480 (b) Thin section, toluidine blue × 480

The conventional method of studying the structure of the alveolar wall in light microscopy has been to use relatively thick (5– 8μm) wax-embedded tissues, stained by routine methods as in micrograph (a); however the resolution obtained by such methods is limited. In contrast, thin resin sections, as shown in micrograph (b), reveal much greater structural detail since they permit better resolution.

In general terms, the alveolar wall consists of three tissue components: surface epithelium, connective tissue and blood vessels.

1. Epithelium forms a continuous alveolar lining and consists of cells of two types. Most of the alveolar surface area is covered by large, extremely flattened cells called *Type I pneumocytes*; since the cytoplasm of these cells covers such an extensive area the characteristic, densely stained nuclei of Type I pneumocytes P_1 are relatively infrequently seen in histological section. A second epithelial cell type, known as the *Type II pneumocyte*, is present in larger numbers in the lining epithelium; these cells are rounded in shape and thus occupy a much smaller proportion (about 3%) of the alveolar surface area. Type II pneumocytes P_2 have large, rounded nuclei with a prominent nucleolus and extensive, vacuolated cytoplasm. Type I pneumocytes constitute part of the extremely thin gaseous diffusion barrier, whereas Type II pneumocytes are thought to secrete a surface-active material called *surfactant* which reduces surface tension within the alveoli preventing alveolar collapse during expiration.

2. Connective tissue forms an attenuated, supporting layer beneath the epithelium and surrounding the blood vessels of the alveolar wall. This layer primarily consists of fine reticular, collagenous and elastic fibres and occasional fibroblasts.

3. Blood vessels, mainly capillaries **C** (7 to 10μm in diameter) form an extremely rich plexus around each alveolus. In most of the alveolar wall, the basement membrane which supports the capillary endothelium is directly applied to the basement membrane supporting the surface epithelium; in such sites the two basement membranes are fused and the connective tissue layer is absent. This arrangement provides an interface of minimal thickness between alveolar air and blood. Note in these micrographs the nuclei of capillary endothelial cells **E** and the close proximity of erythrocytes to the alveolar air spaces.

Although the defence mechanisms of the conducting passages filter most particulate matter from inspired air, small particles such as carbon reach the alveoli and are engulfed by phagocytic cells found in the alveolar wall or free in the alveolar space. These phagocytes **M**, known as *alveolar macrophages* or *dust cells*, are derived from circulating blood monocytes and are usually recognisable by their content of engulfed, particulate material.

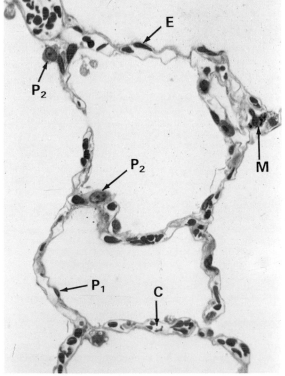

(b)

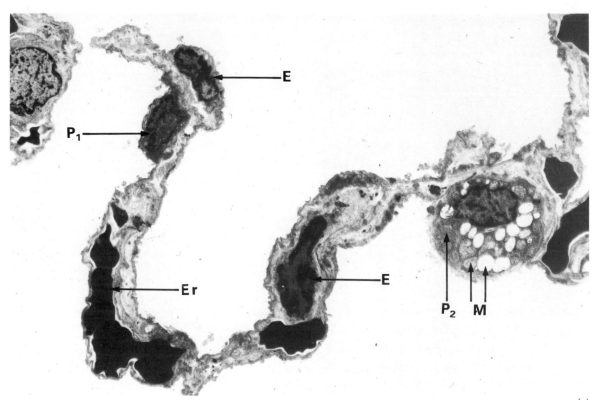

(a)

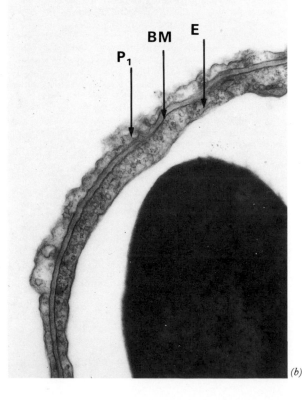

(b)

Fig. 12.14 Alveolar wall

(EM (a) × 3230 (b) × 30 000)

These micrographs illustrate some of the ultra-structural features of the alveolar wall. Micrograph (a) shows the alveolar wall between two alveoli at fairly low magnification. Capillaries make up the bulk of the wall being identified by the uniformly electron-dense erythrocytes which almost fill the lumina; as seen here, the erythrocytes undergo considerable deformation as they pass through the pulmonary capillaries.

Type I pneumocytes, which cover most of the alveolar surface, and capillary endothelial cells are both extremely flattened and distinction between them is best made by tracing their basement membranes; alveolar lining cells lie outside the membrane whilst endothelial cells are enclosed. The nuclei of two capillary endothelial cells **E** and one Type I pneumocyte **P₁** can be identified in this field.

Also in micrograph (a), a Type II pneumocyte **P₂** is seen, typically located at a branching point of the interalveolar septum; the cytoplasm is filled with vesicles containing phospholipid in the form of multilamellate bodies **M**. It is believed that these bodies are discharged into the alveolar air space where they contribute to a surfactant layer on the epithelium-air interface; Clara cells of the respiratory bronchioles (see Fig. 12.12) may synthesise other components of surfactant.

Recent evidence strongly suggests that Type II pneumocytes may differentiate into Type I pneumocytes in response to damage to the alveolar lining.

At high magnification in micrograph (b) the components of the gaseous diffusion barrier between blood and alveolar air are seen to consist of the extremely attenuated cytoplasm of a Type I pneumocyte **P₁**, a common basement membrane **BM**, and the thin cytoplasm of a capillary endothelial cell **E**. Note the erythrocyte in the capillary lumen.

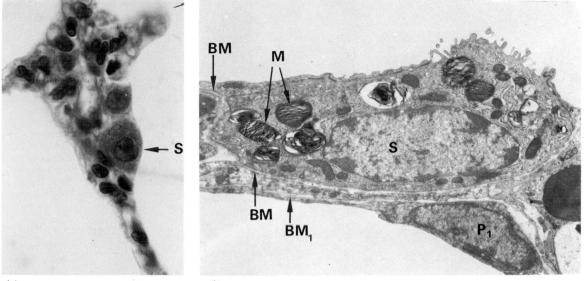

(a)   (b)

Fig. 12.15 Surfactant cells

(a) H & E × 400 (b) EM × 12 000

Micrograph (a) shows, at very high magnification, the light microscopic appearance of Type II pneumocytes, the cells responsible for surfactant production.

Surfactant cells **S** have large plump nuclei with dispersed chromatin and prominent nucleoli. In comparison, the nuclei of Type I pneumocytes (alveolar lining cells) and capillary endothelial cells are small, dense and flattened. The cytoplasm of surfactant cells is bulky and eosinophilic and filled with fine, unstained vacuoles representing multilamellate bodies, the phospholipid of which is dissolved out during tissue preparation.

Electron-dense multilamellate bodies **M** are seen in micrograph (b). Note also the basement membrane **BM** underlying the surfactant cell. On the other side of the alveolar septum shown here is the nucleus of a Type I pneumocyte P_1, its extremely attenuated cytoplasm spreading out to line the alveolus. The basement membrane of this cell BM_1 can also be delineated, and between this and the basement membrane of the surfactant cell lies a shred of fibroblast cytoplasm belonging to the connective tissue element of the alveolar wall.

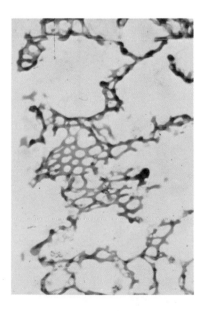

Fig. 12.16 Pulmonary capillaries

(Dye perfused preparation × 420)

The pulmonary arterial system terminates at the alveolar ducts where arterioles ramify to form a widely interconnected capillary basket surrounding each alveolus; the capillaries are of relatively large diameter (7–10 μm). Control of blood flow in the pulmonary capillary bed is predominantly effected by the partial pressure of gases within the alveoli. In poorly ventilated alveoli, the partial pressure of oxygen is low and that of carbon dioxide high; this causes local vasoconstriction, thus directing blood away from the poorly ventilated alveoli.

The lung tissue illustrated in this micrograph was prepared by perfusion of the pulmonary vasculature with a blue dye. This procedure outlines the pulmonary capillary bed; no other histological detail can be seen. In the centre of the field the richly anastomosing capillary network of part of an alveolar wall is demonstrated. This type of technique, in combination with the study of very thick histological sections, provided early microscopists with valuable information about the structure, function and vascular system of the lungs.

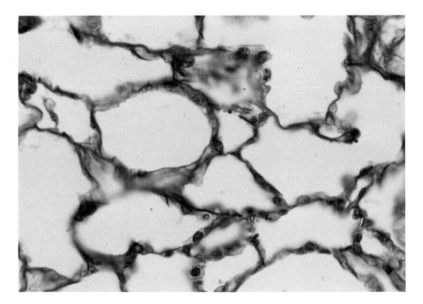

Fig. 12.17 Pulmonary elastic tissue

(Elastic van Gieson × 480)

This staining method demonstrates the large amount of elastin (stained black) in the alveolar walls. At the margins of the openings into the alveoli (arrowed), the elastin is condensed to form a ring. This elastin is continuous with that of adjacent alveoli, the whole forming an elastic framework for the lung parenchyma. The elastic tissue of the lung allows for expansion during inspiration; should air be admitted to the pleural space, a condition known as *pneumothorax*, the lung collapses due to the elasticity of the parenchyma.

Fig. 12.18 Visceral pleura

(H & E × 198)

The cavities containing the lungs, the *pleural cavities*, are lined by a thin, flattened epithelium (mesothelium) called the *pleura* which is analogous in structure to the pericardium surrounding the heart, and the peritoneum lining the abdominal cavity. The pleura lining the thoracic wall, called the *parietal pleura*, is reflected at the hilum over the surface of the lungs to form a continuous layer called the *visceral pleura*. The visceral and parietal pleura are directly applied to one another but separated by a potential space containing a minute amount of serous fluid. The two pleural layers adhere to one another such that movements of the thoracic wall during ventilation result in corresponding expansion and contraction of the lungs. Pleural fluid is rarely present in discernible amounts in the absence of inflammation or other disease processes.

This micrograph illustrates visceral pleura. The outer surface is lined by a layer of flattened mesothelium **M** which is supported by a thin basement membrane. The underlying fibrous connective tissue **F** is particularly prominent in the human lung and consists primarily of collagen and elastic fibres; smooth muscle cells are occasionally seen. The fibrous layer of visceral pleura extends into the lung as fibrous septa **S** which are continuous with the fibroelastic framework of the lung parenchyma.

The visceral pleura contains a superficial plexus of lymph vessels which drain via the connective tissue septa into a deep plexus surrounding the pulmonary blood vessels and airways. Lymph from the deep plexuses drains into the thoracic duct via several prominent lymph nodes in the hilar region. Lymph capillaries are not found in alveolar walls. Several lymph vessels **L** can be seen in the pleura in this micrograph. The visceral pleura also contains numerous small blood vessels and capillaries. Nerves are seen infrequently and are believed to originate from the parasympathetic and sympathetic systems supplying the airways and pulmonary vessels, and from pulmonary stretch receptors.

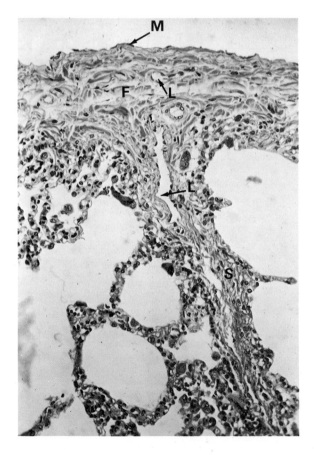

13. Oral tissues

Introduction

The digestive process commences in the oral cavity with the ingestion, fragmentation and moistening of food but in addition to its digestive role, the oral cavity is involved in speech, facial expression, sensory reception and breathing. The major structures of the oral cavity, the *lips, teeth, tongue* and *oral mucosa*, and the associated *salivary glands*, participate in all these functions.

Mastication is the process by which ingested food is made suitable for swallowing. Chewing not only involves co-ordinated movements of the mandible and the cutting and grinding action of the teeth but also activity of the lips and tongue, which continually redirect food between the *occlusal surfaces* of the teeth. The watery component of saliva moistens and lubricates the masticatory process whilst salivary mucus helps to bind the food bolus ready for swallowing.

The entire oral cavity is lined by a protective mucous membrane, the oral mucosa, which contains many sensory receptors, including the taste receptors of the tongue. The epithelium of the oral mucosa is of the stratified squamous type which tends to be keratinised in areas subject to considerable friction such as the palate. The oral epithelium is supported by dense connective tissue, the *lamina propria*. In highly mobile areas such as the soft palate and floor of the mouth, the lamina propria is connected with the underlying muscle by loose submucosal connective tissue. In contrast, in areas where the oral mucosa overlies bone, such as the hard palate and tooth-bearing ridges, the lamina propria is tightly bound to the periosteum by a relatively thin, dense fibrous submucosa. Throughout the oral mucosa, numerous small accessory salivary glands of both serous and mucous types are distributed in the submucosa.

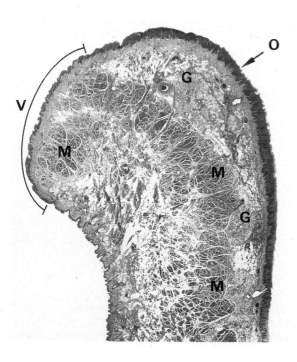

Fig. 13.1 Lip
(H & E × 6)

This micrograph illustrates a midline section through a human lower lip, the bulk of which is made up of bundles of circumoral skeletal muscle **M** seen in transverse section.

The external surface of the lip is covered by hairy skin which passes through a transition zone to merge with the oral mucosa **O** of the inner surface. The transition zone constitutes the free *vermilion border* of the lip **V**, and derives its colour from the richly vascular dermis which here has only a thin, lightly keratinised epidermal covering. The free border is highly sensitive due to its rich sensory innervation. Since the vermilion border is devoid of sweat and sebaceous glands, it requires continuous moistening by saliva to prevent cracking.

The oral mucosa covering the inner surface of the lip has a thick stratified squamous epithelium and the underlying submucosa contains numerous accessory salivary glands **G** of serous, mucous and mixed sero-mucous types.

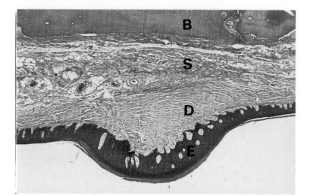

Fig. 13.2 Palatal mucosa
(H & E × 28)

Like the rest of the mouth, the palate is covered by a thick stratified squamous epithelium **E** supported by a tough, densely collagenous dermis **D**. To assist mastication, the palatal mucosa is thrown up into transverse folds or *rugae*, one of which is shown in this micrograph.

The mucosa of the hard palate is bound down to the underlying bone **B** by relatively dense submucosal connective tissue **S** containing a few accessory salivary glands.

In rodents and many other mammals with a coarse diet, the surface epithelium of particularly exposed areas is keratinised for extra protection as in this specimen taken from a monkey.

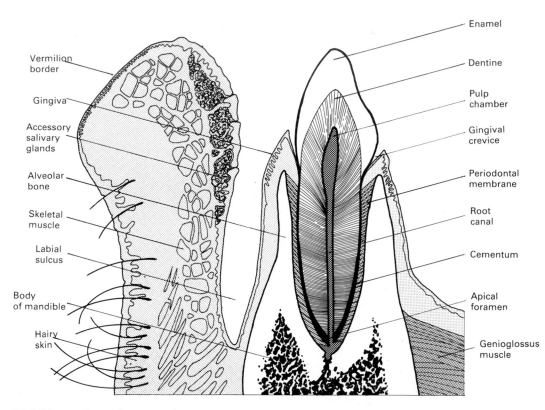

Fig. 13.3 Lip and tooth

This drawing of a section through the lower jaw near the midline illustrates the general arrangement of the lip and a tooth with its supporting structures.

Each tooth may be grossly divided into two segments, the *crown* and the *root*: the crown is that portion which projects into the oral cavity and is protected by a layer of highly mineralised *enamel*, which covers it entirely. The bulk of the tooth is made up of *dentine*, a mineralised tissue which has a similar chemical composition to bone. The dentine has a central *pulp cavity* containing the *dental pulp* which consists of specialised connective tissue containing many sensory nerve fibres. The tooth root is embedded in a bony ridge in the jaw called the *alveolar ridge*; the tooth socket is known as the *alveolus*, and at the lip or cheek aspect of the alveolus,

the bony plate is generally thinner than at the tongue or palatal aspect. The root of the tooth is invested by a thin layer of *cementum* which is connected to the bone of the socket by a thin, fibrous layer called the *periodontal ligament* or *periodontal membrane*.

The oral mucosa covering the upper part of the alveolar ridge is called the *gingiva* and at the junction of the crown and root of the tooth (the *neck of the tooth*) the gingiva forms a tight protective cuff around the tooth. The potential space between the gingival cuff and the enamel of the crown is called the *gingival crevice*. All of the tissues which surround and support the tooth are collectively known as the *periodontium*.

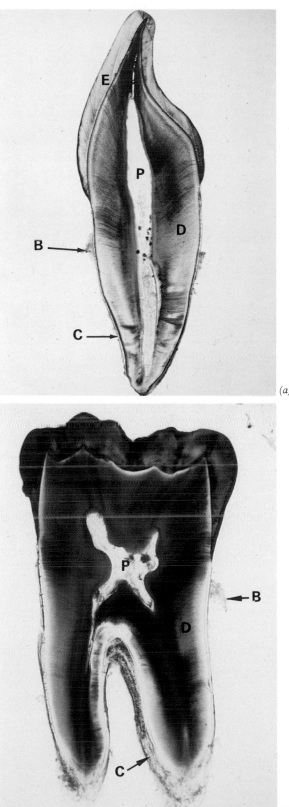

(a)

(b)

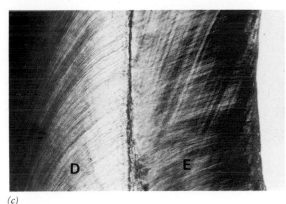

(c)

Fig. 13.4 Tooth structure

(Undecalcified sections, unstained (a) × 5 (b) × 5 (c) × 50)

These undecalcified sections cut with a diamond wheel demonstrate the arrangement of the calcified tissues of an upper central incisor tooth in micrograph (a) and a lower molar tooth in micrograph (b). Micrograph (c) demonstrates the tissues of the crown at high magnification.

The dentine **D** which forms the bulk of the crown and root is composed of a calcified organic matrix similar to that of bone. The inorganic component constitutes a somewhat larger proportion of the matrix of dentine than that of bone and exists mainly in the form of hydroxyapatite crystals. From the pulp cavity **P**, minute parallel tubules, called *dentine tubules*, radiate to the periphery of the dentine; in longitudinal sections of teeth, the tubules appear to follow an S-shaped course.

The crown of the tooth is covered by enamel **E**, an extremely hard, translucent substance composed of parallel rods or prisms of highly calcified material cemented together by an almost equally highly calcified interprismatic material.

The root is invested by a thin layer of cementum **C** which is generally thicker towards the apex of the root. The cementum is an amorphous calcified tissue into which the fibres of the periodontal membrane are anchored. Fragments of alveolar bone **B** have remained attached to the roots after extraction of these specimens.

The morphological form of the tooth crown and roots varies considerably in different parts of the mouth, nevertheless the basic arrangement of the dental tissues is the same in all teeth.

In humans, the *primary (deciduous) dentition* consists of 20 teeth, two *incisors*, one *canine* and two *molars* in each quadrant. These begin to be formed at 6 weeks during fetal development and erupt between the ages of 6 and 30 months after birth. From the age of 6 years, the deciduous teeth are succeeded by permanent teeth namely two incisors, one canine and two *premolars* in each arch; distal to these, three permanent molars (having no primary precursors) develop in addition. The sharp points found on the posterior teeth are known as *cusps*.

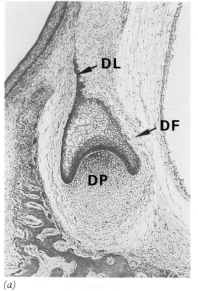

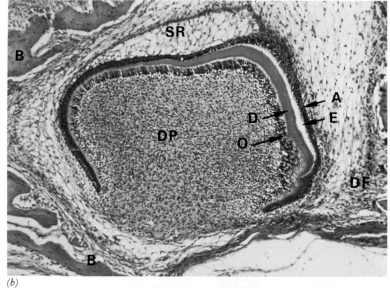

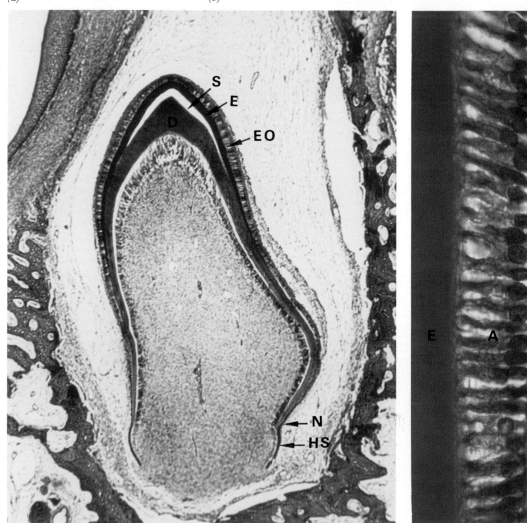

Fig. 13.5 Tooth development *(illustrations opposite)*

(H & E (a) cap stage × 28 (b) bell stage × 96 (c) onset of root development × 45 (d) ameloblasts × 640)

This series of micrographs illustrates the important stages of tooth development.

The tissues of the teeth are derived from two embryological sources. The enamel is of epithelial (ectodermal) origin whilst the dentine, cementum, pulp and periodontal ligament are of mesenchymal (mesodermal) origin. The first evidence of tooth development in humans occurs at 6 weeks of fetal life with the proliferation of a horseshoe-shaped epithelial ridge from the basal layer of the primitive oral epithelium into the underlying mesoderm in the position of the future jaws; this is known as the *dental lamina*. In each quadrant of the mouth, the lamina then develops four globular swellings which will become the *enamel organs* of the future deciduous central and lateral incisors, canines and first molar teeth. Subsequently, the dental lamina proliferates backwards in each arch successively giving rise to the enamel organs of the future second deciduous molar and the three permanent molars. The permanent successors of the deciduous teeth will later develop from enamel organs which bud off from the inner aspect of the enamel organs of their deciduous predecessors.

The primitive mesenchyme immediately subjacent to the developing enamel organ proliferates to form a cellular mass whilst at the same time, the enamel organ becomes progressively cap-shaped, as seen in micrograph (a), enveloping the mesenchymal mass which becomes known as the *dental papilla* **DP**. During the cap stage, the cells lining the concave face of the enamel organ in contact with the dental papilla begin to differentiate into tall columnar cells, the future *ameloblasts*, which will be responsible for the production of enamel. This, in turn, induces the differentiation of a layer of columnar *odontoblasts*, the future dentine-producing cells, in the apical region of the dental papilla. The interface between the differentiating ameloblast and odontoblast layers marks the position and shape of the future junction between enamel and dentine.

As the enamel organ develops further, it assumes a characteristic bell shape, as seen in micrograph (b), the free edge of the 'bell' proliferating so as to determine the eventual shape of the tooth crown.

Meanwhile, the cells forming the main bulk of the enamel organ become large and star-shaped forming the *stellate reticulum* **SR**, the extracellular matrix of which is rich in glycosaminoglycans. Between the stellate reticulum and ameloblast layer, two or three layers of flattened cells form the *stratum intermedium* whilst the outer surface of the enamel organ consists of a simple cuboidal epithelium called the *external enamel epithelium*. By the cap stage of development, the dental lamina **DL** connecting the enamel organ with the oral mucosa has become fragmented, and around the whole developing tooth bud, a condensation of mesenchyme forms the *dental follicle* **DF** which will eventually become the periodontal ligament.

As ameloblasts and odontoblasts differentiate at the tip of the crown, a layer of dentine matrix is progressively laid down between the ameloblast and odontoblast layers. As the odontoblasts retreat, each leaves a long cytoplasmic extension, the *odontoblastic process*, embedded within the dentine matrix thereby forming the dentine tubules (see Fig. 13.6). Dentine matrix has a similar biochemical composition to that of bone and undergoes calcification in a similar fashion. Deposition of dentine induces the production of enamel by the adjacent ameloblasts. Each retreating ameloblast lays down a column of enamel matrix which then undergoes mineralisation resulting in the formation of a dense prismatic structure as described below. With the deposition of dentine and enamel, the overlying stellate reticulum disappears and the enamel organ is much reduced in thickness. These changes are well demonstrated in micrograph (b). A thin layer of dentine **D** has been laid down by the underlying odontoblastic layer **O** of the highly cellular dental papilla **DP**. The ameloblastic layer **A** is about to lay down enamel in the area of the artefactual space **E**; note that in this area, the stellate reticulum has disappeared. Note also the surrounding dental follicle **DF** and early formation of cancellous bone **B**.

By the time that dentine and enamel formation is well under way at the incisal edge or tips of the cusps, as the case may be, the enamel organ will have fully outlined the shape of the whole tooth crown. This is the case in micrograph (c), the neck of the tooth **N** marking the junction of crown and root. A thin, densely-stained layer of poorly mineralised enamel **E** can be seen covered at its external surface by the now much thinned enamel organ **EO**. The unstained space **S** between this and the underlying dentine **D** represents fully mineralised enamel laid down earlier but dissolved away during tissue preparation. Although enamel production is confined to the crown, the rim of the 'bell' of the enamel organ nevertheless continues to proliferate, inducing dentine formation and thereby determining the shape of the tooth root. This part of the enamel organ, known as the *epithelial sheath of Hertwig* **HS**, disintegrates once the outline of the root is completed. The cementum which later forms on the root surface is derived from the dental follicle which, as previously stated, is of mesenchymal origin. As the dentine of the crown and root are progressively laid down, the dental papilla shrinks and eventually becomes the dental pulp contained within the pulp chamber and root canals (see Fig. 13.7).

Growth of the tooth root is one of the principal mechanisms of tooth eruption and root formation is not completed until some time after the crown has fully erupted into the oral cavity.

Micrograph (d), taken from the same specimen as micrograph (c) at much higher magnification, illustrates the characteristic appearance of ameloblasts. Active ameloblasts **A** are tall, columnar, epithelial cells which form a single layer apposed to the forming surface of the enamel **E**. Each ameloblast elaborates a column of organic enamel matrix which undergoes progressive mineralisation by the deposition of calcium phosphate mainly in the form of hydroxyapatite crystals. Fully formed enamel contains less than 1% organic material and is the hardest and most dense tissue in the body.

The structure of mature enamel is not fully understood, but it appears that the process of mineralisation of the enamel matrix is not uniform and, as a result, mature enamel consists of highly calcified prisms separated by so-called *interprismatic material* which may differ only in the orientation of its crystals. Each prism extends from the dentino-enamel junction to the enamel surface and may represent the enamel laid down by a single ameloblast.

Underlying the ameloblast layer are several layers of cells, also of epithelial origin, which constitute the remainder of the enamel organ **EO**. As enamel formation progresses, the enamel organ becomes much reduced in thickness compared with earlier stages of its development. At tooth eruption, the enamel organ, including the ameloblasts, degenerates leaving the enamel exposed to the hostile oral environment, completely incapable of regeneration.

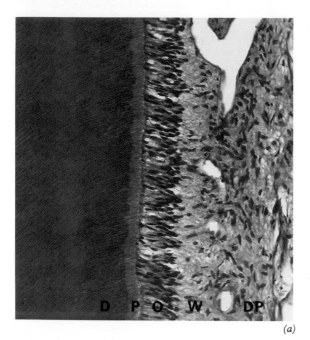

(a)

Fig. 13.6 Odontoblasts and dentine

(Decalcified sections, H & E (a) × 200 (b) × 128)

Dentine, the dense calcified tissue which forms the bulk of the tooth, is broadly similar to bone in composition but is more highly mineralised and thus much harder than bone. The cells responsible for dentine formation, the odontoblasts, differentiate as a single layer of tall, columnar cells on the surface of the dental papilla, apposed to the ameloblast layer of the enamel organ. The odontoblasts initiate tooth formation by deposition of organic dentine matrix between the odontoblastic and ameloblastic layers; calcification of this dentine matrix then induces enamel formation by ameloblasts (see Fig. 13.5). Dentine formation proceeds by continuing odontoblastic deposition of dentine matrix and its subsequent calcification; unlike ameloblasts, each odontoblast leaves behind a slender cytoplasmic process, the odontoblastic process, within a fine dentinal tubule. When dentine formation is complete, the dentine is thus pervaded by parallel odontoblastic processes radiating from the odontoblast layer on the dentinal surface of the reduced dental papilla which now constitutes the dental pulp. After tooth formation is complete, a small amount of less organised *secondary dentine* continues to be laid down resulting in the progressive obliteration of the pulp cavity with advancing age.

These micrographs illustrate active odontoblasts **O** forming a pseudostratified layer of columnar cells at the dentine surface. Parallel dentine tubules containing odontoblastic processes extend through a narrow, pale-stained zone of uncalcified dentine matrix called *predentine* **P** into the mature dentine **D**; the dentine tubules are best seen in micrograph (b). Underlying the odontoblastic layer, a relatively acellular layer, called the *cell free zone of Weil* **W**, gives way to the highly cellular dental pulp **DP**.

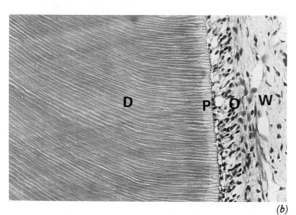

(b)

Fig. 13.7 Dental pulp

(Decalcified section, H & E × 198)

The dental pulp consists of a delicate connective tissue resembling primitive mesenchyme (see Fig. 4.2); it contains numerous stellate fibroblasts, reticulin fibres, fine poorly organised collagen fibres and much ground substance. The pulp contains a rich network of thin-walled capillaries supplied by arterioles which enter the pulp canal from the periodontal membrane, usually via one foramen at each root apex. The pulp is also richly innervated by a plexus of myelinated nerve fibres from which fine, unmyelinated branches extend into the odontoblastic layer. Despite the acute sensitivity of dentine, nerve fibres are rarely demonstrable in dentine and the mechanism of sensory reception is unknown; it has been suggested that the odontoblastic processes may act as sensory receptors.

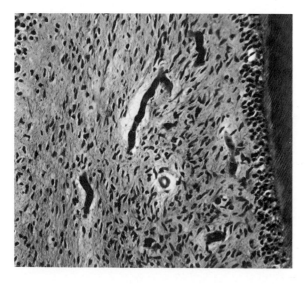

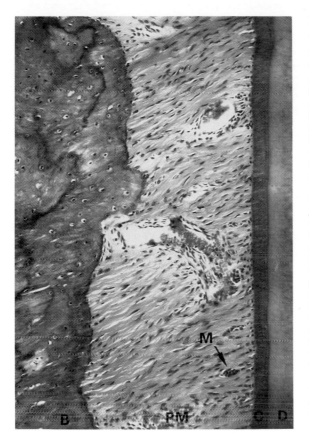

Fig. 13.8 Periodontal membrane and cementum

(Decalcified section, H & E × 200)

The periodontal membrane **PM** forms a thin fibrous attachment between the tooth root and the alveolar bone. The dentine **D**, comprising the root, is covered by a thin layer of cementum **C** which is elaborated by cells called *cementocytes* lying on the surface of the cementum. Cementum consists of a dense, calcified organic material similar to the matrix of bone, and is generally acellular. Towards the root apex, the cementum layer becomes progressively thicker and irregular and cementocytes are often entrapped in lacunae within the cementum.

The periodontal membrane consists of dense, fibrous connective tissue. The collagen fibres, known as *Sharpey's fibres*, run obliquely downwards from their attachment in the alveolar bone **B** to their anchorage in the cementum at a more apical position on the root surface. The periodontal membrane thus acts as a sling for the tooth within its socket, permitting slight movements which cushion the impact of masticatory forces. The points of attachment of the collagen fibres in both cementum and bone are in a constant state of reorganisation to accommodate changing functional stresses upon the teeth. Osteoclastic resorption (see Fig. 10.14) is often seen at one aspect of a tooth socket and complementary osteoblastic deposition (see Fig. 10.13) at the opposite side, thus indicating bodily movement of the tooth through the bone; this is the mechanism which permits tooth movement during orthodontic treatment.

The periodontal membrane is richly supplied by blood vessels and nerves from the surrounding alveolar bone, the apical region and the gingiva. Small clumps of epithelial cells are often found scattered throughout the periodontal membrane; these cells are remnants of Hertwig's sheath (see Fig. 13.5) and are known as *epithelial rests of Malassez* **M**.

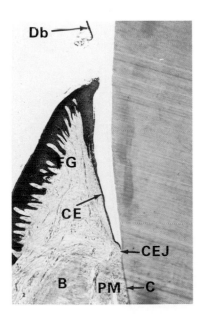

Fig. 13.9 Gingival attachment

(Decalcified section, H & E × 20)

This micrograph shows the relationship of the gingiva or gum to the neck of the tooth. During tissue preparation the enamel has been completely dissolved from the surface of the crown, but the extent of the outer surface of the enamel can be visualised by shreds of remaining organic debris **Db** which had been adherent to the tooth surface.

The gingiva may be divided into the *attached gingiva* which provides a protective covering to the upper alveolar bone **B**, and the *free gingiva* **FG** which forms a cuff around the enamel at the neck of the tooth. Between the enamel and the free gingiva is a potential space, the gingival crevice, which extends from the tip of the free gingiva to the cemento-enamel junction **CEJ**.

The thick, stratified squamous epithelium, which constitutes the oral aspect of the gingiva, undergoes abrupt transition at the tip of the free gingiva to form a thin layer of epithelial cells tapering to only two or three cells thick at the base of the gingival crevice. This crevicular epithelium **CE** is easily breached by pathogenic organisms and the underlying connective tissue is thus frequently infiltrated by lymphoid cells.

Collagen fibres of the periodontal membrane **PM** radiate from the cementum **C** near the cemento-enamel junction into the dense connective tissue of the free gingiva; these fibres, together with circular fibres surrounding the neck of the tooth, maintain the role of the gingiva as a protective cuff.

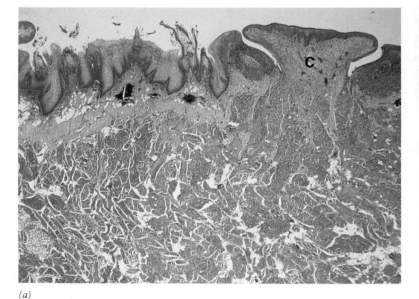

(a)

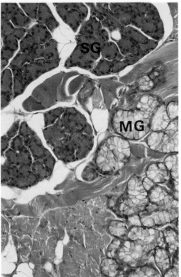

(b)

Fig. 13.10 Tongue

(H & E (a) × 6 (b) × 100)

The tongue is a muscular organ covered by oral mucosa which is specialised for manipulating food, general sensory reception and the special sensory function of taste.

A V-shaped groove, the *sulcus terminalis* demarcates the anterior two-thirds of the tongue from the posterior one-third. The mucosa of the anterior two-thirds is formed into papillae of three types. The most numerous, the *filiform papillae*, appear as short 'bristles' macroscopically. Among them are scattered the small, red, globular *fungiform papillae*; details of both types are shown in Figure 13.11. 12–20 large *circumvallate papillae* form a row immediately anterior to the sulcus terminalis and these papillae contain most of the taste buds (see Figs. 13.12 and 21.1); a circumvallate papilla **C** and numerous filiform papillae are seen in micrograph (a).

The body of the tongue consists of a mass of interlacing bundles of skeletal muscle fibres which permit an extensive range of tongue movements. The mucous membrane covering the tongue is firmly bound to the underlying muscle by a dense, collagenous lamina propria which is continuous with the epimysium of the tongue muscle.

Numerous small serous and mucous accessory salivary glands are scattered throughout the muscle and lamina propria of the tongue and are seen at higher magnification in micrograph (b); in these preparations the serous glands **SG** are stained strongly whereas the mucous glands **MG** are poorly stained. Note bundles of skeletal muscle cut in both transverse and longitudinal section.

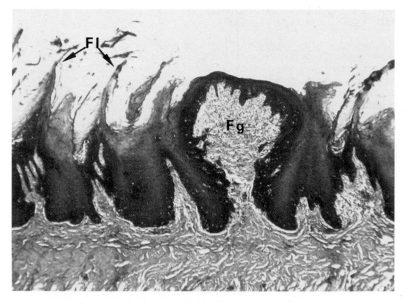

Fig. 13.11 Filiform and fungiform papillae

(H & E × 30)

This micrograph illustrates several filiform papillae **Fl** and a fungiform papilla **Fg**. Filiform papillae are the most numerous type and consist of a dense, connective tissue core and a heavily keratinised surface projection. Fungiform papillae have a thin, non-keratinised epithelium and a richly vascularised connective tissue core giving them a red appearance macroscopically amongst the much more numerous, whitish, filiform papillae.

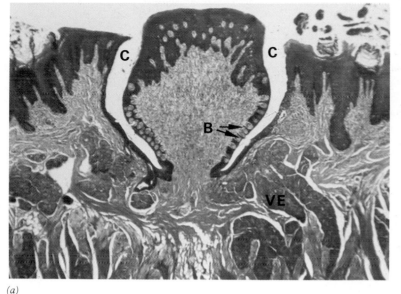

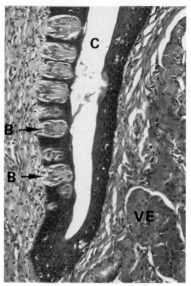

(a)

(b)

Fig. 13.12 Circumvallate papilla

(H & E (a) × 30 (b) × 100)

Circumvallate papillae are the largest and least common type of papilla on the tongue. They are set into the tongue surface and encircled by a deep cleft **C** as seen at higher magnification in micrograph (b). The stratified epithelium lining the papillary wall of the cleft contains numerous taste buds **B**, the detail of which is shown in Figure 21.1.

Aggregations of serous glands, called von Ebner's glands **VE**, open into the base of the circumvallate clefts secreting a watery fluid which dissolves food constituents thus facilitating taste reception.

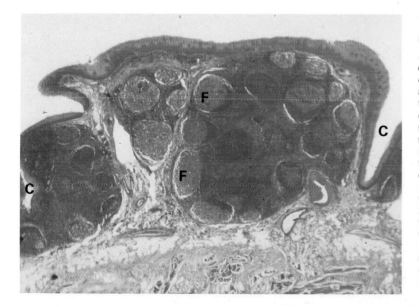

Fig. 13.13 Lingual tonsil

(H & E × 30)

Apart from being of different embyrological origin and having different sensory innervation to the anterior two-thirds, the posterior one-third of the tongue has a distinctly different mucosal surface. The posterior surface has a relatively smooth stratified squamous epithelium under which lies masses of lymphoid tissue containing typical lymphoid follicles **F**. This mass of lymphoid tissue is known as the *lingual tonsil* and with the palatine tonsils and adenoids completes a ring of lymphoid tissue guarding the entrance to the gastrointestinal and respiratory tracts. Like the palatine tonsils (see Fig. 11.14), the lingual lymphoid aggregations are penetrated by epithelial crypts **C** which function in a similar manner to those of the palatine tonsil.

Salivary glands

Saliva is produced by three pairs of major salivary glands, the *parotid, submandibular* and *sublingual glands,* and numerous minor accessory glands scattered throughout the oral mucosa. The minor salivary glands secrete continuously and are, in general, under local control, whereas the major glands mainly secrete in response to parasympathetic activity which is produced by physical, chemical and psychological stimuli.

Saliva is a hypotonic, watery secretion containing variable amounts of mucus, enzymes (principally *amylase* and the antibacterial enzyme *lysozyme*), antibodies and inorganic ions. Two types of secretory cells are found in the salivary glands: serous cells and mucous cells. The parotid glands consist almost exclusively of serous cells and produce a thin, watery secretion rich in enzymes and antibodies. The sublingual glands have predominantly mucous secretory cells and produce a viscid secretion. The submandibular glands contain both serous and mucous secretory cells and produce a secretion of intermediate consistency. The overall composition of saliva varies according to the degree of activity of each of the major gland types.

Traditionally, the role of salivary amylase has been considered to be the initiation of starch digestion in the oral cavity; its primary role, however, is more likely to be as a cleansing agent for starch debris retained around the teeth. The protective role of salivary antibodies is poorly understood; they may be associated functionally with leucocytes also found in saliva.

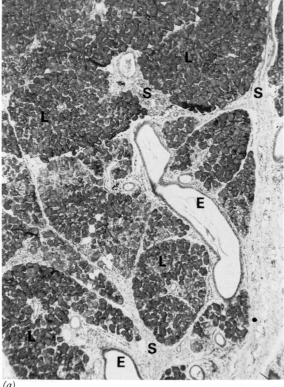

(a)

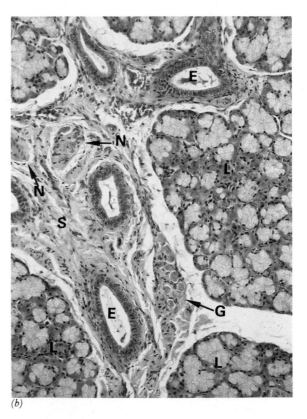

(b)

Fig. 13.14 Salivary gland

(a) PAS/Iron haematoxylin × 10 (b) H & E × 120

The general architecture of all the major salivary glands follows the pattern shown in micrograph (a). The glands are divided into numerous lobules **L** each containing many secretory units. Connective tissue septa **S** radiate between the lobules from an outer capsule and convey blood vessels, nerves and large excretory ducts **E**.

Micrograph (b) shows part of an interlobular septum from a submandibular gland. It contains several excretory ducts; note that these have a stratified cuboidal epithelial lining. Small parasympathetic nerves **N** and a tiny ganglion **G** are also visible in this specimen.

The surrounding secretory lobules contain a mixture of serous and mucous secretory cells, the former staining strongly with H & E, the latter almost unstained.

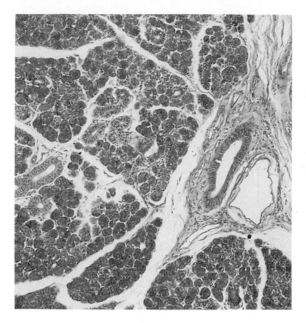

Fig. 13.15 Parotid gland

(H & E × 42)

The parotid gland is almost solely composed of serous secretory acini giving it a strongly stained appearance in H & E preparations.

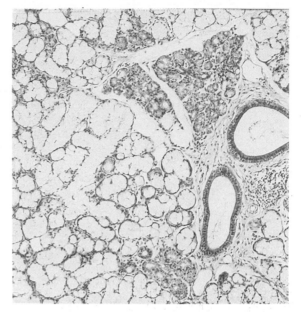

Fig. 13.16 Sublingual gland

(H & E × 42)

Mucous acini predominate in the sublingual glands making them stain very poorly with H & E; with methods such as PAS shown in Figure 13.14 (a), the mucin stains strongly.

Fig. 13.17 Salivary secretory unit

The salivary secretory unit consists of a terminal, branched, tubulo-acinar structure composed exclusively of either serous or mucous secretory cells or a mixture of both types. In mixed secretory units where mucous cells predominate, serous cells often form semilunar caps called *serous demilunes* surrounding the terminal part of the mucous acini.

The terminal secretory units merge to form larger, so-called *intercalated ducts* which are also lined by secretory cells. The intercalated ducts drain into larger ducts called *striated ducts* which are named for their striated appearance in light microscopy. The striations result from the presence of numerous, deep infoldings of the basal plasma membranes of the large cuboidal cells which line these ducts.

In addition to the salivary proteins, the serous cells are involved in active secretion of a watery fluid containing a variety of inorganic ions; this basic secretion is isotonic with plasma. In the striated ducts, the ionic content of the basic secretion is modified by active reabsorption and further secretion of ions to produce saliva which is hypotonic with respect to plasma. The ionic composition of saliva varies at different flow rates, but in general, the concentrations of sodium and chloride ions are below that of plasma, and the concentrations of potassium and bicarbonate ions are above that of plasma. The transport processes in the striated ducts are facilitated by the large surface area offered by the basal infoldings of the lining cells and fuelled by their numerous associated mitochondria.

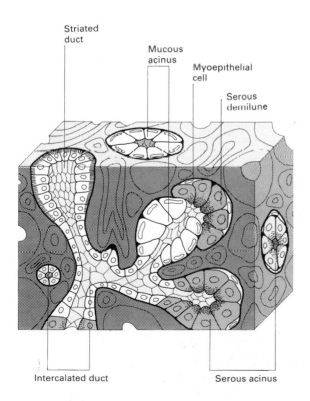

Striated duct

Mucous acinus

Myoepithelial cell

Serous demilune

Intercalated duct

Serous acinus

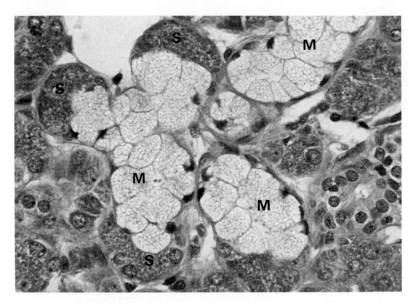

Fig. 13.18 Mixed sero-mucous secretory unit

(H & E × 480)

This micrograph of a mixed sero-mucous secretory unit shows several mucous acini **M** with serous demilunes **S**. In H & E stained preparations, mucigen granules within mucous acini are poorly stained whereas the enzyme-containing (zymogen) granules of serous acini are strongly stained. The nuclei of mucous cells are characteristically condensed and flattened against the basement membrane whereas the nuclei of serous cells are rounded, with dispersed chromatin, and usually occupy a more central position within the cell.

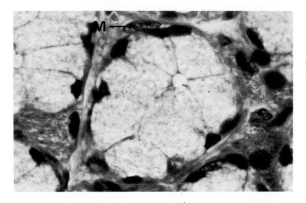

Fig. 13.19 Mucous acinus

(H & E × 800)

Both serous and mucous acini are embraced by the processes of contractile cells called *myoepithelial cells* which, on contraction, force secretion from the acinar lumen into the duct system. Myoepithelial cells are located between the basal plasma membranes of secretory cells and the epithelial basement membrane. These cells are flattened and have long processes which extend around the secretory acinus but in section they can only be recognised by their large, flattened nuclei lying within the basement membrane surrounding the acinus. This micrograph shows the typical appearance of a myoepithelial cell **M** embracing a mucous acinus.

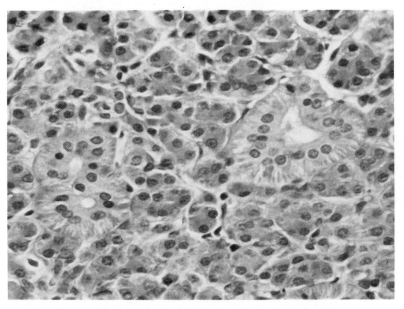

Fig. 13.20 Striated ducts

(H & E × 480)

The striated ducts are lined by large cuboidal cells with large nuclei located between the centre and luminal surface of the cell. The basal cytoplasm appears striated, reflecting the presence of deep basal infoldings of the plasma membrane and associated columns of mitochondria; the apical cytoplasm is uniformly stained and not striated. In predominantly serous salivary glands, the striated ducts are larger than in predominantly mucous glands, a feature associated with the role of the striated duct in modifying isotonic basic saliva to produce hypotonic saliva.

Note in this micrograph that the two striated ducts are surrounded by serous secretory units. Note also the rich capillary network in the sparse supporting tissue between the secretory acini.

14. Gastrointestinal tract

Introduction

The gastrointestinal system is primarily involved in reducing food for absorption into the body. This process occurs in five main phases within defined regions of the gastrointestinal system: ingestion, fragmentation, digestion, absorption and elimination of waste products. The gastrointestinal system is essentially a muscular tract lined by a mucous membrane which exhibits regional variations in structure reflecting the changing functions of the system from the mouth to the anus.

Ingestion and initial fragmentation of food occur in the oral cavity, resulting in the formation of a bolus of food which is then conveyed to the *oesophagus* by the action of the tongue and pharyngeal muscles during swallowing *(deglutition)*. Fragmentation and swallowing are facilitated by the secretion of saliva from three pairs of major salivary glands and numerous small accessory glands within the oral cavity. The oesophagus conducts food from the oral cavity to the *stomach* where fragmentation is completed and digestion initiated. Digestion is the process by which food is progressively broken down by enzymes into molecules which are small enough to be absorbed into the circulation; for example, ingested proteins are first broken down into polypeptides then further degraded to small peptides and amino-acids which can then be absorbed. Initial digestion accompanied by intense muscular action of the stomach wall, reduces the stomach contents to a semi-digested liquid called *chyme*. Chyme is squirted through a muscular sphincter, the *pylorus*, into the *duodenum*, the short, first part of the *small intestine*, where it is neutralised partly by an alkaline secretion from the duodenal mucosa. Digestive enzymes from a large exocrine gland, the *pancreas*, enter the duodenum together with *bile* from the *liver* via the *common bile duct*; bile contains excretory products of liver metabolism, some of which act as emulsifying agents necessary for fat digestion. The duodenal contents pass onwards along the small intestine where the process of digestion is completed and the main absorptive phase occurs. After the duodenum, the next segment of the small intestine, where the major part of absorption occurs, is called the *jejunum*; the rest of the small intestine is called the *ileum*, but there is no distinct junction between these parts of the tract.

The unabsorbed liquid residue from the small intestine passes through a valve, the *ileo-caecal valve*, into the *large intestine*. In the large intestine, water is absorbed from the liquid residue which becomes progressively more solid as it passes towards the anus. The first part of the large intestine is called the *caecum*, from which projects a blind-ended sac, the *appendix*. The next part of the large intestine, the *colon*, is divided anatomically into *ascending, transverse, descending* and *sigmoid* segments although histologically the segments are similar. The terminal portion of the large intestine, the *rectum*, is a holding chamber for faeces prior to defaecation via the *anal canal*.

Food is propelled along the gastrointestinal tract by two main mechanisms: voluntary muscular action in the oral cavity, pharynx and upper third of the oesophagus is succeeded by involuntary waves of smooth muscle contraction called *peristalsis*. Peristalsis and the secretory activity of the entire gastrointestinal system are modulated by the autonomic nervous system and a variety of hormones, some of which are secreted by endocrine cells located within the gastrointestinal tract itself. These cells constitute a diffuse endocrine organ, called the *gastrointestinal endocrine system*, which not only regulates gastrointestinal functions but also has a wide range of metabolic influences; this system is discussed in Chapter 17.

Because of its continuity with the external environment, the gastrointestinal system is a potential portal of entry for pathogenic organisms. Thus the system incorporates a number of defence mechanisms which include prominent aggregations of lymphoid tissue distributed throughout the tract.

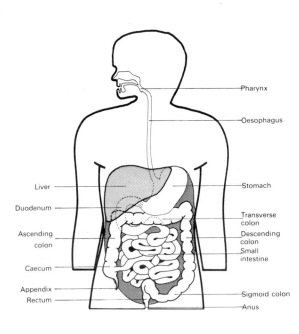

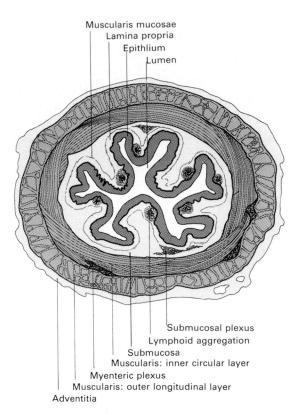

Fig. 14.1 Structure of the gastrointestinal tract

The structure of the gastrointestinal tract conforms to a general plan which is clearly evident from the oesophagus to the anus.

The tract is essentially a muscular tube lined by a mucous membrane. The arrangement of the major muscular component remains relatively constant throughout the tract whereas the mucosa shows marked variations in the different regions of the tract.

The gastrointestinal tract has four distinct functional layers: *mucosa, submucosa, muscularis* and *adventitia.*

1. The mucosa: the mucosa is divided, histologically, into three layers: an epithelial lining, a supporting connective tissue lamina propria and a thin smooth muscle layer, the *muscularis mucosae,* which produces local movements and folding of the mucosa. At several points along the tract the mucosa undergoes abrupt transition from one form to another: these points are the oesophageo-gastric junction, the gastro-duodenal junction, the ileo-caecal junction and the recto-anal junction.

2. The submucosa: this layer of loose connective tissue supports the mucosa and contains the larger blood vessels, lymphatics and nerves.

3. The muscularis propria: the muscular wall proper consists of smooth muscle which is subdivided usually into two histological layers: an inner circular layer and an outer longitudinal layer. The action of these smooth muscle layers, opposed at right angles to one another, is the basis of peristaltic contraction.

4. The adventitia: this outer layer of connective tissue conducts the major vessels and nerves. In the abdominal cavity it is continuous with the connective tissue of the mesenteries and in other sites it is continuous with the surrounding connective tissues. Where the adventitia is exposed to the abdominal cavity it is referred to as the *serosa*

and is lined by a simple squamous epithelium called mesothelium.

The smooth muscle of the bowel has its own inherent rhythmicity which is modulated by the autonomic nervous system, in particular the parasympathetic nervous system. As in other organs of the body, parasympathetic efferent fibres synapse with effector neurones in small ganglia located in or close to the organ involved. In the gastrointestinal tract, parasympathetic ganglia are concentrated in so-called plexuses in the wall of the tract. In the submucosa, isolated or small clusters of parasympathetic ganglion cells give rise to post-ganglionic fibres which supply the mucosal glands and the smooth muscle of the muscularis mucosae; this submucosal plexus is sometimes referred to as *Meissner's plexus.* Larger clusters of parasympathetic ganglion cells are found between the two layers of the muscularis; the post-ganglionic fibres mainly supply the surrounding smooth muscle. This plexus is known as the *myenteric plexus* or *Auerbach's plexus.*

Glands are found throughout the tract at various depths in the tract wall. Firstly, in some parts of the tract, the mucosal lining is arranged into glands which have a variety of secretory functions. Secondly, in some regions, glands penetrate the muscularis mucosa to lie in the submucosa. Thirdly, the pancreas and liver are large glands draining into the gastrointestinal lumen but lying entirely outside the tract wall.

Lymphoid tissue is distributed throughout the gastrointestinal tract both as diffusely-scattered cells particularly in the lamina propria and as dense aggregations which may form follicles; in toto, this mass of lymphoid tissue constitutes the gut associated lymphoid tissue (GALT) described in Chapter 11.

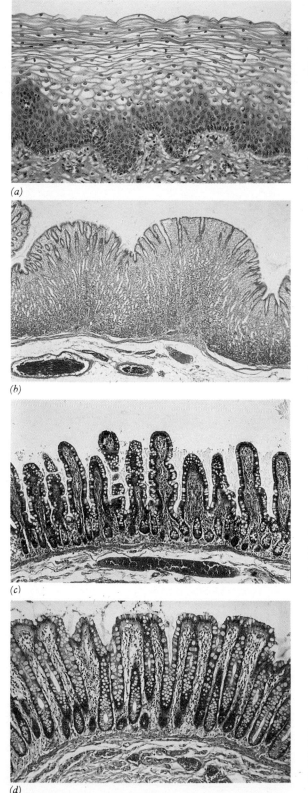

(a)

(b)

(c)

(d)

Fig. 14.2 Basic mucosal forms in the gastrointestinal tract

(a) × 128 (b) × 100 (c) × 128 (d) × 128

There are four basic musocal types found in the gastrointestinal tract which can be classified according to their main function:

(a) **Protective:** this is found in the oral cavity, pharynx, oesophagus and anal canal. The surface epithelium is stratified squamous which is keratinised in animals which have a coarse diet, e.g. rodents, herbivores.

(b) **Secretory:** this occurs only in the stomach. The mucosa consists of long, closely packed, tubular glands which are simple or branched depending on the region of stomach.

(c) **Absorptive:** this mucosal form is typical of the entire small intestine. The mucosa is folded into finger-like projections called villi (to increase surface area) with intervening short glands called crypts.
Note: in the duodenum the crypts extend through the muscularis mucosae to form submucosal mucous glands.

(d) **Absorptive/Protective:** this form lines the whole of the large intestine. The mucosa is arranged into closely packed, straight glands consisting of cells specialised for water absorption and mucus-secreting goblet cells which lubricate the passage of faeces.

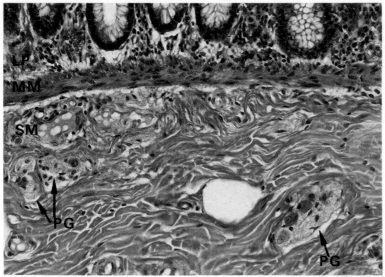

(a)

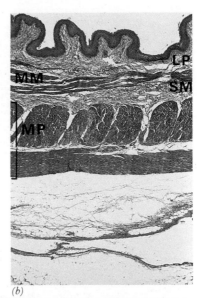

(b)

Fig. 14.3 Components of the wall of the gastrointestinal tract

(H & E (a) × 480 (b) × 28 (c) × 320)

This series of micrographs illustrates the layers of the wall of the tract deep to the surface epithelium.

Micrograph (a) illustrates the deep part of the large bowel mucosa, the muscularis mucosae **MM**, clearly demarcating the delicate lamina propria **LP** from the more robust underlying submucosa **SM**; this arrangement is fairly typical of the whole of the gastrointestinal tract.

The *lamina propria* consists of loose areolar connective tissue which appears highly cellular due to the presence of considerable numbers of leucocytes and other cells of the general defence system (see Fig. 4.16) which deal with any microorganisms which might breach the intestinal epithelium. The lamina propria also contains numerous lymphocytes of the immune system (GALT) which in some areas form dense aggregations. The lamina propria is also typically rich in blood and lymphatic capillaries necessary to support the secretory, absorptive and other highly active functions of the mucosa.

The *muscularis mucosae* consists of several layers of smooth muscle fibres, those in the deeper layers oriented parallel to the luminal surface. The more superficial fibres are oriented at right angles to the surface and extend up into the lamina propria between the glands; in the case of the small intestine, the fibres extend up into the villi as seen in Figure 14.21. Activity of the muscularis mucosae keeps the mucosal surface and glands in a constant state of gentle agitation which expels secretions from the deep glandular crypts, prevents clogging and enhances contact between epithelium and luminal contents for absorption.

The *submucosa* consists of fairly dense, collagenous connective tissue which binds the mucosa to the main bulk of the muscular wall. The submucosa contains the larger blood vessels and lymphatics as well as the nerves supplying the mucosa. Tiny parasympathetic ganglia **PG** are scattered throughout the submucosa forming the submucosal (Meissner's) plexus from which postganglionic fibres supply the muscularis mucosae.

The typical arrangement of the two layers of the muscular wall proper is seen in micrograph (b) which shows a

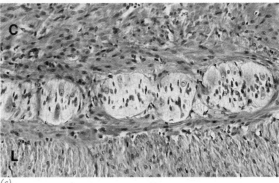

(c)

longitudinal section of the oesophagus, the *muscularis propria* **MP** being made up of an outer longitudinal layer and a somewhat broader, inner circular layer; there has been some artefactual separation of the layers making them easier to visualise. The submucosa **SM** is separated from the lamina propria **LP** by the muscularis mucosae **MM**. In the oesophagus, where the function of the mucosa is to protect against friction, the lamina propria is more collagenous than elsewhere and the muscularis mucosae is more prominent.

Micrograph (c) illustrates, at high magnification, the junction of outer longitudinal **L** and inner circular **C** layers of the muscularis propria in the large intestine; between the layers are clumps of parasympathetic ganglion cells of the myenteric (Auerbach's) plexus. The two layers of the muscularis propria undergo synchronized rhythmic contractions which pass in peristaltic waves down the tract propelling the contents distally. Peristalsis is inherent in the smooth muscle itself but the level of activity is modulated by the autonomic nervous system (especially the parasympathetic system), locally produced gastrointestinal tract hormones and other environmental factors.

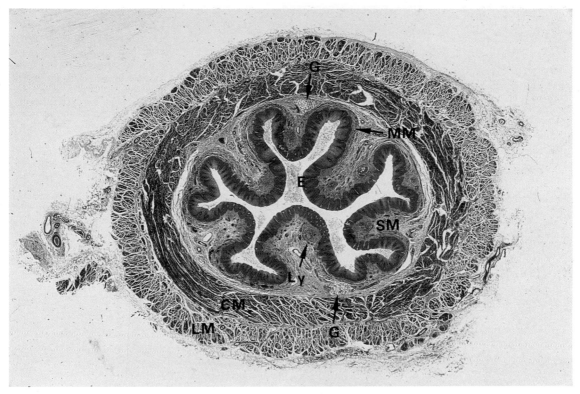

(a)

Fig. 14.4 Oesophagus

(Masson's trichrome (a) × 9 (b) × 320)

The oesophagus is a strong muscular tube which conveys food from the oropharynx to the stomach. The initiation of swallowing is a voluntary act involving the skeletal musculature of the oropharynx which is then succeeded by a strong peristaltic reflex which conveys the bolus of food or drink to the stomach. Food and drink do not normally remain in the oesophagus for more then a few seconds and reflux and regurgitation are normally prevented by a physiological sphincter at the oesophageo-gastric junction. Below the diaphragm, the oesophagus passes for a short distance in the abdominal cavity before joining the stomach at an acute angle. Sphincter control appears to involve diaphragmatic contraction, an excess of intra-abdominal pressure over intragastric pressure being exerted upon the abdominal part of the oesophagus, unidirectional peristalsis and maintenance of correct anatomical arrangements of the structures.

Micrograph (a) shows the lower third of the oesophagus. In the relaxed state, the oesophageal mucosa is deeply folded, an arrangement which permits gross distension during the passage of a food bolus.

The lumen of the oesophagus is lined by a thick protective stratified squamous epithelium **E** which, in some animals with coarse diets, e.g. rodents, may be keratinised. The underlying lamina propria is relatively condensed and contains scattered lymphoid aggregations **Ly**; the underlying muscularis mucosae **MM** is barely visible at this magnification.

The submucosa **SM** is highly vascular and relatively loose allowing for considerable distension during passage of a food bolus. The submucosa also contains small mucous glands **G**

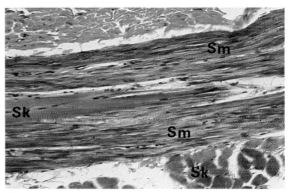

(b)

which aid lubrication and are mainly confined to the lower third of the oesophagus.

The muscularis propria is thick and inner circular **CM** and outer longitudinal **LM** layers of smooth muscle are clearly distinguishable. Since the first part of swallowing is under voluntary control, fasciculi of skeletal muscle predominate in the muscularis of the upper third of the oesophagus. Micrograph (b) shows part of the muscularis propria of the upper oesophagus at high magnification. A bundle of skeletal muscle **Sk**, is seen cut in transverse section. The longitudinal muscle here consists mainly of smooth muscle **Sm** with a couple of skeletal muscle fibres **Sk** in their midst.

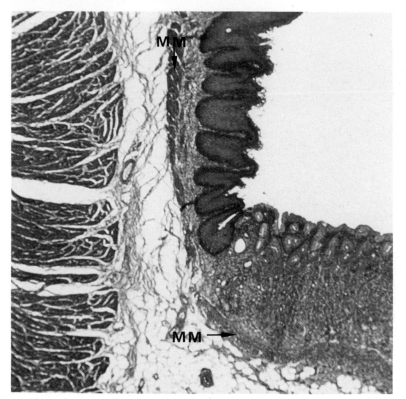

Fig. 14.5 Oesophageo-gastric junction

(H & E × 40)

At the junction of the oesophagus with the stomach, the mucosa of the tract undergoes an abrupt transition from a protective, stratified squamous epithelium to a highly glandular mucosa. The muscularis mucosae **MM** is continuous across the junction though it becomes less clearly visible in the stomach where it lies immediately beneath the base of the gastric glands. The underlying submucosa and muscularis propria continue uninterrupted beneath the mucosal junction. The muscularis propria does not form a thick anatomical sphincter but rather there is a physiological sphincter mechanism which is described with Figure 14.4.

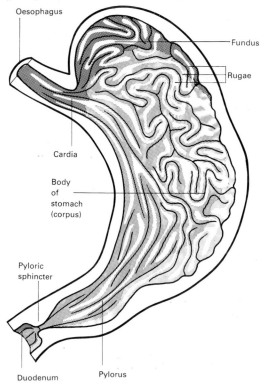

Fig. 14.6 Stomach

The stomach is a dilated part of the gastrointestinal tract in which ingested food is retained for 2 hours or longer so as to undergo mechanical and chemical reduction to form chyme. Mechanical reduction is produced by a strong, muscular, churning action whilst chemical reduction is produced by gastric juices secreted by the glands of the stomach mucosa. There is little absorption of food products from the stomach, although alcohol is a notable exception. Once chyme formation is completed, the pyloric sphincter relaxes and allows the liquid chyme to be squirted into the duodenum. In the non-distended state, the stomach mucosa is thrown into prominent longitudinal folds called *rugae* which permit great distension after eating.

Anatomically the stomach is divided into four regions: the *cardia, fundus, body (corpus)* and *pylorus (pyloric antrum)*. The pylorus terminates in a strong muscular sphincter surrounding the gastroduodenal junction.

The mucosa of the whole stomach is glandular and there are three distinctly different histological zones:

1. The cardia is a small area of predominantly mucus-secreting glands surrounding the entrance of the oesophagus (see Fig. 14.5).

2. The mucosa of the fundus and body forms the major histological region and consists of glands which secrete gastric juices as well as some protective mucus.

3. The pylorus has a different glandular conformation; here the glands secrete mucus, and associated endocrine cells secrete the hormone *gastrin*.

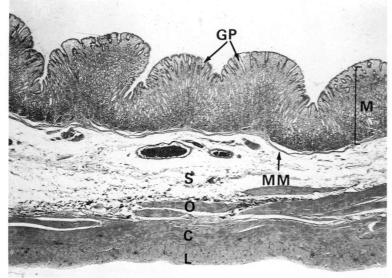

Fig. 14.7 Body of the stomach
(H & E × 12)

This micrograph illustrates the body of the stomach in the non-distended state. The mucosa **M** is thrown into prominent folds or rugae and consists of *gastric glands* which extend from the level of the muscularis mucosae **MM** to open into the stomach lumen via *gastric pits* **GP**.

The muscularis comprises the usual inner circular **C** and outer longitudinal **L** layers but the inner circular layer is reinforced by a further inner oblique layer **O**. The submucosa **S** is relatively loose and distensable and contains the larger blood vessels. The serosal layer which covers the peritoneal surface is thin and barely visible at this magnification.

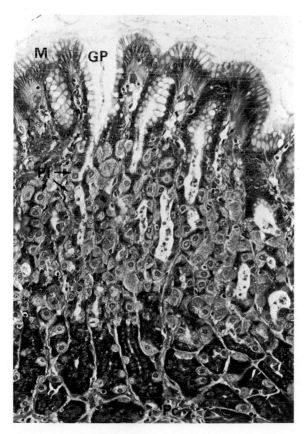

Fig. 14.8 Gastric glands
(H & E × 120)

The mucosa of the fundus and body of the stomach consists of straight, tubular glands which synthesise and secrete gastric juice. Gastric juice is a watery secretion containing hydrochloric acid (pH 0.9–1.5) and the digestive enzyme *pepsin* which hydrolyses proteins into polypeptide fragments. The stomach mucosa is protected from self-digestion by a thick surface covering of mucus.

The gastric glands contain a mixed population of cells of three main types:

1. Mucus-secreting cells **M** cover the luminal surface of the stomach and line the gastric pits **GP** into which the gastric glands open; the cytoplasmic mucigen granules which pack these cells are stained poorly by H & E. Another type of mucous cell, the *neck mucous cell*, is found in the necks of the glands.

2. Hydrochloric acid-secreting cells, called *parietal* **Pl** or *oxyntic cells*, are distributed along the length of the glands but tend to be most numerous in the middle portion. These large, rounded cells have an extensive eosinophilic (oxyntic) cytoplasm and a centrally located nucleus.

3. Pepsin-secreting cells, called *peptic* **Pc**, *chief*, or *zymogenic cells*, tend to be clustered at the base of the gastric glands. Peptic cells are recognised by their condensed, basally located nuclei and strongly basophilic granular cytoplasm which reflects their huge content of ribosomes.

Thin strands of the muscularis mucosae extend between the gastric glands from the base; contraction of this muscle expels gastric secretions into the stomach lumen.

In addition to the exocrine cells of the gastric mucosa, endocrine secretory cells are found scattered throughout the gastric mucosa as in the mucosa of the rest of the gastrointestinal tract.

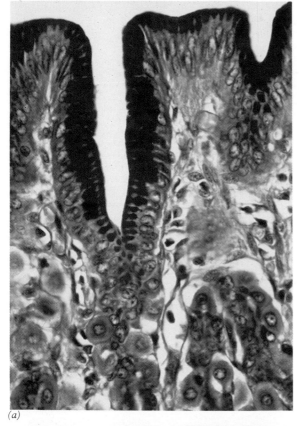

(a)

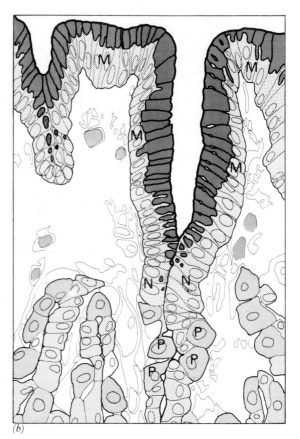

(b)

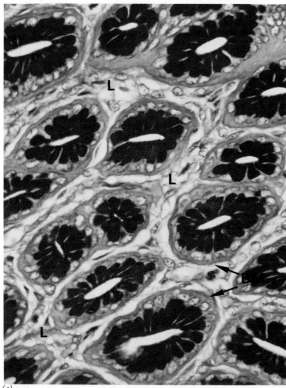

(c)

Fig. 14.9 Gastric pits

(PAS/Haematoxylin/Orange G (a) LS × 480 (b) explanatory diagram (c) TS × 200)

The PAS method has been used in these preparations to highlight the mucus-secreting cells of the gastric mucosa; mucus is PAS-positive because it is a polysaccharide. The stomach surface is lined by a single layer of tall columnar, mucus-secreting cells **M** which are shed continuously and replaced by cells which migrate from the gastric pits. Other mucus-secreting cells in the necks of the gastric glands, called neck mucous cells **N**, secrete a less viscous mucus which may protect the gland duct from autodigestion.

In transverse section as seen in micrograph (c), the tubular nature of the gastric pits is clearly evident. One or more gastric glands may open into each gastric pit. Note the richly vascularised, loose connective tissue of the lamina propria **L** which supports the gastric pits and glands. Note also in micrograph (c), the basement membrane **BM**, lightly PAS-positive, which lies between the epithelium and connective tissue.

Parietal (acid-secreting) cells **P** in the upper parts of the gastric glands can be recognised by their characteristic 'fried egg' appearance; in this preparation their acidophilic cytoplasm is stained strongly with Orange G.

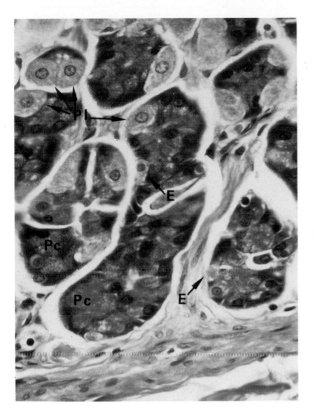

Fig. 14.10 Base of gastric gland
(H & E × 320)

Peptic **Pc** (chief) cells which synthesize and secrete the proteolytic enzyme pepsin, are the principal cell type in the basal third of the gastric glands, although parietal cells **Pl** are also found at this level. Peptic cells have a basally-located nucleus and extensive, granular cytoplasm packed with rough endoplasmic reticulum, the ribosomes of which account for the marked cytoplasmic basophilia. The inactive pepsin precursor, *pepsinogen* is synthesized by the ribosomes and stored in numerous secretory granules located towards the luminal surface. Pepsinogen remains inactive until it reaches the lumen of the stomach where it is activated by the gastric juices; this mechanism prevents destruction of the gastric glands by autodigestion.

In contrast to the peptic cells, the parietal cells are rounded with large centrally-located nuclei and eosinophilic (pink-stained) cytoplasm; the eosinophilia is due to the numerous mitochondria which are a feature of these metabolically highly active cells. Whereas peptic cells tend to occur in clusters at the base of the gastric glands, parietal cells are scattered throughout the glands from neck to base.

The secretory activity of both parietal and peptic cells is controlled by the autonomic nervous system and the gastrointestinal hormone *gastrin* secreted by endocrine cells mainly located in the pylorus. A variety of other APUD cells of the gastrointestinal endocrine system are also scattered in the gastric mucosa and elsewhere in the gastrointestinal tract. Occasionally, the endocrine cells **E** can be identified in sections fixed with chromium containing fixatives as in this example.

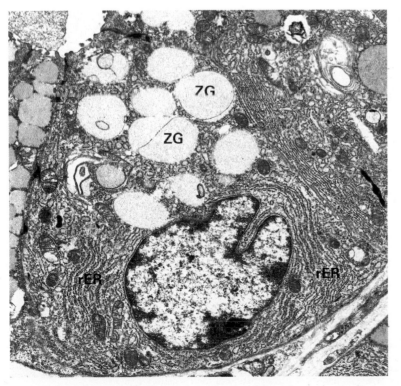

Fig. 14.11 Peptic cell
(Rat: EM × 7200)

This electron micrograph illustrates a peptic cell at the base of a gastric gland. The ultrastructural features of peptic cells are those of protein secreting (zymogenic) cells in general; these features include an extensive rough endoplasmic reticulum **rER** and membrane bound secretory vesicles **ZG** (zymogen granules) crowded in the apical cytoplasm, thus restricting the nucleus to the base of the cell. The extensive rough endoplasmic reticulum accounts for the intense basophilia of peptic cells seen with light microscopy.

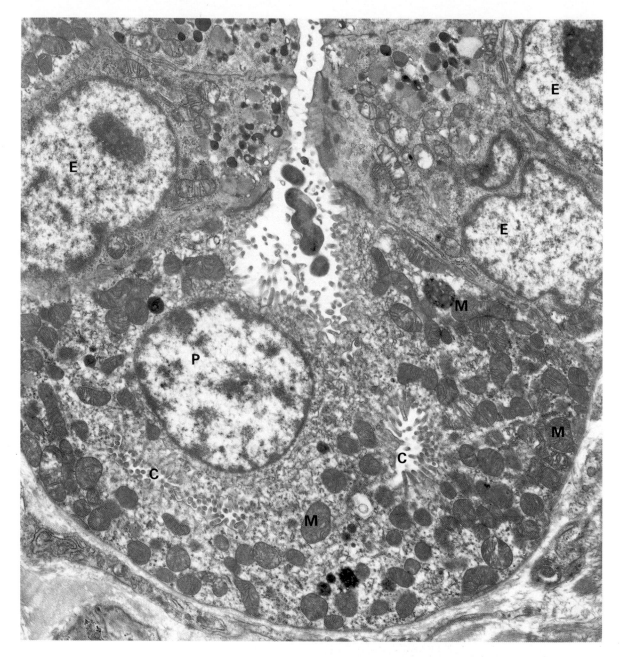

Fig. 14.12 Parietal cell

(Rat: EM × 9600)

This micrograph shows a parietal cell **P** within a gastric gland. The luminal plasma membrane of the parietal cell forms deep, branching canaliculi **C** which extend throughout the cytoplasm. Numerous short microvilli project into the lumina of the intracellular canaliculi greatly increasing the surface area. The cytoplasm is crowded with mitochondria **M** which have closely packed cristae.

An extensive labyrinth of smooth endoplasmic reticulum pervades the cytoplasm. The mechanism by which parietal cells produce hydrochloric acid is poorly understood. The concentration of hydrogen ions, by the order of one million

times compared with plasma, and the equivalent concentration of chloride ions, is a highly energy-dependent process; this energy is provided by the extremely numerous mitochondria. Parietal cells are also thought to secrete the substance called *intrinsic factor* which is essential for the absorption of vitamin B_{12} in the terminal ileum.

Also seen in this micrograph are several endocrine cells **E** of the gastrointestinal endocrine series which are recognised by their small electron-dense secretory granules. Special histochemical techniques must be used to identify the precise nature of their secretory product.

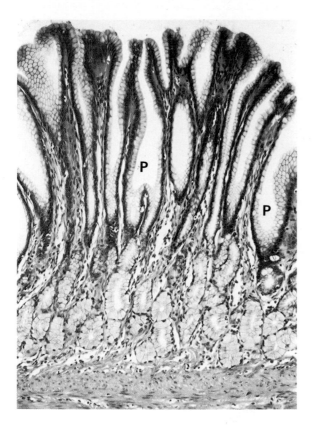

Fig. 14.13 Pyloric stomach

(H & E × 120)

In contrast to the simple tubular glands of the fundus and body, the pyloric glands are branched, and are composed almost exclusively of mucus-secreting cells which stain poorly with standard histological methods. The glands open into deep, irregularly shaped pits **P** giving a characteristic frond-like appearance in histological sections. The function of the mucus secreted by the pyloric glands is to lubricate and protect the entrance to the duodenum.

Scattered amongst the pyloric mucous cells are endocrine cells which secrete the peptide hormone gastrin and are thus called 'G' cells. Demonstration of G cells requires special histochemical methods as shown in Figure 14.14.

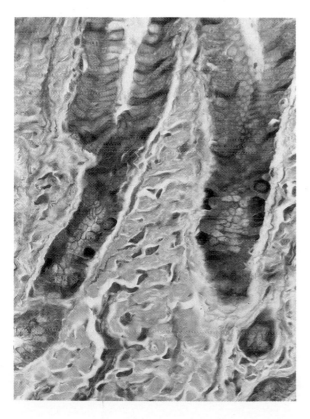

Fig. 14.14 Gastrin cells

(Frozen section, modified aldehyde fucsin × 480)

Throughout the gastrointestinal mucosa are numerous APUD cells of the gastrointestinal endocrine system which is described in detail in Chapter 17. These cells secrete a variety of peptide hormones usually in response to some local stimulus and most of these hormones then act on the same or some functionally-related parts of the gastrointestinal tract to produce a complementary response.

Gastrin cells were amongst the earliest of the gastrointestinal endocrine cells to be recognised. Since they are found in fairly large numbers and their distribution is more or less restricted to the pyloric region of the stomach, their secretion product and its actions have been relatively easy to elucidate, unlike that of many of the newfound APUD cells.

The presence of food in the stomach stimulates the secretion of gastrin into the blood stream; gastrin then promotes secretion of pepsin and acid by the gastric glands of the fundus and body as well as enhancing gastric motility.

This empirical staining method demonstrates gastrin cells in the pyloric mucosa, the cytoplasm of the G cells being stained a dark purple colour.

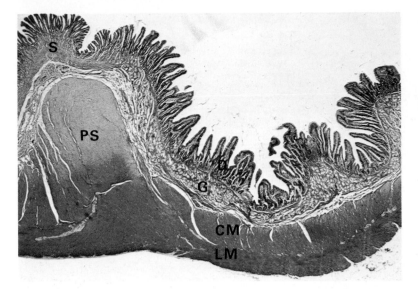

Fig. 14.15 Gastroduodenal junction

(Monkey: H & E × 12)

The pyloric sphincter **PS** marks a dramatic transition in the gastrointestinal mucosa from the glandular arrangement of the stomach **S** to the villous arrangement which characterises the duodenum **D** and the rest of the small intestine. In addition, the duodenum is characterised by the presence of numerous mucus-secreting glands **G** which lie in the submucosa. These submucosal glands are called *Brunner's glands* and are not found elsewhere in the small intestine.

The pyloric sphincter consists of an extreme thickening of the circular layer of the muscularis at the gastroduodenal junction. Note the continuity of both the circular **CM** and longitudinal **LM** layers of the muscularis between the pylorus and duodenum.

Fig. 14.16 Duodenum *(illustrations opposite)*

(H & E (a) monkey × 20 (b) human × 15 (c) Brunner's glands of monkey × 50)

The duodenum, which represents the first part of the small intestine, receives partly digested food in the form of acidic chyme from the stomach via the pyloric canal. The main function of the duodenum is to neutralise gastric acid and pepsin and to initiate further digestive processes.

Micrograph (a) illustrates monkey duodenum. The mucosa **M** has the characteristic villous form of the whole of the small intestine with glandular crypts between the villi extending down to the muscularis mucosae **MM**. The feature unique to the duodenum is the extensive mass of coiled, branched, tubular glands in the submucosa **SM**. The ducts of these *Brunner's glands* pass up to the muscularis mucosae to open into the crypts between the mucosal villi. Beneath the mass of submucosal glands, the smooth muscle wall consists of an inner circular layer **CM** and an outer longitudinal layer **LM** as in the rest of the small intestine.

A specimen of human duodenum is shown for comparison in micrograph (b). Note the extraordinary thickness of the layer of glands in the submucosa **SM** and the thin layer of glands in the lamina propria **LP** above the muscularis mucosae **MM**. The mucosal form is almost indistinguishable from that of the monkey.

Micrograph (c) shows a Brunner's gland from the distal part of the duodenum where the glands tend to be smaller and less branched than in the proximal section. The tall, columnar cells of Brunner's glands have extensive, poorly stained, mucigen-filled cytoplasm and dense, basally located nuclei. The presence of chyme in the duodenum stimulates Brunner's glands to secrete a thin, alkaline mucus which helps to neutralise the acidic chyme and to protect the duodenal mucosa from autodigestion.

Chyme also stimulates the release of two peptide hormones, *secretin*, and *cholecystokinin-pancreozymin (CCK)* from APUD cells of the gastrointestinal endocrine system scattered throughout the duodenal mucosa. Secretin and CCK promote pancreatic secretion into the pancreatic duct, and CCK also stimulates contraction of the gall bladder thus propelling bile into the common bile duct. The pancreatic and bile ducts merge to empty their contents into the duodenum via a single short duct.

Pancreatic juice is highly alkaline due to a high content of bicarbonate ions and thus helps to neutralise the acidic gastric contents entering the duodenum. The pancreas also secretes a variety of digestive enzymes including the proteolytic enzymes *trypsin* and *chymotrypsin*; like the pepsin of the stomach, these are secreted in an inactive pro-enzyme form. On entering the duodenal lumen, trypsin is activated by the enzyme *enterokinase* secreted by the duodenal mucosa; activated trypsin then in turn activates the chymotrypsin. The pancreatic enzymes, which also include amylase and lipases initiate the processes of luminal digestion described overleaf. The biliary secretions contain bile acids which act as emulsifying agents and are particularly important in the digestion of lipids.

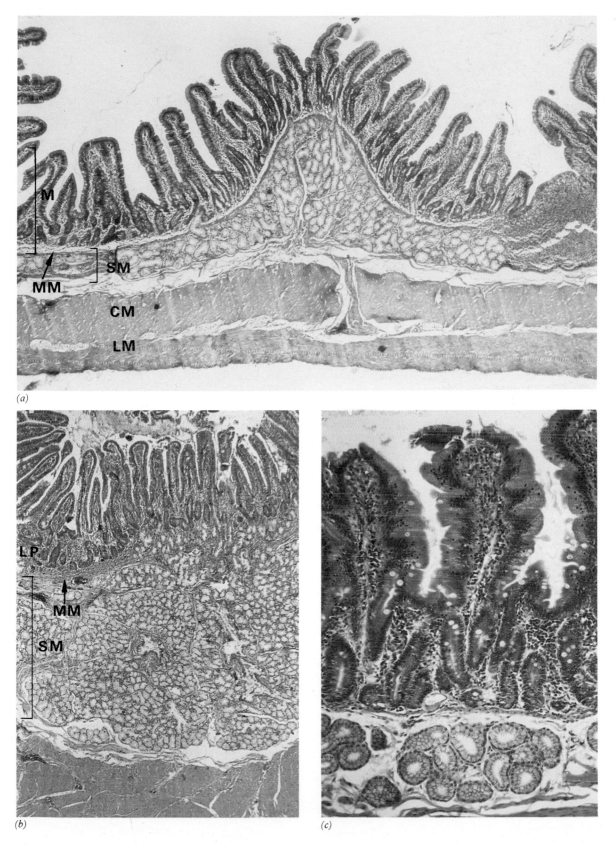

(a)

(b)

(c)

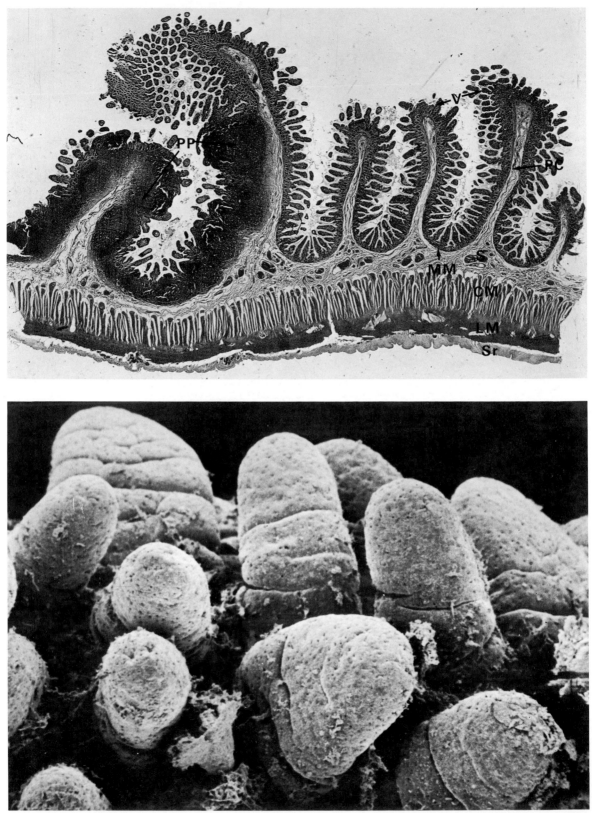

(a)

(b)

Fig. 14.17 Small intestine *(illustrations opposite)*

(a) H & E × 16 (b) Scanning EM × 100

The small intestine, comprising the duodenum, jejunum and ileum, is the principal site for absorption of digestion products from the gastrointestinal tract. Digestion begins in the stomach and is completed in the small intestine in intimate association with the absorption process.

Digestion and absorption are enhanced by the provision of an enormous surface area in the small intestine by virtue of four main features:

1. The great length of the small intestine (4–6 m long in man);

2. The presence of circularly arranged folds of the mucosa and submucosa called *plica circulares* or *valves of Kerckring*; the plica are particularly numerous in the jejunum;

3. The arrangement of the mucosa into extremely numerous finger-like projections, called *villi*, and the invagination of the mucosa between the bases of the villi into crypts, called *crypts of Lieberkuhn*;

4. The presence of extensive microvilli on the surface of each intestinal lining cell.

Micrograph (a) taken at very low magnification, shows a section of small intestine. The mucosa is thrown into transverse folds, the plica circulares **PC**, covered with villi **V**. The muscularis mucosae **MM** immediately underlies the intervening crypts and is difficult to identify at this magnification. The vascular submucosa **S** extends into, and forms the core of, the plica circulares. The inner circular **CM** and outer longitudinal **LM** layers of the muscularis produce continuous peristaltic activity of the small intestine. The peritoneal aspect of the muscularis is invested by the loose connective tissue serosa **Sr** which is lined on its peritoneal surface by mesothelium.

A prominent feature of the small intestine is the presence of lymphoid aggregations of various size within the lamina propria; the larger aggregations are known as *Peyer's patches* **PP**. The functional significance of the gastrointestinal lymphoid tissues is discussed in Chapter 11.

Micrograph (b) taken from the same specimen demonstrates, in three dimensions, the intestinal villi along the crest of a plica circularis. Crypts of Lieberkuhn open into the spaces between the bases of the villi but are obscured by residual mucus. Surface openings of scattered goblet cells give each villus the appearance of a pepper pot in this type of preparation.

The mechanisms of digestion and absorption

The process of digestion occurs within the lumen proper or at the mucosal surface, the latter usually being intimately linked with a complementary absorptive process.

Luminal digestion involves the mixing of chyme with pancreatic enzymes with subsequent molecular breakdown occurring within the intestinal lumen. Luminal digestion is greatly facilitated by adsorption of pancreatic enzymes onto the mucosal surface. *Membrane digestion* involves enzymes located within the luminal plasma membranes of the cells lining the small intestine; these digestive enzymes do not occur freely in the intestinal lumen. The following is a brief summary of the principal means of digestion and absorption of the main food constituents, i.e. proteins, carbohydrates and lipids.

Proteins are initially denatured by the acidic gastric juice before being hydrolysed to polypeptide fragments by the enzyme pepsin. In the duodenum, pancreatic enzymes including trypsin, chymotrypsin, elastase and carboxypeptidases mediate further luminal digestion to small peptide fragments. Membrane-bound oligopeptidases complete the process leading to amino acid absorption; this involves active transport with different carrier systems for each amino acid. In young infants, some proteins can be absorbed undigested by the process of endocytosis, colostrum having been shown to have some anti-digestive properties.

Carbohydrates occur in the diet mainly in the form of starches and the disaccharides sucrose and lactose. Pancreatic amylase hydrolyses starch to glucose and the disaccharide maltose in the small intestinal lumen. This process is commenced by salivary amylase in the mouth though its contribution to digestion is probably insignificant. Membrane-bound disaccharidases and oligosaccharidases convert the sugars to monosaccharides, mainly glucose, galactose and fructose, which are actively absorbed against concentration gradients.

Lipids, predominantly triglycerides, are converted by the mechanical action of the stomach into a coarse emulsion which is further reduced in the duodenum to a fine emulsion by bile acids synthesised in the liver. Each triglyceride molecule is broken down into a monoglyceride and two free fatty acids by pancreatic lipases though some glycerol and diglycerides are also produced. These smaller lipid molecules are now absorbed but most are then resynthesised back into triglycerides in which form they are transported from the gut into the general circulation.

The products of protein and carbohydrate digestion, namely amino acids and monosaccharides respectively, enter the intestinal capillaries and pass via the portal vein to the liver. In contrast, the reconstituted triglycerides pass into the intestinal lymphatics, known as *lacteals,* and thence via the thoracic duct to the general circulation, bypassing the liver. In the lymphatics, the triglycerides, coated with phospholipids and proteins form fine globules known as *chylomicrons.* A minority of lipid digestion products such as short-chain fatty acids and glycerol pass in the portal system to the liver along with almost all the bile acids which are reabsorbed and recirculated.

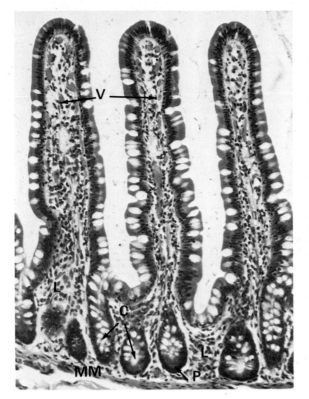

Fig. 14.18 Intestinal villi and crypts
(H & E × 120)

The intestinal villi **V** are lined by a simple, columnar epithelium which is continuous with that of the crypts **C**. The cells of this epithelium are of two main types: *enterocytes* and *goblet cells*. The enterocytes, which are involved in membrane digestion and absorption, are tall columnar cells with basally located nuclei; goblet cells are scattered among the enterocytes. The entire epithelial lining of the intestine is replaced every 3–5 days by the continual shedding of cells from the tips of the villi into the lumen. Mitotic activity in the crypts produces a continuous supply of new cells which progress up the villi where they mature before degenerating and being shed.

A third cell type, with no known digestive or absorptive function, is found in clusters at the base of the crypts. These cells, called *Paneth cells* **P**, are packed with strongly eosinophilic granules and are a prominent feature of the small intestine in man, although absent in some mammals. Paneth cells are known to be a stable population of cells and to have the ultrastructural characteristics of exocrine, protein-secreting cells yet their function remains obscure.

The lamina propria **L** extends between the crypts and into the core of each villus and contains a rich vascular and lymphatic network into which digestive products are absorbed. The muscularis mucosae **MM** lies immediately beneath the base of the crypts.

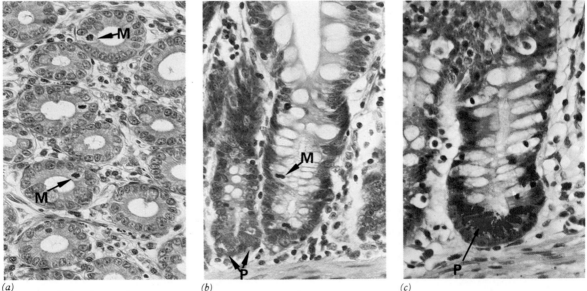

(a)   *(b)*   *(c)*

Fig. 14.19 Crypts of Lieberkuhn
(H & E (a) TS × 32 (b) LS × 320 (c) Phloxine-tartrazine × 320)

At high magnification, mitotic figures **M** can be seen in the crypts. With such a high rate of cell turnover, more mitotic figures might be expected to be seen; the mitotic phase, however, occupies only a small proportion of the cell cycle

(see Fig. 2.1), thus at any one point in time relatively few mitotic figures are seen.

With H & E staining, cells with intensely eosinophilic, cytoplasmic granules are seen in the base of the crypts; these cells, Paneth cells **P**, are more clearly demonstrated by the phloxine-tartrazine method which stains the granules scarlet.

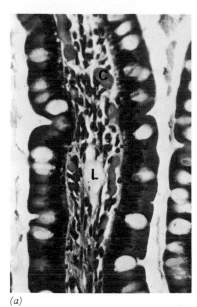
(a)

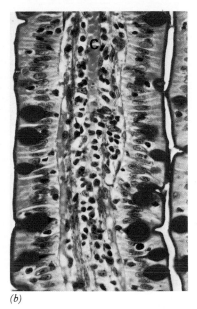
(b)

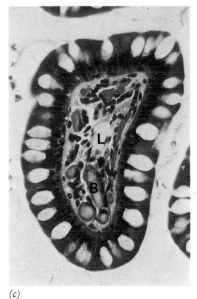
(c)

Fig. 14.20 Intestinal villi

(LS: (a) H & E × 320 (b) PAS/Iron haematoxylin/Orange G × 320 (c) TS: H & E × 320)

In the longitudinal sections of intestinal villi seen in micrographs (a) and (b), the tall columnar nature of enterocytes can be seen. The luminal surface of the enterocytes seen in micrograph (b) is strongly PAS positive due to the presence of a particularly thick glycocalyx (see Fig. 1.2) and a surface layer of goblet cell derived mucus; both these surface features protect against auto-digestion. It has been suggested that the glycocalyx acts as the site for adsorption of pancreatic digestive enzymes.

Lymphocytes and plasma cells are thought to secrete antibodies of the IgA class which pass into the intestinal lumen where they may provide defence against invading pathogens.

Capillaries **C** lie immediately beneath the layer of enterocytes and transport amino acids, monosaccharides and most other digestive products to the hepatic portal vein. Small lymphatic vessels drain into a single, larger vessel called a *lacteal* **L** located in the centre of the core of the villus; lacteals, which often contain lymphocytes, may be difficult to distinguish. The lacteals transport much of the absorbed lipid into the circulatory system via the thoracic duct, thus bypassing the liver.

In transverse section in micrograph (c), the arrangement of the blood and lymphatic systems within a villus can be seen. Blood capillaries **B** tend to be disposed at the periphery, immediately beneath the enterocyte lining. Lymph drains into a single, central lacteal **L** via minute lymphatic tributaries.

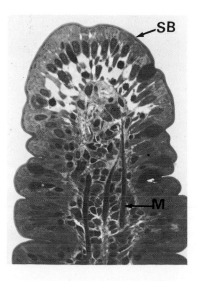

Fig. 14.21 Tip of intestinal villus

(LS: thin section, toluidine blue × 320)

This method of tissue preparation shows several features of the intestinal villus which are more difficult to demonstrate in thicker, conventional paraffin wax-embedded sections.

Firstly, degenerating enterocytes and goblet cells are seen about to be shed from the tip of the villus. Secondly, a striated or brush border **SB** can be seen on the luminal surface of the enterocytes; this represents the tall microvilli present on each enterocyte. Individual microvilli are too small to be resolved by light microscopy. Thirdly, occasional smooth muscle fibres **M** are seen within the connective tissue core of the villus; these muscle cells are extensions of the muscularis mucosae from beneath the base of the crypts. Contraction of the smooth muscle strands enhances drainage of lymph from the lacteals.

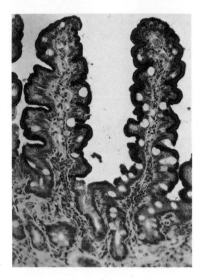

Fig. 14.22 Intestinal villi

(LS: Enzyme histochemical method for alkaline phosphatase × 128)

This frozen section from an intestinal biopsy has been stained for the enzyme alkaline phosphatase which is one of the many membrane-bound enzymes characteristic of enterocyte microvilli; alkaline phosphatase activity is represented by a red deposit. Alkaline phosphatase is thought to be involved in the transport of calcium ions from the intestinal lumen. Other membrane enzymes are involved in the breakdown of peptides and disaccharides to amino-acids and monosaccharides respectively. The membrane-bound enzymes of the striated border are structurally integrated into the plasma membrane and are synthesised by enterocytes, in contrast to those enzymes adsorbed on to the surface which are synthesised by the pancreas. Note that the relatively immature enterocytes in the intestinal crypts show little alkaline phosphatase activity.

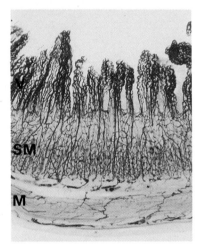

Fig. 14.23 Intestinal villi

(Carmine perfused × 10)

This specimen of small intestine has been perfused before fixation with a red dye and demonstrates the blood supply of the mucosa. From a dense capillary network in the submucosa **SM**, long loops of branching capillaries extend up to the tips of the villi **V**. Note also the capillary network supplying the muscular wall **M**. Most of the absorbed food products, with the exception of triglycerides, enter the capillaries and pass via the portal vein to the liver.

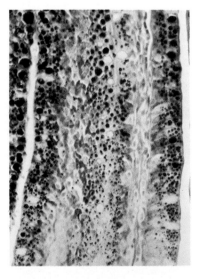

Fig. 14.24 Intestinal villus

(LS: Sudan black × 320)

This frozen section from the intestine of a rat fed with milk has been stained to demonstrate the presence of absorbed lipids within a villus. Ingested triglycerides are emulsified by bile and hydrolysed by the pancreatic enzyme, *lipase*; the degradation products, mainly free fatty acids and monoglycerides, are absorbed by enterocytes where they are resynthesised into triglycerides.

The triglycerides, with the addition of protein and phospholipid components, are packaged into membrane-bound vesicles called *chylomicrons* by the enterocyte Golgi apparatus, then passed towards the base of the cell where they are released by exocytosis into intercellular clefts; from here they pass into the lacteals from which they enter the general circulation. Note the high concentration of black-stained lipid in the enterocyte cytoplasm and in chylomicrons within the central lacteal.

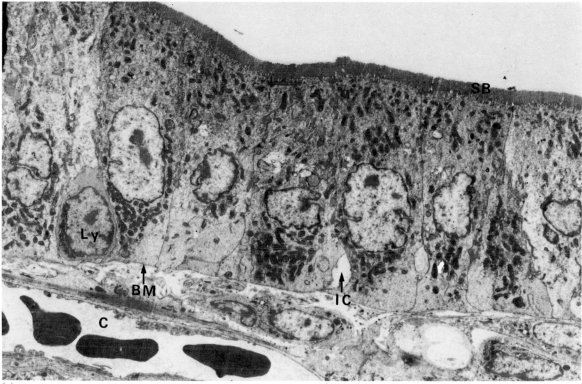

(a)

Fig. 14.25 Intestinal epithelium: enterocytes

(EM (a) × 4540 (b) × 50 000)

These micrographs illustrate the main ultrastructural features of the absorptive cells of the small intestine, the enterocytes. Enormous numbers of microvilli, up to 3000 per cell, increase about thirtyfold the surface area of the plasma membrane exposed to the lumen. The microvilli are of uniform length, approximately 1 μm, and constitute the striated border **SB** of light microscopy. The glycocalyx of the enterocyte microvilli is usually prominent and is thought not only to provide protection against autodigestion but also to act as the site for adsorption of pancreatic digestive enzymes. Note in micrograph (b) the filamentous cytoskeleton of the microvilli **Mv** extending into the terminal web **TW**. Enterocytes are tightly bound near their luminal surface by junctional complexes (see Fig. 5.24) which prevent direct access of luminal contents into the intercellular spaces.

Most absorption in the small intestine is thought to occur by direct passage of low molecular weight digestion products across the luminal plasma membrane. Mitochondria are particularly abundant within enterocytes reflecting the high energy demands of active absorptive processes. In actively absorbing enterocytes, endocytotic vesicles are often seen between the bases of microvilli. The importance of this mode of absorption in the small intestine is not well understood although endocytosis may be a minor pathway of lipid absorption.

Between the bases of the enterocytes are intercellular clefts **IC** into which chylomicrons are first passed after

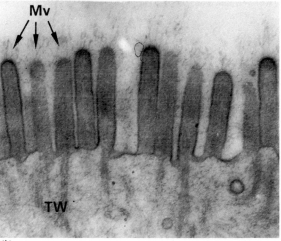

(b)

processing by the Golgi apparatus. From the clefts, the chylomicrons pass across the thin basement membrane **BM** to be preferentially absorbed into the lacteals. Lymphocytes **Ly** and plasma cells are commonly found in the intercellular clefts between enterocytes where they play an important part in the immunological defence of the tract. Note the close proximity of a blood capillary **C** to the enterocyte basement membrane.

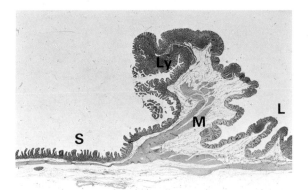

Fig. 14.26 Ileo-caecal junction

(H & E × 5)

Unabsorbed and indigestible food residues from the ileum are forced, by peristalsis, into the distended first part of the large intestine, the caecum, through a simple cone-shaped valve which marks the ileo-caecal junction. There is an abrupt transition in the lining of the valve from the villiform pattern in the small intestine **S** to the glandular form in the large intestine **L**.

The ileo-caecal valve consists of a thickened extension of the muscularis **M** which provides robust support for the mucosa. Variable quantities of lymphoid tissue **Ly** are found in the mucosa.

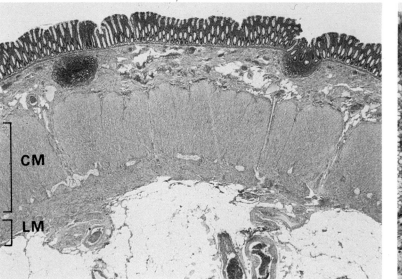

(a)

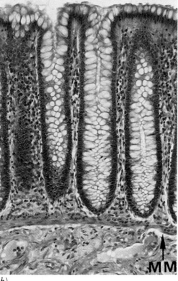

(b)

Fig. 14.27 Colon

(H & E (a) × 4 (b) × 100)

The principal functions of the large intestine are the recovery of water from the liquid residue of the small intestine and the propulsion of increasingly more solid faeces to the rectum prior to defaecation.

As shown in micrograph (a), the muscular wall is consequently thick and capable of powerful peristaltic activity. As in the rest of the gastrointestinal tract, the muscularis propria of the large intestine consists of inner circular **CM** and outer longitudinal layers **LM**, but except in the rectum, the longitudinal layer does not completely surround the tract but, rather, forms three separate longitudinal bands called *taeniae coli*.

Consistent with its functions of water absorption and faecal lubrication, the mucosa is lined by cells of two types, absorptive cells and mucus-secreting goblet cells. As seen in micrograph (b), these are arranged in closely packed straight tubular glands, an arrangement which greatly enhances the functional surface area. As faeces pass along the large intestine and become progressively dehydrated, the mucus becomes increasingly important in protecting the mucosa from trauma. The glands are analogous to the crypts of Lieberkuhn of the small intestine and this term may also be applied to the glands of the large intestine. Like the stomach and small intestine, the epithelium undergoes continual turnover at the luminal surface, the cells being replaced by mitosis at the base of the glands. The thick, glandular mucosa is highly folded in the non-distended state, but it does not exhibit distinct plica circulares like those of the small intestine (see Fig. 14.17). Immediately above the anal valves, the mucosa forms longitudinal folds called the *columns of Morgagni*. The muscularis mucosae **MM** is a prominent feature of the large intestinal mucosa and its activity prevents clogging of the glands and enhances expulsion of mucus.

As protection from ingress of microorganisms, the large intestinal wall contains numerous leucocytes and cells of the immune system, the latter forming large aggregations in the lamina propria and submucosa as seen in micrograph (a).

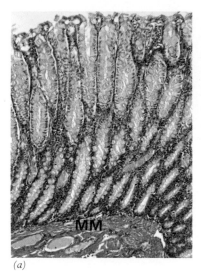
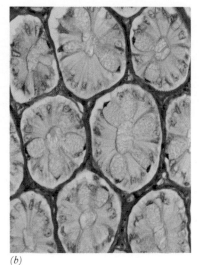
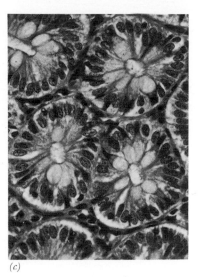

(a)   *(b)*   *(c)*

Fig. 14.28 Colonic glands

(Alcian blue/van Gieson (a) LS × 80 (b) TS × 320 (c) H & E, TS × 320)

The alcian blue staining method permits ready differentiation of the two major cell types which comprise the glands of the large intestine; goblet cell mucus is stained a greenish-blue colour while the absorptive cells remain poorly stained. As seen in longitudinal section in micrograph (a), the simple tubular glands extend from the luminal surface to the muscularis mucosae **MM** and are separated from each other by thin plates of lamina propria, the collagen of which is stained red in this preparation. Thin strands of the muscularis mucosae extend into the lamina propria between the glands, contraction facilitating the expulsion of mucus into the bowel lumen. Goblet cells predominate in the base of the glands whereas the luminal surface is almost entirely lined by columnar absorptive cells; the middle part of the glands represents the transition between the two.

Micrographs (b) and (c) show transverse sections through the upper part of the large intestinal glands highlighting the closely packed arrangement of the glands in the mucosa. The absorptive cells are tall columnar with large, ovoid, basally-located nuclei, in contrast, goblet cell nuclei are small and condensed. Lamina propria fills the spaces between the glands and contains numerous blood and lymphatic vessels into which water is absorbed by passive diffusion.

The large intestine is inhabited by a variety of commensal bacteria which further degrade food residues. Bacterial degradation is an important mechanism for the digestion of cellulose in ruminants but in man this function is of little importance. Small quantities of fat-soluble vitamins derived from bacterial activity are absorbed in the large intestine.

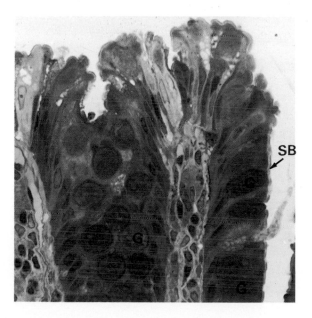

Fig. 14.29 Colonic mucosa

(Thin section, toluidine blue × 480)

This micrograph illustrates the similarity of the epithelium in the large intestine to that of the small intestine as shown in Figure 14.21. As in the small intestine, the absorptive cells of the large intestine have a striated border **SB** formed by microvilli which increase greatly the surface area exposed to the lumen, thus enhancing passive water absorption. The epithelial lining of the large intestine is replaced every 3–5 days like that of the small intestine; note several degenerating cells in the process of being shed from the luminal surface. Goblet cells **G** are seen in different phases of secretory activity.

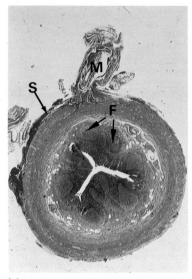

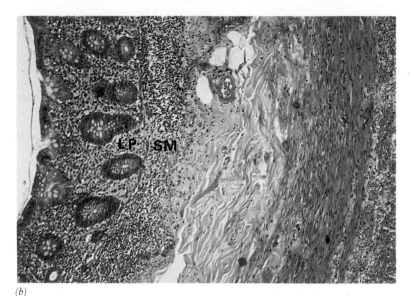

(a)   *(b)*

Fig. 14.30 Appendix

(H & E (a) × 5 (b) × 42)

The appendix is a small blind-ended sac extending from the caecum just below the ileo-caecal junction. Although not known to have any digestive or absorptive function in man, the general structure of the appendix conforms to that of the rest of the large intestine as can be seen in these specimens taken from a young person. Micrograph (a) also illustrates the suspensory mesentery **M** which becomes continuous with the outer serosal layer and is a feature of all parts of the gastrointestinal tract which lie free in the peritoneal cavity. In this specimen, the serosa **S** contains a moderate amount of haemorrhage resulting from surgical removal. The mesenteries conduct blood vessels, lymphatics and nerves to and from the gastrointestinal tract.

The most characteristic feature of the appendix, particularly of a young person, is the presence of masses of lymphoid tissue in the mucosa and submucosa. As seen in micrograph (b), the lamina propria **LP** and upper submucosa **SM** are diffusely infiltrated with lymphocytes which are also seen to a lesser extent in the deeper submucosa and muscularis propria. Note that the mucosal glands are much less closely packed than elsewhere in the large intestine. As seen in micrograph (a), the lymphoid tissue also forms follicles **F** often containing germinal centres.

Undoubtedly, the appendix contains a significant part of the gut-associated lymphoid tissue, especially in the young, but no specific function has yet been ascribed to it.

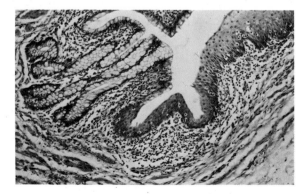

Fig. 14.31 Recto-anal junction

(H & E × 128)

The rectum is the short, dilated, terminal portion of the large intestine, the main function of which is to store semi-solid faeces immediately prior to defaecation. The mucosa of the rectum, which is similar to that of the rest of the large bowel except that it has even more numerous goblet cells, undergoes an abrupt transition at the recto-anal junction to become stratified squamous epithelium in the anal canal. The anal canal forms the last 2 or 3 cm of the gastrointestinal tract and is surrounded by an external skeletal muscle mass which constitutes the anal sphincter. At the anal sphincter, the stratified squamous epithelium undergoes a gradual transition to that of skin containing sebaceous glands and large apocrine sweat glands (see Fig. 9.13).

15. Liver and pancreas

Liver and biliary system

The liver, like the pancreas, develops embryologically as a glandular outgrowth of the primitive gut. The major functions of the liver may be summarised as follows:

1. Detoxification of metabolic waste products;
2. Destruction of spent red cells and reclamation of their constituents (in conjunction with the spleen);
3. Synthesis and secretion of bile into the duodenum via the biliary system; bile contains many of the end products of the processes described in (1) and (2) above, thus bile may be considered as both an excretory product and an exocrine secretion;
4. Synthesis of the plasma proteins including the clotting factors but excluding the immunoglobulins;
5. Synthesis of plasma lipoproteins;
6. Metabolic functions eg glycogen synthesis, gluconeogenesis.

Many of these biosynthetic funtions directly utilise the products of digestion. With the exception of most lipids, absorbed food products pass directly in venous blood from the small intestine to the liver via the *hepatic portal system* before entering the general circulation. Thus the vascular bed of the liver is perfused by blood rich in amino acids, simple sugars and other products of digestion but relatively poor in oxygen. Oxygen required to support the intense metabolic activity of the liver is supplied in arterial blood via the *hepatic artery*. The liver, therefore, is unusual in that it has a dual blood supply that is both arterial and venous. Venous drainage of the liver occurs via the *hepatic vein* and lymph from the liver is drained directly into the thoracic duct.

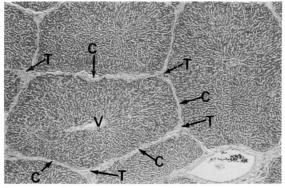

(a)

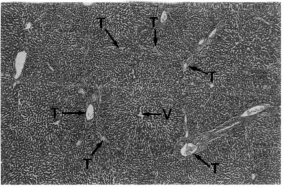

(b)

Fig. 15.1 Liver

(H & E (a) Pig liver × 20 (b) Human liver × 20)

The principal cells of the liver, the *hepatocytes*, are arranged into structures called *lobules*, the structure of which maximises contact of hepatocytes with blood flowing through the liver. In pigs, the 'classical' liver lobule is particularly well delineated by connective tissue boundaries **C** as seen in micrograph (a). The liver lobules are roughly hexagonal in shape when seen in any section, reflecting their regular, polyhedral three-dimensional shape. Branches of the hepatic artery and hepatic portal vein ramify throughout the liver within the connective tissue bounding the liver lobules, the larger vessels tending to be concentrated at the angles of

the lobule margins in the so-called *portal tracts* **T**. Blood from the portal tracts percolates towards a central vein **V** of each lobule via sinusoids which pass between plates of hepatocytes. The central vein drains into the hepatic vein.

The human liver has a similar lobular pattern to that of the pig but the boundaries of the lobules are not defined by distinct connective tissue. As seen in micrograph (b), portal tracts **T** define the angles of the lobule margins and a central vein **V** defines the centre of each lobule. Note that each portal tract and its branches supplies more than one lobule whereas each central vein drains only a single lobule.

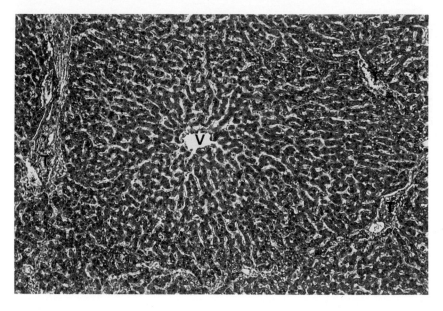

Fig. 15.2 Hepatic lobule
(H & E × 75)

This micrograph illustrates a single human liver lobule. The irregular, hexagonal boundary of the lobule is defined by the sparse connective tissue and vessels of the portal tracts **T**. Sinusoids originate at the lobule margin and course between anastomosing plates of hepatocytes to converge upon the central vein **V**.

The plates of hepatocytes are usually only one cell thick and each hepatocyte is thus bathed by blood on at least two sides giving a huge surface area for exchange of metabolites. The plates of hepatocytes branch and anastomose to form a three-dimensional structure like a honeycomb.

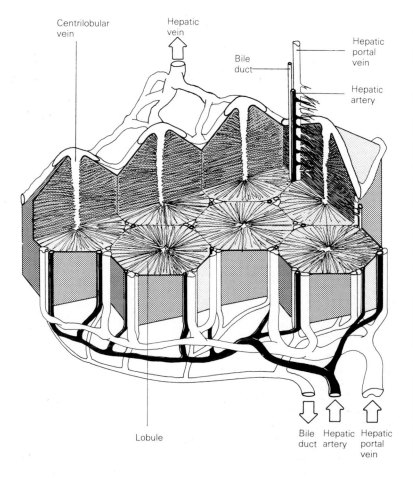

Centrilobular vein

Hepatic vein

Bile duct

Hepatic portal vein

Hepatic artery

Lobule

Bile duct   Hepatic artery   Hepatic portal vein

Fig. 15.3 Hepatic lobule

This diagram summarises in schematic form the gross arrangement of the liver lobules, the vascular system and the bile collecting system. The hepatic portal vein and hepatic artery branch repeatedly within the liver, the branches running within the portal tract regions at the angles of the polygonal shaped lobules. Blood from both supply systems then percolates between the branching plates of hepatocytes in the sinusoids which converge to drain into a central vein. These so-called *centrilobular veins* merge with each other to form the hepatic vein which drains into the inferior vena cava.

In contrast, bile is secreted into a network of minute *bile canaliculi* which pass between the hepatocytes within the plates; these canaliculi are too small to be represented in this diagram. The bile canaliculi then drain into a system of collecting ducts which also run in the portal tracts but in the opposite direction to the two blood supply systems. The biliary system then drains into the common bile duct and ultimately to the duodenum.

In certain pathological conditions, it is more useful to subdivide the liver into *portal lobules*, each made up of a portal tract and the parts of the three surrounding hepatic lobules; the boundaries of the portal lobule are defined by lines joining surrounding centrilobular veins.

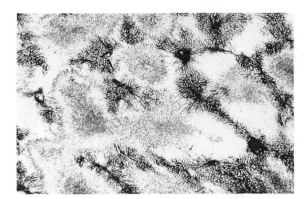

Fig. 15.4 Liver

(Perfusion method × 20)

This preparation illustrates one of the techniques which was used by early histologists in mapping blood flow within the liver. The hepatic portal vein (supplying the liver) has been perfused with a red dye and the hepatic vein (draining the liver) has been back-perfused with a blue dye. It is thus evident from this micrograph that blood enters each lobule from several portal tracts (stained red) and then converges upon a centrilobular vein (stained blue) to drain ultimately into the hepatic vein.

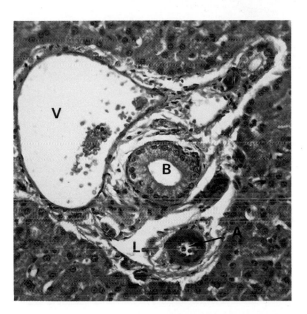

Fig. 15.5 Portal tract

(H & E × 200)

This micrograph focuses on a portal tract between three adjacent liver lobules. Each portal tract contains vessels of three main types. Firstly, the largest diameter vessels are branches of the hepatic portal vein **V** which have the typical, thin-walled structure and irregular outline of all veins. Secondly, the smaller diameter, thick-walled vessels, with the typical structure of arterioles and arteries, are branches of the hepatic artery **A** which supplies oxygenated blood to the liver. Thirdly, ducts of variable size lined by simple cuboidal or columnar epithelium are the bile-collecting ducts **B** which ultimately drain into the common bile duct. Because vessels of these three types are always found in the portal tracts, the tracts are often referred to as *portal triads*. A fourth type of vessel, lymphatics **L**, are also present in the portal tracts, but since their walls are delicate and often collapsed they are not readily seen.

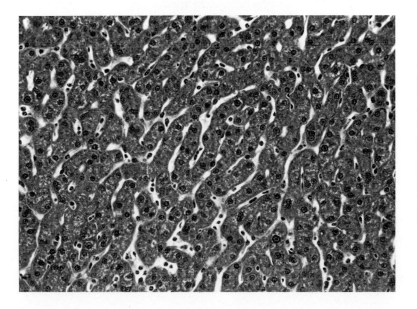

Fig. 15.6 Liver parenchyma

(H & E × 198)

The arrangement of hepatocytes within the liver parenchyma can be readily seen at this magnification. The hepatocytes form flat, anastomosing plates usually only one cell thick between which blood passes sluggishly towards the centre of the lobule. This arrangement maximises the contact between hepatocytes and blood. The sinusoids are lined by a discontinuous layer of cells, analogous to the endothelial cells lining all other blood vessels; this lining layer is thought to pose little barrier to the interaction of blood elements with hepatocytes.

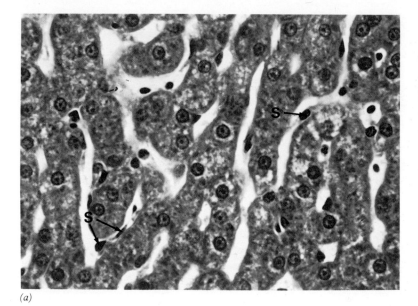

(a)

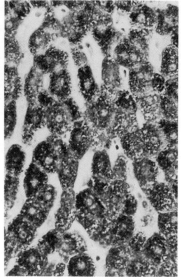

(b)

Fig. 15.7 Hepatocytes

(a) H & E × 480 (b) Glycogen method × 400

Hepatocytes are large, polyhedral cells which have a variable cytoplasmic appearance depending on the nutritional status of the body. In well-nourished individuals, hepatocytes store significant quantities of glycogen and process large quantities of lipid; both these metabolites are partially removed during routine histological preparation thereby leaving irregular, unstained areas within the cytoplasm. The remaining cytoplasm is strongly eosinophilic due to a high content of organelles. The nuclei of hepatocytes are large with peripherally dispersed chromatin and prominent nucleoli. The nuclei, however, vary greatly in size, reflecting an unusual cellular feature; more than half the hepatocytes contain twice the normal (diploid) complement of

chromosomes within a single nucleus (i.e. they are tetraploid) and some contain four or even eight times this amount (polyploid). Occasional binucleate cells are seen in section although up to 25% of all hepatocytes are binucleate.

Micrograph (a) shows the typical appearance of hepatocytes in standard preparations. Sinusoid lining cells **S** are readily distinguishable from hepatocytes by their flattened, condensed nuclei and attenuated, poorly stained cytoplasm.

In micrograph (b), a histochemical method has been used to demonstrate the presence within the hepatocytes of glycogen which stains magenta.

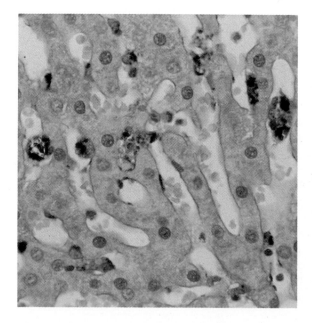

Fig. 15.8 Sinusoid lining cells

(Perls' Prussian blue × 48)

The nature and function of the sinusoid lining cells has been in dispute ever since the liver was first studied. At least a proportion of these cells can be shown to be highly phagocytic when 'fed' either artificially or under pathological conditions with appropriate particulate matter. The animal used for this preparation was injected intravenously with a particulate iron-sugar compound which, with this staining method, is demonstrated as a dark deposit within the sinusoid lining cells. Some authorities believe that all sinusoid lining cells are capable of intense phagocytosis when appropriately stimulated whereas others believe that a distinct population of phagocytic cells exists amongst endothelial-like sinusoid lining cells. In either case, the intensely phagocytic cells probably represent cells analogous to, or identical with, the cells of the monocyte-macrophage defence system (see Ch. 3 and 4). The phagocytic cells of the liver are commonly referred to as *Kupffer cells*. Kupffer cells participate, with the spleen, in the removal of spent erythrocytes and other particulate debris from the circulation.

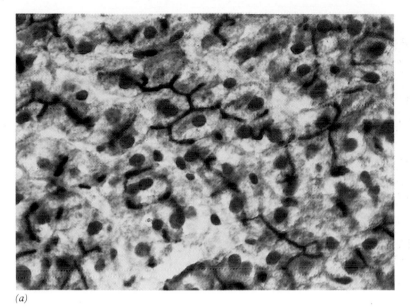

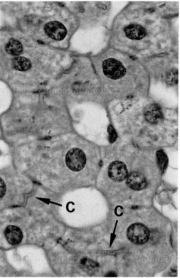

(a)   *(b)*

Fig. 15.9 Bile canaliculi

(a) Enzyme histochemical method for ATP-ase × 480 (b) Iron haematoxylin × 480

Bile is synthesised by all hepatocytes and secreted into a system of minute canaliculi which form an anastomosing network between hepatocytes. The canaliculi have no discrete structure of their own but consist merely of fine channels running between adjacent hepatocytes, the walls of the canaliculi being formed by the plasma membranes of adjacent hepatocytes; the ultrastructural features are shown in Figure 15.11. Thus within each plate of hepatocytes, which is one cell thick, the canaliculi form a regular, hexagonal network in the plane of the plate, each mesh enclosing a single hepatocyte.

From within each lobule, bile canaliculi drain towards bile collecting vessels of the portal tracts. The hepatocyte plasma membranes forming the walls of the canaliculi contain the enzyme ATP-ase on the basis of which it has been suggested that bile secretion is an energy-dependent process. In micrograph (a), a histochemical method for ATP-ase has been used to demonstrate bile canaliculi (stained brown) which are difficult to demonstrate with routine methods for light microscopy. In micrograph (b) iron has been deposited in the walls of the canaliculi C.

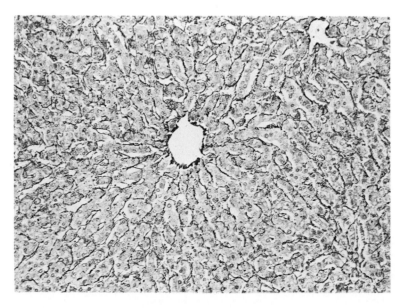

Fig. 15.10 Liver

(Reticulin method × 250)

Hepatocytes and sinusoid lining cells are supported by a fine meshwork of reticulin fibres which radiate from around the central vein of each lobule to merge with the reticular and sparse connective tissue framework of the portal tracts and lobule boundaries. Reticulin is thus almost the only connective tissue element supporting the liver. This framework becomes continuous with a thin but tough connective tissue capsule, called *Glisson's capsule*, which invests the external surface of the liver.

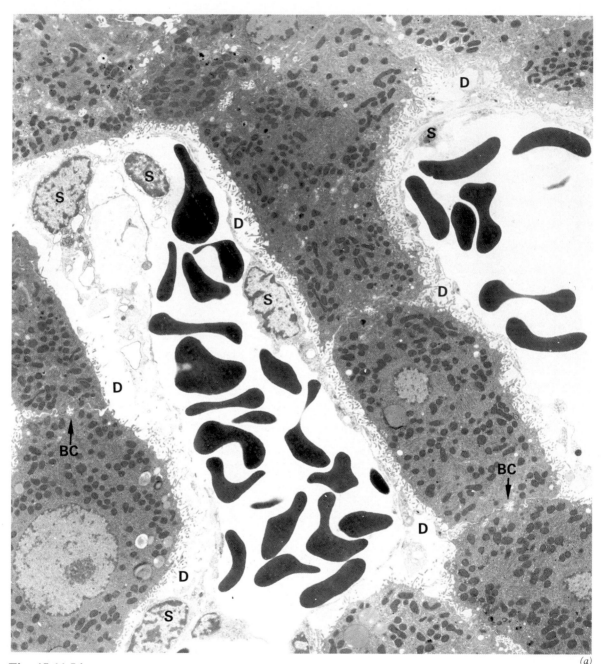

(a)

Fig. 15.11 Liver

EM (a) × 4400 (b) × 15 200 (opposite)

These micrographs demonstrate the main ultrastructural features of the liver. Each hepatocyte is bathed on at least two sides by blood within the sinusoids which are lined by a discontinuous layer of sinusoid lining cells **S**. Sinusoid lining cells are supported by the fine reticular framework of the liver (see Fig. 15.10) such that a space, known as the *space of Disse* **D**, remains between the lining cells and the hepatocyte surface. Since the sinusoid lining cells form a discontinuous layer, the space of Disse is continuous with the sinusoid lumen. Numerous irregular microvilli **Mv** extend from the hepatocyte surface into the space of Disse thus greatly increasing the plasma membrane surface available for

bidirectional exchange of metabolites between liver and blood.

Reflecting the extraordinary range of biosynthetic and degradative activities, the hepatocyte cytoplasm is crowded with organelles, particularly rough and smooth endoplasmic reticulum, mitochondria **M** and lysosomes **Ly**. Lipid droplets and glycogen rosettes are present in variable numbers depending on nutritional status (see Fig. 1.14).

Bile canaliculi **BC** are seen to be formed from the plasma membranes of adjacent hepatocytes, the plasma membranes being tightly bound by junctional complexes; small microvilli project into the canaliculi.

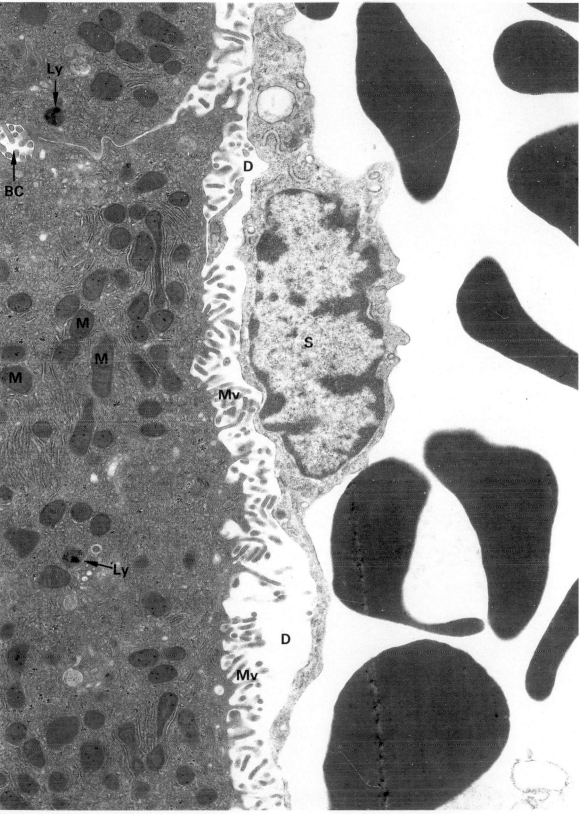

(b)

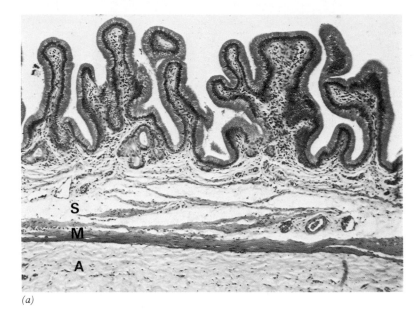

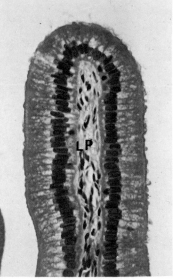

(a)   *(b)*

Fig. 15.12 Gall bladder

(H & E (a) × 30 (b) × 480)

The intrahepatic bile collecting system merges to form a
single large duct, the *common bile duct*, which joins the
pancreatic duct to form the short *ampulla of Vater* before
entering the duodenum. The duodenal opening is guarded
by the muscular *sphincter of Oddi*. Immediately after leaving
the liver, the common bile duct has a major branch, the
cystic duct, which connects the common bile duct to the *gall
bladder*.

Most of the bile does not pass directly down the common
bile duct but is shunted into the gall bladder where it is
temporarily stored and concentrated. A well developed
biliary sphincter regulates bile flow from the common bile
duct into the ampulla of Vater. The tonus of this smooth
muscle also controls the flow of bile into the gall bladder.

The gall bladder is a muscular sac lined by a simple
columnar epithelium; it has a capacity of about 100 ml in
man. The presence of lipid in the duodenum promotes the
secretion of the hormone cholecystokinin-pancreozymin
(CCK) by endocrine cells of the duodenal wall. CCK
stimulates contraction of the gall bladder smooth muscle
thus forcing bile along the biliary tract into the duodenum.

Bile is essentially an emulsifying agent which facilitates the
hydrolysis of dietary lipids by pancreatic lipases.

Micrograph (a) shows the wall of a gall bladder in the
non-distended state in which the lining mucosa is thrown up
into many folds. The relatively loose submucosal connective
tissue **S** is rich in elastic fibres and contains many blood and
lymphatic vessels which drain water reabsorbed from bile
during the concentration process. The muscle layer **M** is
seen to separate the submucosa from the outer adventitial
connective tissue **A**. In the neck of the gall bladder, mucous
glands are often found in the submucosa; this mucus may
provide a protective surface film for the biliary tract.

As seen in micrograph (b) at high magnification, the
simple epithelial lining of the gall bladder consists of very
tall columnar cells with basally located nuclei. Although not
usually evident with light microscopy, the luminal surface of
the cells is formed into very numerous, short irregular
microvilli. Bile is concentrated 5- to 10-fold by an active
process, mediated by the lining cells, which involves
absorption of water into the vessels of the lamina
propria **LP**.

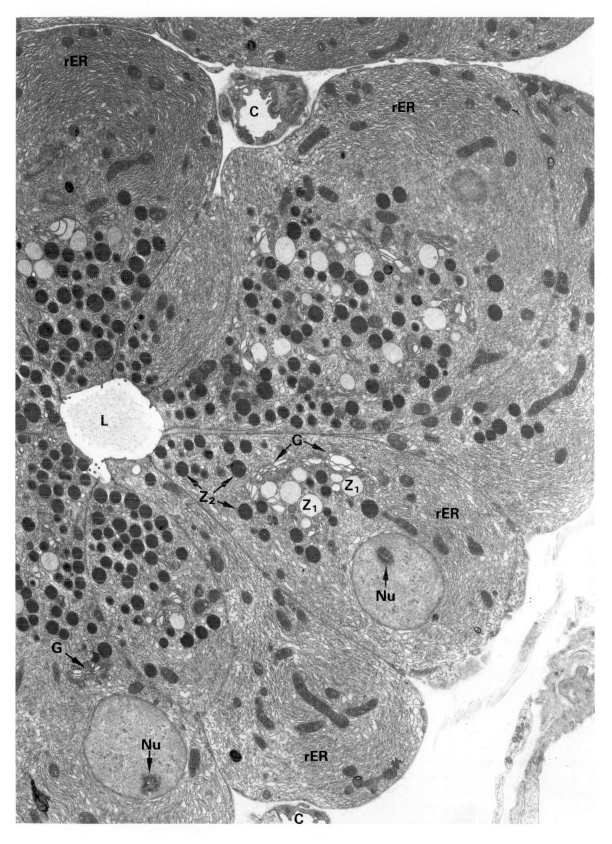

16. Urinary system

Introduction

The urinary system is the principal organ system responsible for water and electrolyte homeostasis. The maintenance of homeostasis requires that any input into a system is balanced by an equivalent output; the urinary system provides the mechanism by which excess water and electrolytes are eliminated from the body. A second major function of the urinary system is the excretion of many toxic metabolic waste products, particularly the nitrogenous compounds urea and creatinine; this excretory function is intimately related to water and electrolyte elimination which provides an appropriate fluid vehicle. The end product of these processes is *urine*. Since all body fluids are maintained in dynamic equilibrium with one another via the circulatory system, any adjustment in the composition of the blood is reflected in complementary changes in the other fluid compartments of the body. Thus regulation of the osmotic concentration of blood plasma ensures the osmotic regulation of all other body fluids. The process, primarily performed by the urinary system, is called *osmoregulation*.

The functional units of the urinary system are the *nephrons*, of which there are approximately one million in each human kidney. Nephrons perform the functions of osmoregulation and excretion by the following processes:

1. Filtration of most relatively small molecules from blood plasma to form a filtrate;
2. Selective reabsorption of most of the water and other molecules from the filtrate, leaving behind excess and waste materials to be excreted;
3. Secretion of some excretory products directly from blood into the filtrate.

The kidney is also involved in two other homeostatic mechanisms which are mediated via hormones. The *renin-angiotensin-aldosterone mechanism* contributes to the maintenance of blood pressure, and the hormone *erythropoietin* stimulates erythrocyte production in bone marrow and hence contributes to the maintenance of the oxygen-carrying capacity of blood.

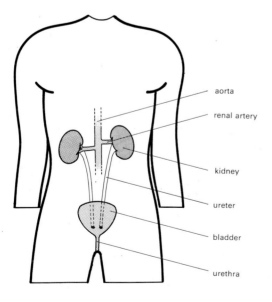

Fig 16.1 The urinary system

The urinary system comprises two *kidneys*, two *ureters*, a *bladder* and a *urethra*. Urine is produced in the kidneys and conducted by the ureters to the bladder where it is stored until voided via the urethra.

Blood is supplied to each kidney by *renal arteries* which arise from the aorta. The total blood volume of the body is circulated through the kidneys about 300 times each day.

aorta

renal artery

kidney

ureter

bladder

urethra

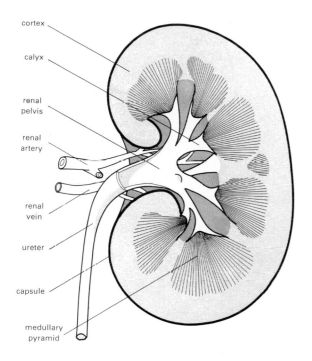

cortex

calyx

renal
pelvis

renal
artery

renal
vein

ureter

capsule

medullary
pyramid

Fig. 16.2 Kidney

The gross structure of the kidney reflects the arrangement of nephrons within it. The substance of the kidney may be divided into an outer *cortex* and an inner *medulla*. A portion of each nephron is located in both the cortex and the medulla, although the major part of each nephron is found in the cortex. The medulla is arranged into pyramid-shaped units called *medullary pyramids* which are separated by extensions of cortical tissue. The medullary pyramids convey ducts which converge to discharge urine at their apices; the apices of the pyramids are known as *renal papillae*. *Calyces* are funnel-shaped spaces into which one or more renal papillae project. The calyces converge to form the larger, funnel-shaped *renal pelvis* from which urine is conducted to the bladder by the ureter.

The kidney is invested in a capsule of tough fibrous tissue. The renal artery and renal vein enter and leave the kidney above the ureter at the region known as the *hilum*.

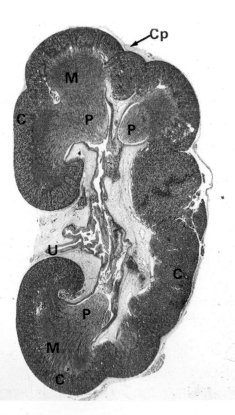

Cp

M

C

P

P

U

C

P

M

C

Fig. 16.3 Kidney

(H & E × 3)

This micrograph of a kidney from a newborn child illustrates the gross features of the kidneys as described in Fig. 16.2. In histological section, only a single plane through the pelvi-calyceal system can be visualised.

The darker-stained cortex **C** can be clearly differentiated from the paler-stained medulla **M**. Note the continuity of the cortex throughout the outer zone of the kidney and the cortical extensions between the medullary pyramids. Three renal papillae **P** are seen projecting into the pelvi-calyceal system which becomes continuous with the ureter **U** at the hilum. Note that the fibrous capsule **Cp** of the kidney is continuous, at the hilum, with connective tissue which packs the spaces between the hilar structures. In later life, the hilum often contains significant quantities of adipose tissue. The kidney is cushioned by a thick pad of adipose tissue, not seen in this preparation, and is protected by the lower ribs retroperitoneally.

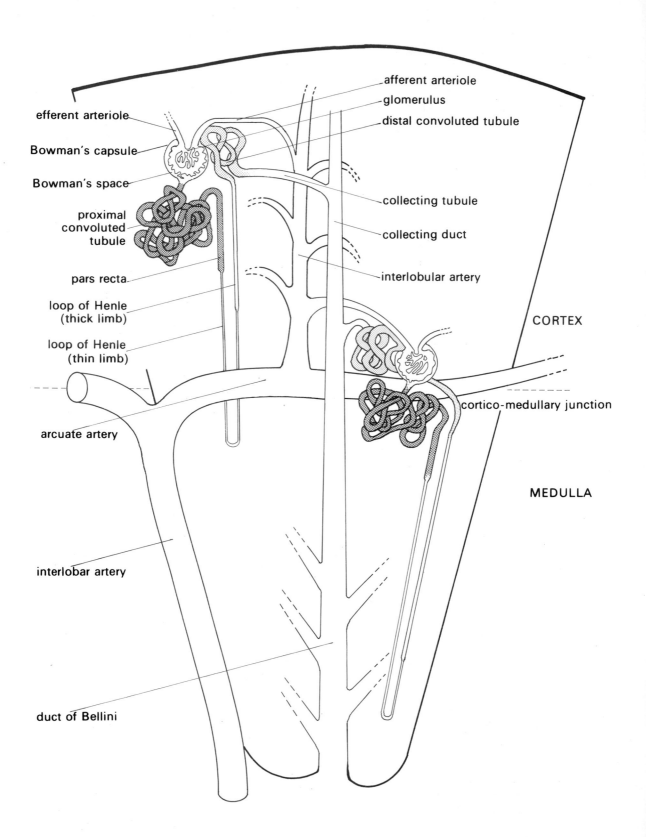

efferent arteriole

Bowman's capsule

Bowman's space

proximal convoluted tubule

pars recta

loop of Henle (thick limb)

loop of Henle (thin limb)

arcuate artery

interlobar artery

duct of Bellini

afferent arteriole

glomerulus

distal convoluted tubule

collecting tubule

collecting duct

interlobular artery

CORTEX

cortico-medullary junction

MEDULLA

Fig. 16.4 The nephron *(illustration opposite)*

The nephron, the functional unit of the kidney, consists of two major components, the *renal corpuscle* and the *renal tubule*.

1. Renal corpuscle: the renal corpuscle is that part of the nephron responsible for the filtration of plasma and is a combination of two structures, *Bowman's capsule* and the *glomerulus*.

(a) Bowman's capsule consists of a single layer of flattened cells resting on a basement membrane; it forms the distended, blind end of an epithelial tubule, the renal tubule.

(b) The glomerulus is a tightly coiled network of anastomosing capillaries which invaginates Bowman's capsule. Within the capsule, the glomerulus is invested by a layer of epithelial cells, called *podocytes*, which constitutes the *visceral layer of Bowman's capsule*; the visceral layer is reflected around the vascular stalk of the glomerulus to become continuous with the *parietal layer*, the Bowman's capsule proper. The space between the visceral and parietal layers is known as *Bowman's space* and is continuous with the lumen of the renal tubule; the parietal epithelium of Bowman's capsule is continuous with the epithelium lining of the renal tubule.

In the renal corpuscle, elements of plasma are filtered from the glomerular capillaries into Bowman's space, and the *glomerular filtrate* then passes into the renal tubule. Thus the filtration barrier between the capillary lumen and Bowman's space consists of the capillary endothelium, the podocyte layer and a common basement membrane, the *glomerular basement membrane*, separating these two cellular layers.

The *afferent arteriole* which supplies the glomerulus, and the *efferent arteriole* which drains the glomerulus, enter and leave the corpuscle at the so-called *vascular pole* which is usually situated opposite the entrance to the renal tubule, the so-called *urinary pole*.

2. Renal tubule: the renal tubule extends from Bowman's capsule to its junction with a *collecting duct*. The renal tubule is up to 55 mm long in man and is lined by a single layer of epithelial cells. The primary function of the renal tubule is the selective reabsorption of water, inorganic ions and other molecules from the glomerular filtrate. In addition, some inorganic ions are secreted directly from blood into the lumen of the tubule. In man, glomerular filtrate is produced at a steady rate of approximately 120 ml per minute; of this, approximately 119 ml per minute are reabsorbed in the renal tubules. The highly convoluted renal tubule has four distinct histo-physiological zones, each of which has a different role in tubular function.

(a) *The proximal convoluted tubule (PCT):* this is the longest, most convoluted section of the tubule; PCTs make up the bulk of the renal cortex. Approximately 75% of all the ions and water of the glomerular filtrate are reabsorbed from the PCT.

(b) *The loop of Henle:* this arises from the PCT as a straight, thin-walled limb (*the thin limb*) which descends from the cortex into the medulla; here it loops closely back on itself to ascend as a straight, thicker-walled limb (*the thick limb*) into the renal cortex. The limbs of the loop of Henle are closely associated with parallel, wide capillary loops, the *vasa recta* (not shown in this diagram). The vasa recta, which arise from glomerular efferent arterioles, descend into the medulla then loop back on themselves to drain into veins at the junction of the medulla and cortex. In man, only a relatively small proportion of the water in glomerular filtrate is absorbed from the loops of Henle into the vasa recta. The main function of the loops of Henle is to generate a high osmotic pressure in the extracellular fluid of the renal medulla; the mechanism by which this is achieved is known as the *counter-current multiplier system*, the details of which are beyond the scope of this discussion.

(c) *The distal convoluted tubule (DCT):* this is shorter and less convoluted than the PCT. Sodium ions are actively reabsorbed from the DCT by a process which is controlled by the adreno-cortical hormone *aldosterone*. Sodium reabsorption is in some way coupled with the secretion of hydrogen or potassium ions into the DCT.

(d) *The collecting tubule:* this is the terminal portion of the DCT and conducts urine to the *collecting ducts* which merge to form the large *ducts of Bellini* in the renal medulla. The collecting tubules and ducts are not normally permeable to water; however, in the presence of antidiuretic hormone (ADH), secreted by the posterior pituitary, the collecting tubules and ducts become permeable to water which is then drawn out by the high osmotic pressure of the medullary extracellular fluid; reabsorbed water is returned to the general circulation via the vasa recta. The activity of the loops of Henle and ADH thus provide a mechanism for the production of urine which is hypertonic with respect to plasma.

This diagram also illustrates the arterial supply of the renal cortex. In the hilum, the renal artery divides into two main branches. Each of these gives rise to several *interlobar arteries* which ascend between the pyramids to the cortico-medullary junction. Here they branch to form the *arcuate arteries* which run parallel to the capsule of the kidney. The arcuate arteries give rise to numerous *interlobular arteries* which extend towards the capsule and branch to form the glomerular afferent arterioles.

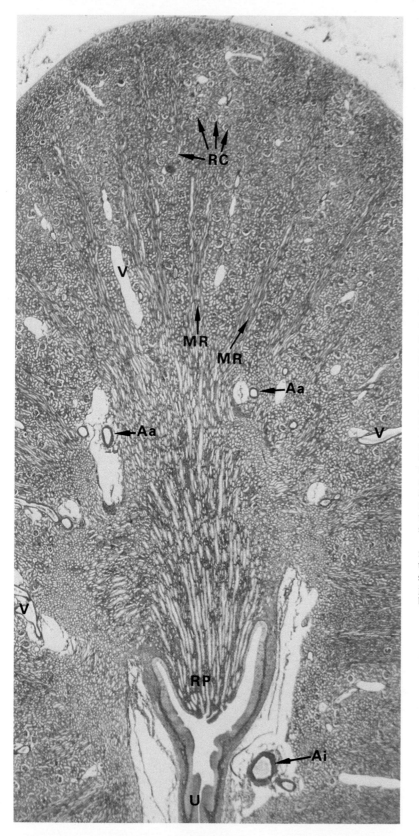

Fig. 16.5 Kidney

(Monkey: TS, Jones' methenamine silver/H & E × 12)

The basic geography of the kidney can be seen in this section through the kidney at the level of the ureter **U**.

In the cortex, numerous renal corpuscles **RC** are just visible at this magnification. The corpuscles tend to be arranged in parallel rows at right angles to the capsule, corresponding to the course of the interlobular arteries from which they derive their blood supply. The venous system, arranged in a similar manner to the arterial system, converges upon the medulla; venous elements appear as thin-walled vessels **V**.

Most of the tissue mass surrounding the renal corpuscles in the cortex consists of proximal and distal convoluted tubules. From the cortex, pale-stained lines appear to radiate towards the medulla and thence to the tip of the renal papilla **RP**. These lines, which are called *medullary rays* **MR**, are bundles of collecting tubules and ducts derived from nephrons located high in the cortex. The collecting ducts merge to form the larger ducts of Bellini which drain urine into the pelvi-calyceal space through the renal papilla. Although not visible at this magnification, the limbs of the loops of Henle dip into the medulla between, and parallel with, the collecting tubules and ducts. The vasa recta, the long, straight vessels into which water is absorbed from the collecting tubules and ducts, also dip down into the medulla alongside the loops of Henle; these vessels are also too small to be seen at this magnification.

Note a large interlobar branch of the renal artery **Ai** in the hilar connective tissue surrounding the pelvi-calyceal space. At the cortico-medullary junction, several arcuate arteries **Aa** can be seen in transverse section.

Fig. 16.6 Renal cortex

(Azan × 80)

Further magnification reveals more details of the cortical tissue. Renal corpuscles **RC** appear as dense, rounded structures, the glomeruli, surrounded by narrow spaces, Bowman's spaces. Even at this magnification, it is evident that the tubules comprising the tissue between the renal corpuscles differ from one another in diameter, staining intensity and shape. The mass of cortical tubules seen in section mainly consists of proximal convoluted tubules with smaller numbers of distal convoluted tubules and a lesser number of other segments of renal tubules.

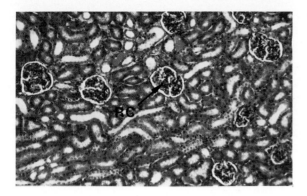

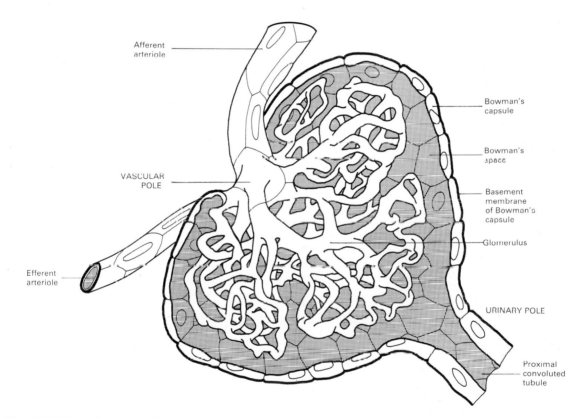

Fig. 16.7 Renal corpuscle

The main structural features of the renal corpuscle are demonstrated in this idealised diagram.

The relatively wide diameter afferent arteriole pierces Bowman's capsule at the vascular pole of the renal corpuscle and then branches to form a tightly anastomosing network of capillaries, the glomerulus. The glomerulus is thus suspended in Bowman's space from the vascular pole. Although not shown in this diagram, the capillary loops are supported by stalks of specialised connective tissue called *mesangium* extending into the glomerulus through the vascular pole. If the capillary loops are likened to the coils of the small bowel lying in the abdominal cavity, then the mesangium forms the equivalent of the mesenteries.

The efferent vessel which drains the glomerulus is unusual in that it has the structure of an arteriole and is thus called the efferent arteriole (rather than the efferent venule). The efferent arteriole is of smaller diameter than the afferent arteriole and a pressure gradient is thus maintained which drives the filtration of plasma into Bowman's space.

The layer of podocytes which invests the glomerular capillaries is not represented in this diagram. At the vascular pole, the podocyte layer is reflected to become continuous with the epithelium of Bowman's capsule which in turn becomes continuous with the first part of the renal tubule, the proximal convoluted tubule.

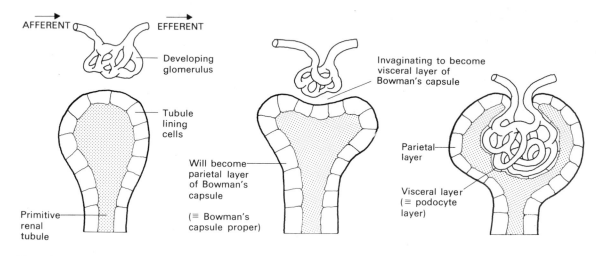

Fig. 16.8 Development of the renal corpuscle

This diagram illustrates in a highly schematic manner the mode of development of the renal corpuscle. The nephrons develop from the embryological metanephros as blind-ended tubules consisting of a single layer of cuboidal epithelium. The ends of the tubules dilate and become invaginated by a tiny mass of tissue which differentiates to form the glomerulus. The layer of invaginated epithelium flattens and differentiates into podocytes which become closely applied to the surface of the knot of glomerular capillaries. The intervening connective tissue disappears so that the basement membrane of glomerular endothelial cells and

podocytes effectively fuse forming the glomerular basement membrane. A small amount of connective tissue nevertheless remains to support the capillary loops and differentiates to form the mesangium. Where the mesangium stretches between the capillary loops, its surface is directly invested by podocyte cytoplasm with podocyte basement membrane lying between the two. When examining ultra-thin light microscope specimens as in Figure 16.11 and electron micrographs as in Figure 16.14, the podocytes, endothelial cells and mesangium are identified most easily by tracing out the podocyte and endothelial cell basement membranes.

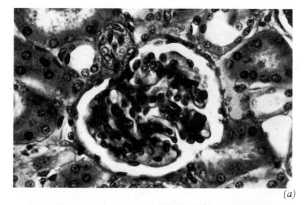

(a)

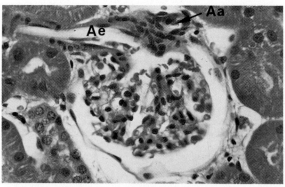

(b)

Fig. 16.9 Renal corpuscle

(a) Azan × 320 (b) H & E × 320

The renal corpuscles in both of these micrographs have been sectioned through the vascular pole and in the case of micrograph (a) through the urinary pole also. At the vascular pole, the afferent arteriole **Aa** is seen entering the corpuscle to supply the glomerulus though in micrograph (a) the lumen of this vessel cannot be seen. In micrograph (b), the efferent arteriole **Ae** is also seen cut longitudinally. Glomerular capillaries are cut in transverse, longitudinal and oblique section but little detail can be resolved in such preparations. The numerous nuclei in the glomerulus are those of capillary endothelial cells, *mesangial cells* of the supporting mesangium, and podocytes.

Note the flattened nuclei of the squamous cells lining Bowman's capsule. In micrograph (a), the basement membranes of the glomerulus and Bowman's capsule are stained a prominent blue. Note the continuity of Bowman's space with the lumen of the proximal convoluted tubule. Due to shrinkage of the glomerulus, inevitable in this type of tissue preparation, Bowman's space appears artefactually enlarged. In vivo, Bowman's space is filled with glomerular filtrate which is at much lower pressure than that of the plasma within the glomerular capillaries; this pressure gradient forces the glomerular filtrate down the renal tubular system.

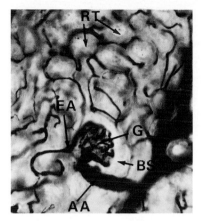

Fig. 16.10 Blood supply of the glomerulus

(Carmine-gelatine perfused × 128)

This is a section of a kidney which has been perfused with a red dye in order to demonstrate the renal blood supply. The kidney tissue remains unstained in this preparation.

An interlobular artery (see Fig. 16.4) can be seen branching to form the afferent arteriole **AA** of glomerulus **G**. Note that the afferent arteriole has a greater diameter than the efferent arteriole **EA**. This arrangement maintains the pressure within glomerular capillaries necessary for blood plasma to be filtered into Bowman's space **BS**. Blood pressure within the glomerulus is controlled by appropriate variation of the diameter of the afferent and efferent arterioles.

The efferent arteriole gives rise to a network of capillaries which surround the renal tubules **RT**. The efferent arterioles also give rise to the vasa recta which loop into the medulla and are therefore not seen in this section of the renal cortex. Molecules reabsorbed from glomerular filtrate are returned to the general circulation via this capillary network which drains into the renal venous system.

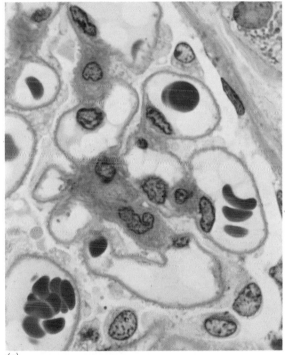

(a)

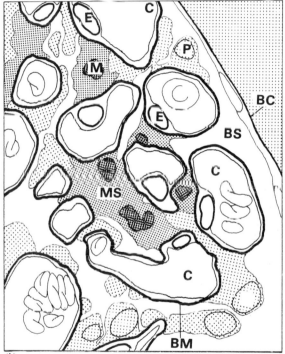

(b)

Fig. 16.11 Glomerulus

(a) Thin section, toluidine blue × 1200 (b) Explanatory diagram

Using resin-embedding techniques it is possible to cut thin sections (approximately 0.5–1.0 μm thick) which permit much greater resolution at high magnification.

In this preparation, the glomerular capillaries **C**, some of which contain erythrocytes, are defined by their prominent basement membranes **BM**. Occasional capillary endothelial cell nuclei **E** are seen bulging into the capillary lumina. Mesangium, which consists of mesangial cells **M** and densely stained extracellular substance called *mesangial substance* **MS**, provides support for the capillary loops particularly at their branching points. Mesangium represents specialised connective tissue but its physiological role is poorly understood.

The surface of the glomerular capillary loops exposed to Bowman's space **BS** is invested by a continuous but irregular layer of podocytes. The podocytes **P** have an extensive, branching, pale-stained cytoplasm and large rounded pale-stained nuclei. Thus, the glomerular filtrate must traverse capillary endothelium, basement membrane and the podocyte layer before reaching Bowman's space. Bowman's space is much less prominent in this type of preparation in which little glomerular shrinkage occurs. Note the nuclei of two squamous cells of Bowman's capsule **BC**, the outline of which may be traced by its prominent basement membrane.

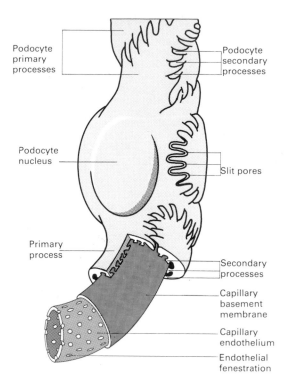

Podocyte primary processes

Podocyte secondary processes

Podocyte nucleus

Slit pores

Primary process

Secondary processes

Capillary basement membrane

Capillary endothelium

Endothelial fenestration

Fig. 16.12 Components of the glomerular filter

During filtration of plasma from glomerular capillaries into Bowman's space, the filtrate passes through three layers:

1. Capillary endothelium: glomerular capillary endothelial cells contain numerous pores or fenestrations which are large enough to permit the passage of all the non-cellular elements of blood.

2. Capillary basement membrane: this layer is continuous and non-fenestrated. Clinical evidence has demonstrated that free haemoglobin (molecular weight 65 000) and smaller molecules pass freely through the glomerular filter, whereas albumin (molecular weight 68 000) and larger molecules are retained. Experimental evidence, based on the use of tracer molecules, suggests that the basement membrane acts as the glomerular *ultrafilter*.

3. Podocytes: these cells, which envelop the glomerular capillaries, have long cytoplasmic extensions called *primary processes*. The primary processes in turn give rise to short *secondary foot processes (pedicels)* which closely interdigitate with those of other primary processes and are directly applied to the glomerular basement membrane. The gaps between these interdigitations are of uniform width (25 nm) and are called *slit pores*. The role of slit pores in the filtration process is poorly understood. Plasma molecules, too large to be filtered, remain within the glomerular capillaries and maintain a colloidal osmotic pressure which prevents filtration of all the water from plasma.

Fig. 16.13 Glomerulus

(micrographs (b) and (c) opposite)
(Scanning EM (a) × 675 (b) × 1500 (c) × 6000)

Scanning electron microscopy readily demonstrates the three-dimensional relationships of podocytes and their processes which extend like octopus tentacles over the whole surface of the glomerulus.

In micrograph (a), part of Bowman's capsule **BC** has been removed to reveal a three-dimensional view of the glomerulus. Note the tightly packed capillary loops **C**.

At higher magnification in micrograph (b), the capillaries can be seen to be enveloped by podocytes which have large, flattened cell bodies and bulging nuclei **N**. Each podocyte has several long primary processes P_1 which embrace one or more capillaries. Each primary process has numerous secondary foot processes.

With further magnification in micrograph (c), the secondary foot processes P_2 can be seen as extensions of the larger processes P_1. The secondary foot processes interdigitate with those of other primary processes.

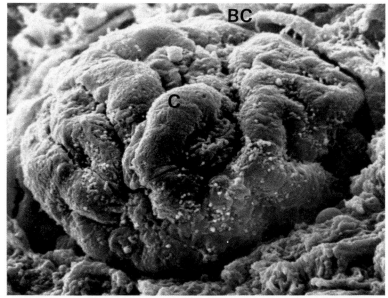

(a)

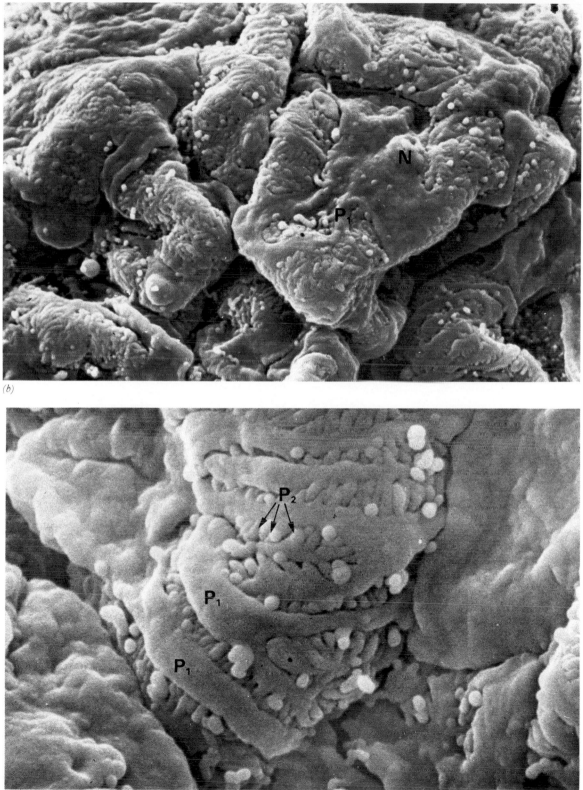

(b)

(c)

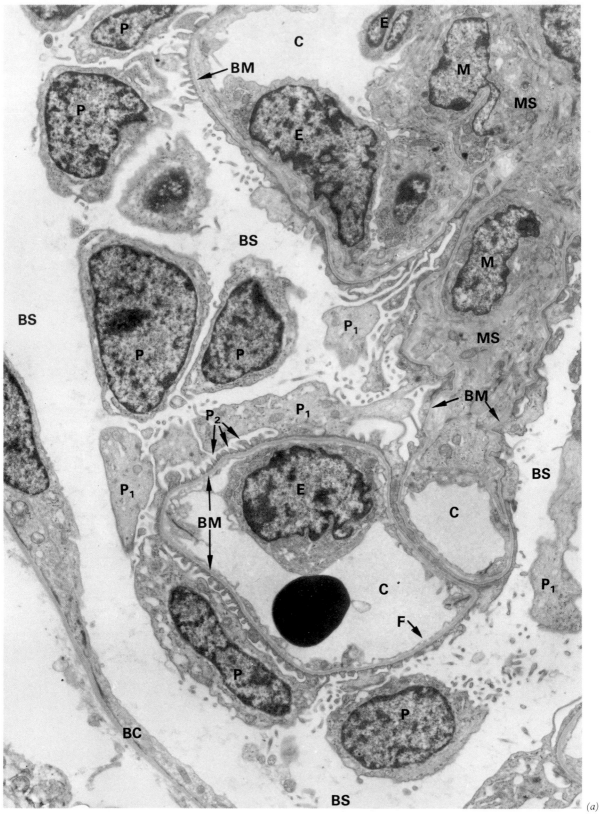

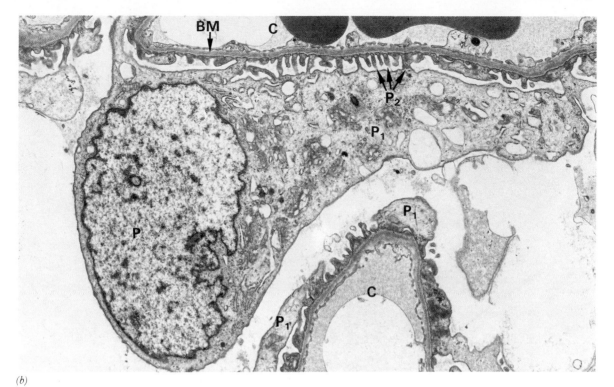

(b)

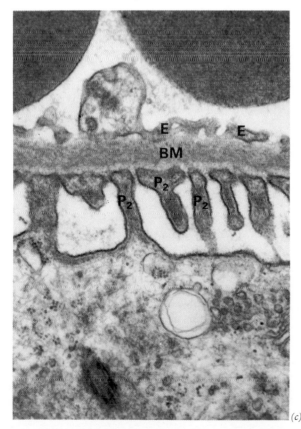

(c)

Fig. 16.14 Glomerulus *(micrograph (a) opposite)*

(EM (a) × 4800 (b) × 8500 (c) × 66 000)

The ultrastructural details of the glomerulus are demonstrated in this series of micrographs; the basement membranes of the capillary endothelial cells and podocytes provide the key to interpretation.

Micrograph (a) shows several capillary loops C, recognised by their content of erythrocytes and precipitated plasma proteins; the capillaries are lined by a thin layer of fenestrated endothelial cytoplasm and endothelial cell nuclei E can be seen bulging into the capillary lumina. Capillary endothelial fenestrations F are better seen at higher magnification in (c). A branched mesangial stalk comprising mesangial cells M and dense mesangial substance MS provides support for the capillary loops. The nuclei of several podocytes P can be seen, their primary processes P_1 giving rise to numerous secondary foot processes P_2 which rest on the glomerular basement membrane BM. Part of Bowman's capsule BC is seen at the periphery. Note the labyrinth of Bowman's space BS which pervades the glomerulus.

In micrograph (b), the relationship of a podocyte P and its primary P_1 and secondary P_2 foot processes with the basement membrane of a glomerular capillary C is demonstrated. With further magnification in micrograph (c), the three components of the glomerular filter are seen. The fenestrated capillary endothelium E is closely applied to the luminal surface of the glomerular basement membrane BM and on the opposite side are podocyte secondary foot processes P_2, separated by slit pores of approximately uniform width.

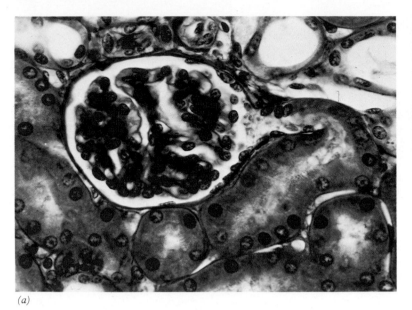

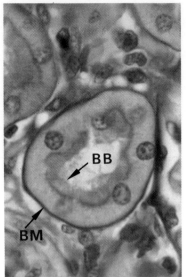

(a)

(b)

Fig. 16.15 Proximal convoluted tubule

(a) Azan × 480 (b) PAS/Haematoxylin × 800

Micrograph (a) shows a proximal convoluted tubule (PCT) arising from a renal corpuscle; convolutions of this PCT are seen in longitudinal, oblique and transverse sections.

Approximately 75% of the glomerular filtrate is reabsorbed from the PCT and this reabsorptive function is reflected in the structure of the epithelial lining. The simple, tall cuboidal epithelium has a prominent brush border which almost completely fills the lumen. The brush border greatly increases the surface area of plasma membrane through which molecules can be reabsorbed from the glomerular filtrate. The cytoplasm of PCT epithelial cells stains intensely due to a high content of organelles, principally mitochondria. The bulk of the renal cortex is composed of proximal tubules since the PCT is the longest and most convoluted part of the nephron.

The PAS staining method has been used in micrograph (b) to demonstrate the prominent brush border **BB** of microvilli projecting into the lumen of the PCT. The brush border is PAS-positive since the surfaces of the microvilli are coated with a particularly dense glycocalyx (see Fig. 1.2). The glycocalyx is thought to afford physical and chemical protection to the microvilli. Like all other basement membranes, the basement membrane **BM** supporting the tubular epithelium is strongly PAS-positive due to its condensed ground substance.

A rich capillary network arising from the efferent arteriole of the glomerulus (see Fig. 16.10) surrounds the PCT and returns molecules reabsorbed from the glomerular filtrate back into the general circulation.

Fig. 16.16 Proximal convoluted tubule *(illustrations opposite)*

(EM (a) × 600 (b) × 8500)

Electron microscopy of the PCT reveals profuse, tall microvilli **Mv** constituting the brush border seen with light microscopy The plasma membrane of the microvilli contains a variety of transport proteins and enzymes involved in selective reabsorption of solutes from the glomerular filtrate. Some of these transport processes are dependent on energy which is supplied in the form of ATP by mitochondria **M** which crowd the cytoplasm of PCT cells. The cytoplasm immediately beneath the brush border contains many pinocytotic vesicles **V** and lysosomes **L** which are thought to be involved in reabsorption and degradation of small amounts of protein which have leaked through the glomerular ultrafilter. Reabsorbed solutes are transported through the basal plasma membrane into surrounding capillaries **C**.

At high magnification, the basal plasma membrane **P** of the PCT is seen to exhibit deep basal infoldings into the cell. These infoldings are closely related to columns of elongated mitochondria **M**. This mitochondrial arrangement may give rise to the appearance of basal striations in light microscopy. The basal infoldings of the plasma membrane increase the surface area for transport of reabsorbed molecules from PCT cells into the extracellular fluid and thence into capillaries. The presence of numerous mitochondria reflects the high energy demands of this process. Note the basement membrane **BM** separating the base of the tubule lining cells from the delicate capillary endothelium **E**.

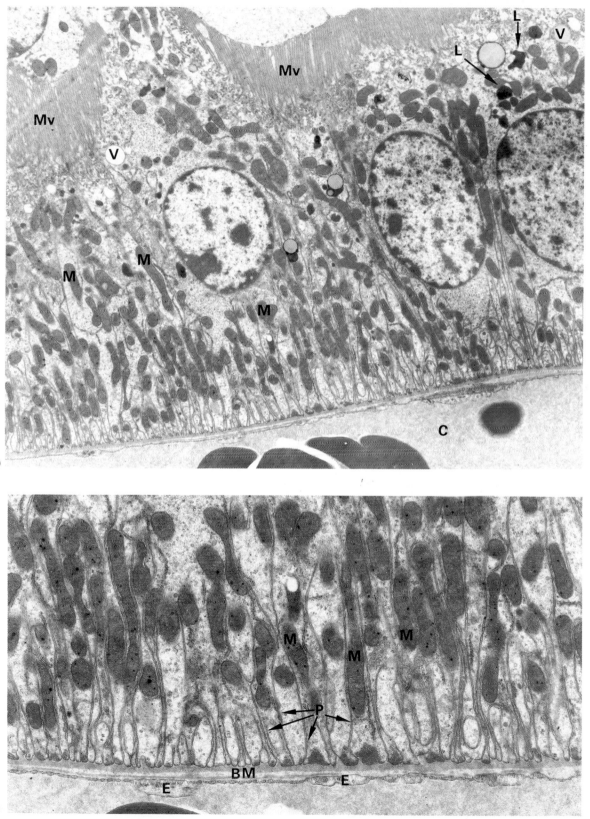

(a)

(b)

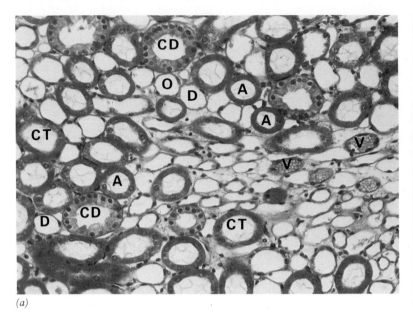

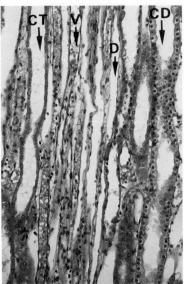

(a)   (b)

Fig. 16.17 Loop of Henle

(H & E (a) TS × 198 (b) LS × 100)

The loop of Henle is a continuation of the PCT and
constitutes the second histo-physiological zone of the renal
tubule (see Fig. 16.4). Each loop of Henle arises in the renal
cortex, dips down into the medulla as the descending limb,
then returns to the cortex as the ascending limb before
becoming continuous with the distal convoluted tubule.
Thus loops of Henle are best seen in sections of renal
medulla. In addition to loops of Henle, the medulla also
contains the vasa recta, collecting tubules and collecting
ducts. All these structures are seen in these micrographs and
may be distinguished by the following features.

The thin descending limbs **D** have a simple squamous
epithelium but may be differentiated from the vasa recta **V**
by their regular, rounded shape, when seen in transverse
section, and the absence of erythrocytes. The thick

ascending limbs **A** are lined by low cuboidal epithelium and
are also round in cross-section. Neither limb of the loop of
Henle has a brush border. Collecting tubules **CT** have a
similar epithelial lining to the ascending limbs but are of
wider and less regular diameter. The collecting ducts **CD**
are easily recognised by their large diameter and columnar,
pale-stained epithelial lining.

The function of the loop of Henle is to produce an
increasing osmotic gradient from the cortex to the deepest
part of the renal medulla. The high osmotic pressure in
medullary extracellular fluid permits the removal of water,
by osmosis, from fluid in the collecting tubules and ducts in
the presence of ADH (see Fig. 16.22). The vasa recta take
up water from the medullary extracellular fluid and return it
to the general circulation.

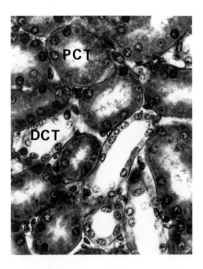

Fig. 16.18 Distal convoluted tubule

(Azan × 320)

The distal convoluted tubule (DCT) extends from the ascending limb of the loop of
Henle after its return to the cortex, and forms the third histo-physiological zone of
the renal tubule. Therefore, DCTs are found mainly within the cortex where they
are entangled with proximal convoluted tubules.

As seen in this micrograph of the renal cortex, distal convoluted tubules **DCT**
may be differentiated from surrounding proximal convoluted tubules **PCT** on the
basis of the following characteristic features: absence of a brush border; a larger,
more clearly defined lumen; more nuclei are seen in transverse section (since DCT
cells are smaller than those of the PCT); less affinity for cytoplasmic stains (due to
a smaller content of organelles). In addition, sections of the DCT are seen much
less frequently than sections of the PCT since the DCT is a much shorter segment
of the renal tubule than the PCT.

The DCT is mainly involved in reabsorption of sodium ions from the tubular
fluid; this process is directly coupled to the secretion of hydrogen and potassium
ions into the tubular fluid. One hydrogen ion or one potassium ion is secreted for
every one sodium ion reabsorbed. This process is controlled by the hormone
aldosterone secreted by the adrenal cortex (see Fig. 17.13).

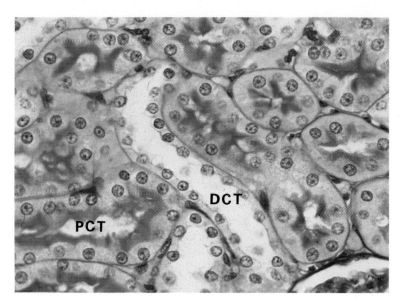

Fig. 16.19 Renal tubules
(PAS/Haematoxylin × 480)

This micrograph demonstrates a method of differentiating between proximal and distal convoluted tubules on the basis of the presence or absence of a brush border. The PCT has a profuse PAS-positive brush border (see Fig. 15.16b) whereas a brush border is almost completely absent from the DCT.

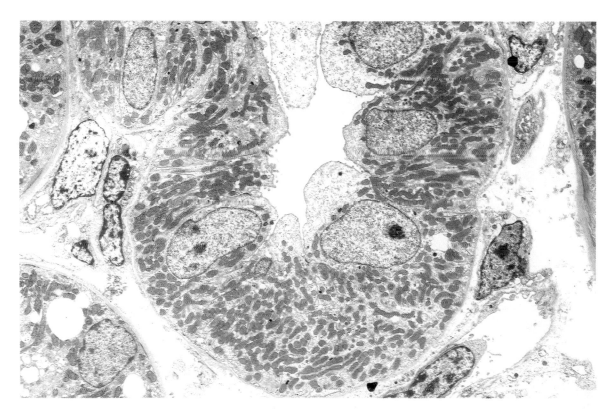

Fig. 16.20 Distal convoluted tubule
(EM × 3000)

The distal convoluted tubule has many ultrastructural features in common with the proximal convoluted tubule, in particular the large number of mitochodria and infolding of the basal plasma membrane. The most striking difference is that the DCT lacks a brush border, having only a few irregular microvilli at the luminal surface. The cells of the DCT have less cytoplasm than those of the PCT although the nucleus is of about the same size and consequently the nucleus takes up much more of the cell. In addition, the nuclei of the DCT cells lie closer to the luminal surface and consequently tend to bulge into the lumen.

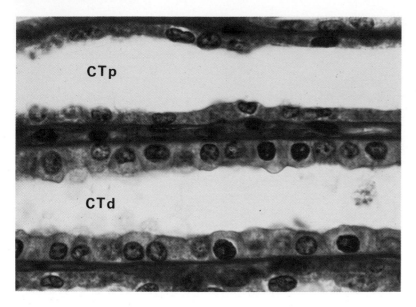

Fig. 16.21 Collecting tubules
(LS: Azan × 750)

The collecting tubule continues from the terminal part of the DCT and constitutes the fourth histo-physiological zone of the nephron. The collecting tubules converge in the renal cortex to form bundles of tubules termed medullary rays (see Fig. 16.5). As the medullary rays approach the medulla, the cuboidal epithelium lining the collecting tubules becomes progressively taller. This micrograph illustrates a proximal section of a collecting tubule **CTp** and a more distal section **CTd** of an adjacent tubule within a medullary ray. The absence of a brush border and a clear cytoplasm are consistent with the evidence that no active reabsorption takes place within collecting tubules.

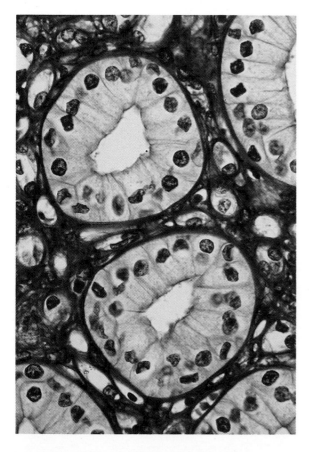

Fig. 16.22 Collecting ducts
(TS: Azan × 480)

The collecting ducts are formed by the fusion of collecting tubules and convey urine into the pelvi-calyceal space. As they converge upon the renal papilla the collecting ducts merge to form progressively larger ducts, the largest ducts being known as the ducts of Bellini.

This micrograph of the renal medulla illustrates two collecting ducts surrounded by thin limbs of the loop of Henle and vasa recta. Collecting ducts are characterised by tall columnar epithelium, well defined cellular outlines, pale-stained cytoplasm and the absence of a brush border.

No active reabsorption takes place from the collecting ducts, but in the presence of anti-diuretic hormone (ADH) secreted by the pituitary, the collecting ducts become permeable to water. Water is drawn out of collecting ducts, by osmosis, into extracellular fluid and thence into adjacent vasa recta. Release of ADH from the pituitary is stimulated by dehydration. This promotes the uptake of water from the collecting tubules thereby producing a reduced volume of hypertonic urine. Conversely, ADH secretion is inhibited by water overloading and an increased volume of hypotonic urine is thus produced.

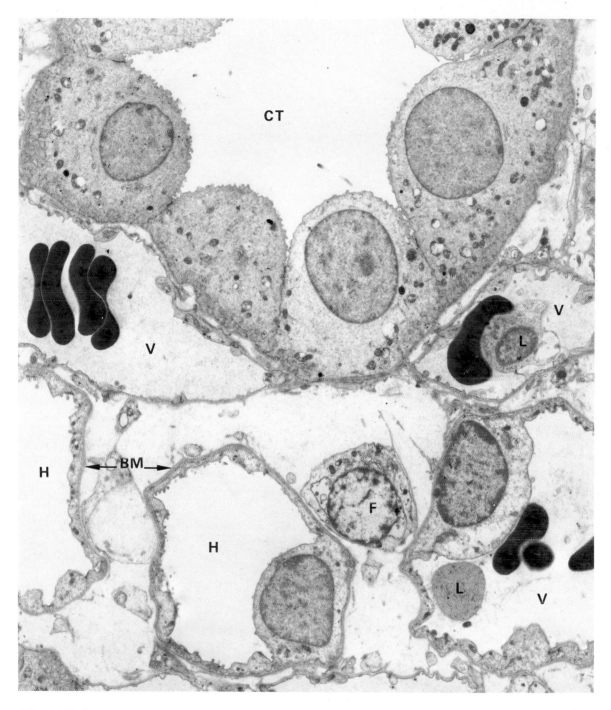

Fig. 16.23 Renal medulla

(EM × 4000)

This electron micrograph illustrates the ultrastructural features of thin limbs of loops of Henle **H**, vasa recta **V** and a collecting tubule **CT**.

The cells of the thin limbs are similar to capillary endothelial cells in structure, most of the wall consisting of a thin irregular layer of cytoplasm with a few very short luminal microvilli and the nucleus bulging into the lumen. Around the tube is a supporting basement membrane **BM**.

The vasa recta can only be readily distinguished from the thin limbs by their content of erythrocytes, occasional leucocytes **L** and precipitated plasma proteins.

The collecting tubules consist of simple cuboidal cells with relatively sparse organelles. Between vessels and nephrons is delicate connective tissue containing a little collagen, scattered fibroblasts **F** and their slender cytoplasmic processes.

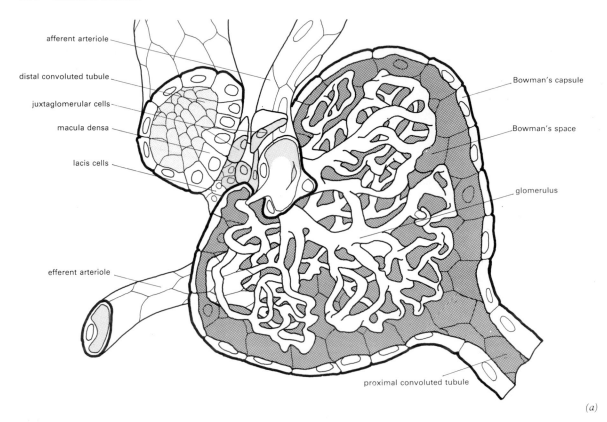

afferent arteriole

distal convoluted tubule

juxtaglomerular cells

macula densa

lacis cells

efferent arteriole

Bowman's capsule

Bowman's space

glomerulus

proximal convoluted tubule

(a)

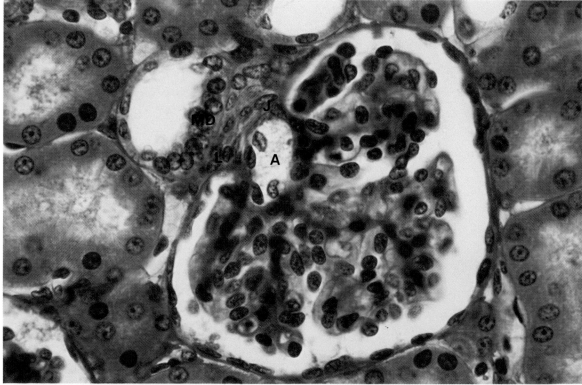

(b)

Fig. 16.24 The juxtaglomerular apparatus *(illustrations opposite)*

(a) Schematic diagram (b) Azan × 640

The juxtaglomerular apparatus (JGA) is involved in the regulation of systemic blood pressure.

The JGA is made up of the part of the afferent arteriole just before it enters Bowman's capsule, and a section of DCT of the same nephron which loops back to lie against the afferent arteriole at this point. The JGA has the following components as seen in the diagram.

1. **Juxtaglomerular cells:** these cells are derived from the smooth muscle of the wall of the afferent arteriole and form a cuff of several layers around the afferent arteriole just before it enters the glomerulus. Juxtaglomerular cells have a prominent nucleus and the cytoplasm contains granules of the enzyme *renin*. It is thought that the juxtaglomerular cells are directly sensitive to the pressure of blood in the afferent arteriole. A decrease in systemic blood pressure stimulates the release of renin granules which activates the *renin-angiotensin-aldosterone mechanism*; this promotes an increase in systemic blood pressure (see Fig. 16.25).

2. **Macula densa:** this consists of modified DCT cells and is found where the juxtaglomerular cells and DCT are closely apposed. The cells of the macula densa are taller and have larger, more prominent nuclei than the other cells lining the DCT. The basement membrane between the macula and juxtaglomerular cells is extremely thin.

It is postulated that the cells of the macula densa are sensitive to the concentration of sodium ions in the fluid within the DCT. A decrease in systemic blood pressure results in decreased production of glomerular filtrate and hence decreased concentration of sodium ions in the fluid of the DCT; this stimulates the release of renin granules into the blood of the afferent arteriole via the juxtaglomerular cells. Consequently the JGA is thought to respond to systemic blood pressure changes via both mechano- and chemoreceptors.

3. **Lacis cells (or polkissen):** this small group of cells lies between the macula densa and Bowman's capsule at the point of entry of the afferent arteriole. These cells are thought to be extra-glomerular mesangial cells but their function is uncertain. Lacis cells may produce the hormone erythropoietin which promotes erythropoiesis in bone marrow. The stimulus for erythropoietin release is postulated to be a low concentration of oxygen in the blood of the afferent arteriole.

The micrograph shows a section through the vascular pole of a renal corpuscle including a juxtaglomerular apparatus; the diagram was based on this micrograph. Note the tall columnar cells of the macula densa **MD** and the thickening of the muscular wall of the adjacent afferent arteriole **A** representing the juxtaglomerular cells **J**. Nearby lies a small clump of lacis cells **L**.

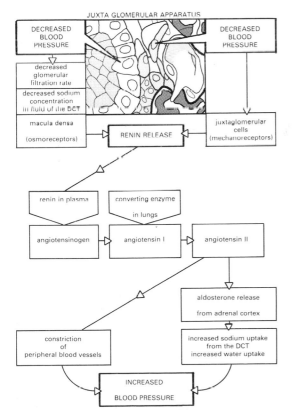

Fig. 16.25 Juxtaglomerular apparatus: control of blood pressure

This diagram summarises the mode of action of the juxtaglomerular apparatus. There are two circumstances in which renin is thought to be released into the bloodstream:

1. A fall in systemic blood pressure; this may be sensed by pressure receptors (the juxtaglomerular cells) in the wall of the afferent arteriole.

2. A decrease in the concentration of sodium ions in the DCT which occurs when the glomerular filtration rate decreases due to a fall in blood pressure. This may be sensed by cells of the macula densa acting as chemoreceptors.

The enzyme renin, when liberated into the bloodstream, acts on the plasma globulin *angiotensinogen* to produce a polypeptide chain of ten amino-acids called *angiotensin I*. A further enzyme, called *converting enzyme*, cleaves two amino-acids from angiotensin I to form *angiotensin II* which is a potent vasoconstrictor.

Angiotensin II brings about an increased blood pressure in two ways: firstly, by constriction of peripheral blood vessels, and secondly by promoting the release of aldosterone from the adrenal cortex. Aldosterone promotes the reabsorption of sodium ions and therefore water from the DCT, thus expanding the plasma volume and hence increasing blood pressure.

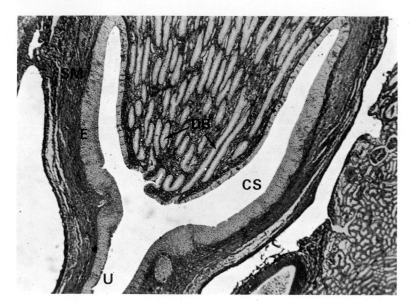

Fig. 16.26 Renal papilla
(Monkey: Azan × 30)

The renal papilla forms the apex of the medullary pyramid where it projects into the calyceal space. The ducts of Bellini **DB**, the largest of the collecting ducts, converge in the renal papilla to discharge urine into the pelvicalyceal space **CS**. The renal pelvis is lined by urinary epithelium **E**, and the wall of the pelvis contains smooth muscle **SM** which contracts to force urine into the ureter **U**.

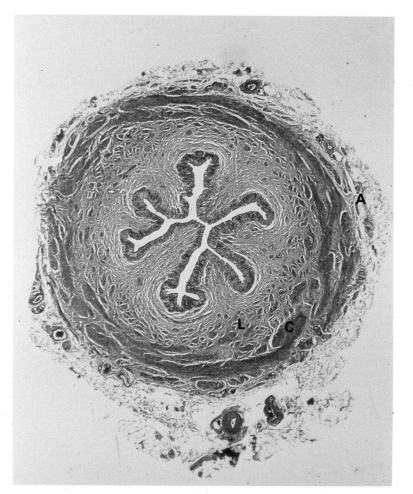

Fig. 16.27 Ureter
(TS: Masson's trichrome × 18)

The ureters are muscular tubes which conduct urine from the kidneys to the bladder. Urine is conducted from the pelvi-calyceal system as a bolus which is propelled by peristaltic action of the ureteric wall. Thus the wall of the ureter contains two layers of smooth muscle arranged into an inner longitudinal layer **L** and an outer circular layer **C**. Another outer longitudinal layer is present in the lower third of the ureter. The lumen of the ureter is lined by urinary epithelium which is thrown up into folds in the relaxed state allowing the ureter to dilate during the passage of a bolus of urine. Surrounding the muscular wall is a loose connective tissue adventitia **A** containing blood vessels, lymphatics and nerves.

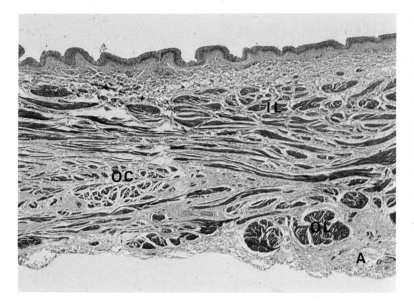

Fig. 16.28 Bladder
(TS: Masson's trichrome × 12)

The general structure of the bladder wall resembles that of the lower third of the ureters. The wall of the bladder consists of three loosely arranged layers of smooth muscle and elastic fibres which contract during micturition. Note the inner longitudinal **IL**, outer circular **OC** and outermost longitudinal **OL** layers of smooth muscle. The urinary epithelium lining the bladder is thrown into many folds in the relaxed state. The outer adventitial coat **A** contains arteries, veins and lymphatics.

The urethra, the final conducting portion of the urinary tract, is discussed as part of the male reproductive tract in Chapter 18.

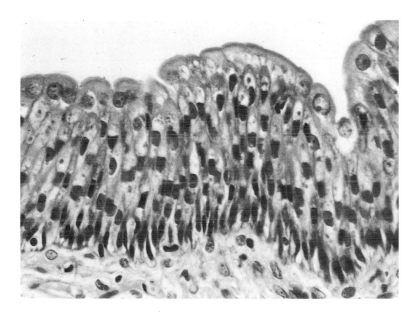

Fig. 16.29 Urinary epithelium
(H & E × 480)

Urinary epithelium, also called transitional epithelium or urothelium, is found only within the conducting passages of the urinary system for which it is especially adapted. The plasma membranes of the superficial cells are much thicker than most cell membranes and have a highly ordered substructure, thus rendering urinary epithelium impermeable to urine which is potentially toxic. This permeability barrier also prevents water from being drawn through the epithelium into hypertonic urine. The cells of urinary epithelium have highly interdigitating cell junctions which permit great distension of the epithelium without

damage to the surface integrity (see also Figs. 5.16 and 5.17).

Urinary epithelium rests on a basement membrane which is often too thin to be resolved by light microscopy and was formerly thought to be absent. The basal layer is irregular and may be deeply indented by strands of underlying connective tissue containing capillaries. This unusual feature led early histologists to believe, mistakenly, that urinary epithelium contradicted the principle that epithelium never contains blood vessels.

17. The endocrine glands

Introduction

Endocrine glands are the sites of synthesis and secretion of substances known as *hormones* which are disseminated throughout the body by the bloodstream where they act on specific *target organs*. In conjuction with the nervous system, hormones co-ordinate and integrate the functions of all the physiological systems.

Endocrine glands are in general composed of secretory cells of epithelial origin supported by connective tissue which is rich in blood and lymphatic capillaries. The secretory cells discharge hormones into the interstitial spaces from which they are rapidly absorbed into the circulatory system. Thus a characteristic feature of all endocrine glands is a very rich vascular supply. Unlike exocrine glands (see Ch. 5), endocrine glands have no duct system and are therefore called the *ductless glands*.

Reflecting their active synthetic function, endocrine secretory cells are generally characterised by prominent nuclei and prolific cytoplasmic organelles, especially mitochondria, endoplasmic reticulum, Golgi bodies and secretory vesicles.

Some endocrine glands exist in the form of discrete organs, e.g. pituitary, thyroid, parathyroid and adrenal glands. Other endocrine tissues are found in association with exocrine glands, e.g. pancreas, or within complex organs, e.g. kidney, testis, ovary, placenta, brain and the gastrointestinal tract. This chapter deals with the pituitary, thyroid, parathyroid, adrenal, endocrine pancreas, pineal and the gastrointestinal endocrine system; other endocrine tissues are discussed with the organs with which they are associated.

Pituitary gland

The *pituitary gland*, also known as the *hypophysis*, is a specialised appendage of the brain which secretes a variety of hormones. The hormones mediate non-nervous mechanisms by which the central nervous system integrates and controls many body functions. The pituitary hormones fall into two functional groups:

1. Hormones which act directly on non-endocrine tissues: growth hormone (GH), prolactin, antidiuretic hormone (ADH), oxytocin and melanocyte stimulating hormone (MSH);
2. Hormones which modulate the secretory activity of other endocrine glands, the so-called *trophic hormones*: thyroid stimulating hormone (TSH), adrenocorticotrophic hormone (ACTH) and the gonadotrophic hormones, follicle stimulating hormone (FSH) and luteinising hormone (LH). Thus the thyroid, adrenal cortex and gonads may be described as *pituitary-dependent endocrine glands*.

The secretion of all pituitary hormones is directly controlled by the hypothalamus; the activity of the hypothalamus, however, is under the influence of nervous stimuli from higher centres in the central nervous system, and is controlled by feedback from the levels of circulating hormones produced by the pituitary-dependent glands. Thus the pituitary gland plays a central role in integrating the nervous and endocrine systems.

The pituitary gland is a small, slightly elongated organ, approximately 1 cm in diameter, lying immediately beneath the third ventricle in a bony cavity in the floor of the skull. The gland is divided structurally into anterior and posterior parts having entirely different embryological origins, functions and control mechanisms.

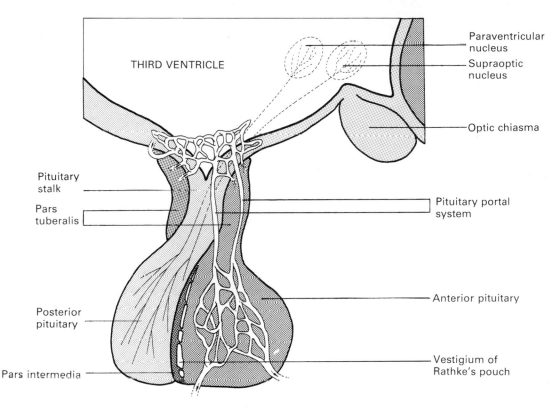

Fig. 17.1 Pituitary gland

The anterior and posterior parts of the pituitary originate from different embryological sources and this is reflected in their structure and function.

1. The posterior pituitary, also called the *neurohypophysis* or *pars nervosa*, is derived from a downgrowth of nervous tissue from the hypothalamus to which it remains joined by the pituitary stalk.

2. The anterior pituitary arises as an epithelial upgrowth from the roof of the primitive oral cavity, known as *Rathke's pouch*. This specialised glandular epithelium is wrapped around the posterior pituitary and is often called the *adenohypophysis*. The adenohypophysis may contain a cleft or group of cyst-like spaces which represent the vestigial lumen of Rathke's pouch. This vestigial cleft divides the major part of the anterior pituitary from a thin zone of tissue lying against the posterior pituitary; this thin zone is known as the *pars intermedia*. An extension of the adenohypophysis surrounds the neural stalk and is known as the *pars tuberalis*.

The type and mode of secretion of the posterior pituitary differs greatly from that of the anterior pituitary. The posterior pituitary secretes two hormones: *antidiuretic hormone* (ADH), also called *vasopressin*, and the hormone *oxytocin*; both these hormones act directly on non-endocrine tissues. ADH is synthesised in the neurone cell bodies of the *supraoptic nucleus*, and oxytocin is synthesised in those of the *paraventricular nucleus* of the hypothalamus. These hormones, bound to glycoproteins, pass down the axons of the hypothalamo-pituitary tract through the pituitary stalk to the posterior pituitary where they are stored in the distended terminal parts of the axons. Release of posterior pituitary hormones into the bloodstream is controlled directly by nervous impulses passing down the axons from the hypothalamus; this process is known as *neurosecretion*.

The anterior pituitary in contrast has the typical structure of epithelial-derived endocrine glands elsewhere in the body. It secretes both trophic and direct action hormones:

1. Trophic hormones: thyroid stimulating hormone (TSH), adrenocorticotrophic hormone (ACTH), and the gonadotrophic hormones, follicle stimulating hormone (FSH) and luteinising hormone (LH).

2. Direct action hormones: growth hormone (GH) and prolactin. (Recent evidence suggests that prolactin has a trophic action on the endocrine tissues of the ovary in some animals.)

Hypothalamic control of anterior pituitary secretion is mediated by specific hypothalamic releasing hormones such as *thyroid stimulating hormone releasing hormone* (TSHRH); an exception to this is prolactin secretion which appears to be under the inhibitory control of dopamine. These releasing hormones are conducted from the *median hypothalamic eminence* to the anterior pituitary by a unique system of portal veins.

The pars intermedia synthesises and secretes melanocyte-stimulating hormone (MSH); in man, the pars intermedia is rudimentary and the physiological importance of MSH and the control of its secretion is poorly understood.

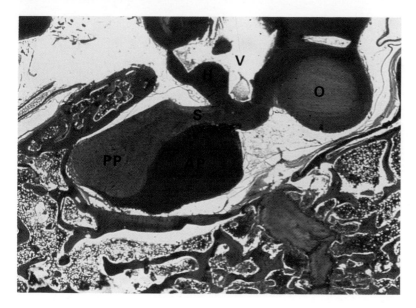

Fig. 17.2 Pituitary gland
(Monkey: H & E × 12)

This micrograph from a mid-line section through the brain and cranial floor illustrates the pituitary gland in situ. The pituitary is almost completely enclosed in a bony depression in the sphenoid bone, called the *sella turcica*. The two major components of the gland, the anterior pituitary **AP** and the posterior pituitary **PP**, are easily seen at this magnification. The posterior pituitary is connected to the hypothalamus **H** by a short stalk, the pituitary stalk **S**, and like the hypothalamus, is composed of nervous tissue. Note the close proximity of the third ventricle **V** above the hypothalamus and the close relationship of the optic chiasma **O** which lies anteriorly.

Fig. 17.3 Anterior pituitary *(illustrations opposite)*
(a) H & E × 480 (b) Modified Azan × 480 (c) EM × 4270

The secretory cells of the anterior pituitary have been traditionally classified into two groups, *chromophils* and *chromophobes*, according to their affinities for histological dyes. The chromophils are subdivided into two groups, *acidophils* and *basophils* because of their staining properties with a variety of histological methods. For example in micrograph (b), acidophils **A** are stained orange and basophils **B** are stained blue. In H & E preparations, the distinction between basophils and acidophils is much less obvious.

The chromophobes **C** are the smallest cell type in the anterior pituitary and contain few cytoplasmic granules; they have little affinity for either acidic or basic dyes and probably represent resting forms of chromophil cells.

All the cells of the anterior pituitary form cords of secretory cells which are surrounded by a rich network of sinusoidal capillaries. The basement membranes surrounding the clumps of epithelial cells are clearly demonstrated as blue-stained structures in preparation (b).

Traditional histological methods of studying the pituitary have been superseded by specific immuno-histochemical techniques by which five types of cells are defined according to their secretory product.

1. Somatotrophs, the cells responsible for growth hormone secretion, are the most numerous, making up almost half of the bulk of the anterior pituitary.

2. Mammotrophs (lactotrophs), the prolactin secreting cells, comprise up to 20% of the anterior pituitary increasing in number during pregnancy and controlling milk production during lactation.

3. Corticotrophs secrete ACTH (corticotrophin) and constitute about 20% of the anterior pituitary mass. ACTH is a polypeptide which becomes split off from a much larger peptide molecule known as *pro-opiocortin*. From the same

molecule can be derived *lipotrophins* (involved in regulation of lipid metabolism), *endorphins* (endogenous opioids) and various species of MSH; the last explains the hyperpigmentation associated with excessive ACTH secretion.

4. Thyrotrophs, which secrete TSH (thyrotrophin), are much less numerous making up only about 5% of the gland.

5. Gonadotrophs, the cells responsible for the secretion of the gonadotrophins FSH and LH, make up the remaining 5% of the anterior pituitary; it seems most likely that there are two distinctive cell types, each responsible for one of the gonadotrophins.

The somatotrophs and mammotrophs represent the acidophils of traditional light microscopy, the basophils being the thyrotrophs, gonadotrophs and probably the corticotrophs (which were formerly thought to be chromophobic).

The secretory granules of each cell type have a characteristic size, shape and electron density by which the different cell types can be recognised with the electron microscope, as in micrograph (c). Somatotrophs **S** are packed with secretory granules of moderate size. Thyrotrophs **T** have considerably smaller granules which tend to be more peripherally located. Gonadotrophs **G** are large cells with secretory granules of moderate and variable size. Corticotrophs **C** have a pale cytoplasm and sparse secretory granules located at the extreme periphery of the cell.

The endothelial lining of capillary sinusoids in endocrine tissues is characteristically fenestrated (see Fig. 8.13). Note the fenestrations **F** in the sinusoid seen in micrograph (c). It is postulated that fenestrations facilitate the passage of hormones into the sinusoids.

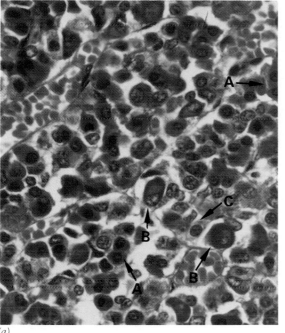

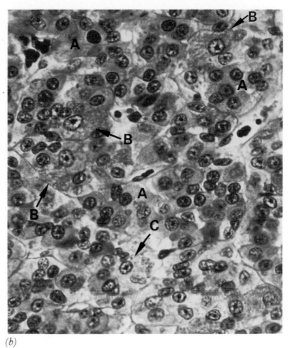

(a)

(b)

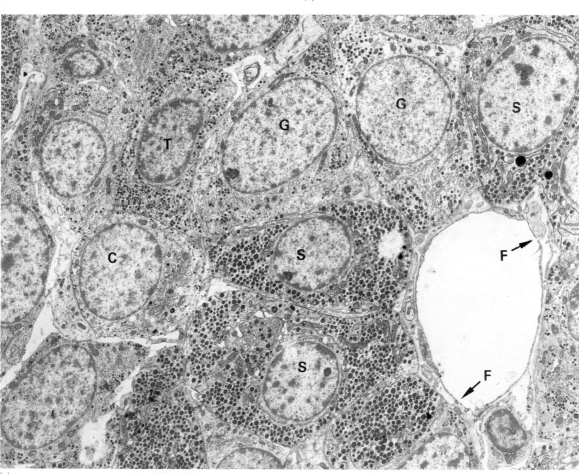

(c)

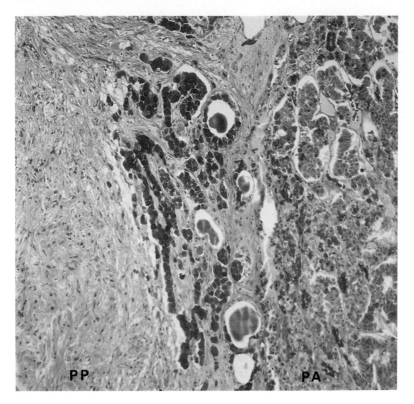

Fig. 17.4 Pituitary: pars intermedia

(Isamine blue/Eosin × 100)

The pars intermedia is a constituent of the anterior pituitary being derived embryologically from the cells lining the cavity of Rathke's pouch; the cells are basophilic, stained blue in this preparation, and form irregular clumps lying between the pars anterior **PA** and pars posterior **PP** but tending to spill out into the neural tissue of the pars posterior.

Small cystic spaces filled with eosinophilic colloid may be seen representing the residuum of Rathke's pouch. The pars intermedia is poorly developed in man as in this specimen but relatively well developed in other mammals and some lower species.

Ultrastructurally, the cells contain secretory granules similar to other anterior pituitary cells. Pro-opiocortin, the same precursor peptide as found in corticotrophs, is synthesised in the pars intermedia where it can be broken into a number of fragments including two species of MSH, endorphins and lipotrophins. MSH promotes melanin synthesis by skin melanocytes thereby increasing skin pigmentation.

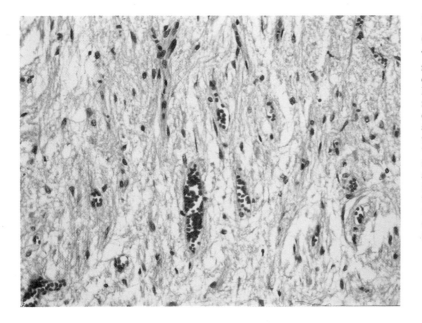

Fig. 17.5 Posterior pituitary

(H & E × 200)

The posterior pituitary contains the non-myelinated axons of neurosecretory cells, the cell bodies of which are located in the hypothalamus. The neurosecretory axons are supported by cells called *pituicytes* similar in structure and function to the neuroglial cells of the central nervous system (see Fig. 7.22). Most of the nuclei seen in this micrograph are those of pituicytes; the axons of the neurosecretory cells are indistinguishable from the cytoplasm of the pituicytes in H & E preparations. A rich network of fine, fenestrated capillaries pervades the posterior pituitary.

Thyroid gland

The thyroid gland is a lobulated endocrine gland lying in the neck in front of the upper part of the trachea. The thyroid gland produces hormones of two types:

1. Iodine-containing hormones *triiodothyronine* (T_3) and *thyroxine (tetra-iodothyronine, T_4)*; T_4 is converted to T_3 in the general circulation by removal of one iodothyronine unit although a small amount of T_3 is secreted directly. T_3 is much more potent than T_4 and appears to be the metabolically active form of the hormone. Thyroid hormone regulates the basal metabolic rate and has an important influence on growth and maturation particularly of nervous tissue. The secretion of these hormones is regulated by TSH secreted by the anterior pituitary.

2. The polypeptide hormone *calcitonin*; this hormone regulates blood calcium levels in conjunction with parathyroid hormone. Calcitonin lowers blood calcium levels by inhibiting the rate of decalcification of bone by osteoclastic resorption and by stimulating osteoblastic activity. Control of calcitonin secretion is dependent only on blood calcium levels and is independent of pituitary and parathyroid hormone levels.

The thyroid gland is unique among the human endocrine glands in that it stores large amounts of thyroid hormone in an inactive form within extracellular compartments called follicles; in contrast, other endocrine glands store only small quantities of hormones in intracellular sites.

The main bulk of the gland develops from an epithelial downgrowth from the fetal tongue whereas the calcitonin-secreting cells are derived from the ultimobranchial element of the fourth branchial pouch.

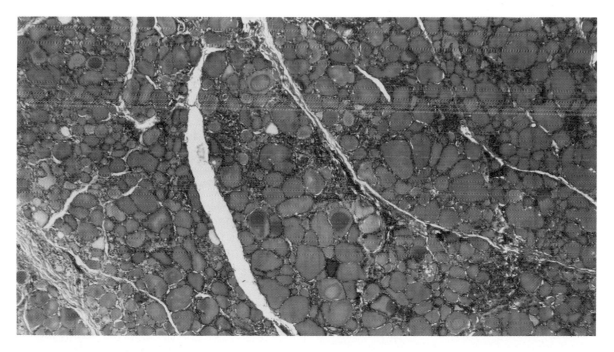

Fig. 17.6 Thyroid gland

(H & E × 12)

The functional units of the thyroid gland are the *thyroid follicles*, irregular, spheroidal structures composed of a single layer of cuboidal epithelial cells bounded by a basement membrane (see also Figs. 5.36 and 5.37). The follicles are variable in size and contain a homogeneous, colloid material which is stained pink in this preparation.

The thyroid gland is enveloped in an outer capsule of loose connective tissue and an inner capsule of fibro-elastic tissue. From the inner capsule, connective tissue septa extend into the gland dividing the gland into lobules, and conveying a rich blood supply, together with lymphatics and nerves.

This micrograph illustrates follicles of widely differing sizes, a characteristic of the normal active thyroid; the size of each follicle reflects its state of synthetic or secretory activity.

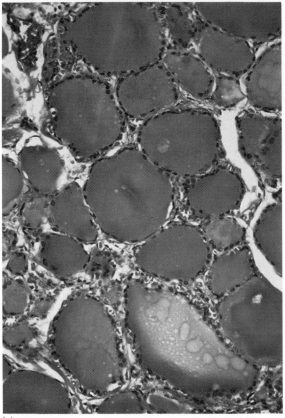

(a)

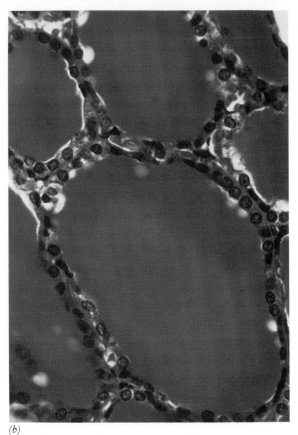

(b)

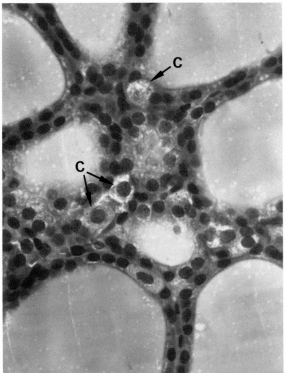

(c)

Fig. 17.7 Thyroid gland

(H & E (a) Human × 240 (b) Human × 480 (c) Dog × 480)

Thyroid follicles are lined by a simple cuboidal epithelium which is responsible for the synthesis and secretion of the iodine-containing hormones T_3 and T_4. Thyroid follicles are filled with a glycoprotein complex called *thyroglobulin* or *thyroid colloid*, which stores the thyroid hormones prior to secretion. In actively secreting thyroid glands, as in these micrographs, the follicles tend to be small and the amount of colloid diminished; the cuboidal lining cells are relatively tall reflecting active hormone synthesis and secretion. Conversely, the follicles of the less active thyroid are distended by stored colloid and the lining cells appear flattened against the follicular basement membrane.

A second secretory cell type is found in the thyroid gland either as single cells among the follicular cells or as small clumps in the interfollicular spaces. These so-called *parafollicular cells* were first described in the dog in which they have an extensive unstained cytoplasm and were therefore also called *'C' (clear cells)* **C**; this characteristic feature is seen in micrograph (c). In other mammals, including man, the cytological characteristics of parafollicular cells are similar to those of the dog but usually much less distinctive. Parafollicular cells synthesise and secrete the hormone calcitonin in direct response to raised blood calcium levels.

Parafollicular cells have a different embryological origin from the follicular cells and in some species constitute a discrete endocrine organ called the ultimo-branchial body.

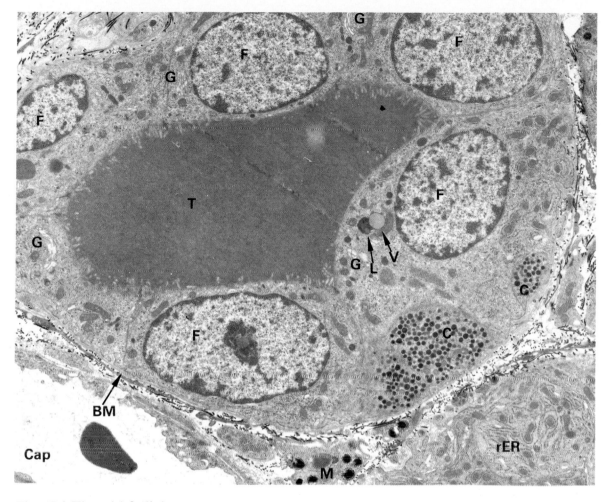

Fig. 17.8 Thyroid follicle

(Rat: EM × 6800)

This micrograph demonstrates a thyroid follicle composed of cuboidal follicular cells **F** surrounding a lumen containing the homogeneous colloid, thyroglobulin **T**. A basement membrane **BM** bounds the follicle. Two portions of the cytoplasm of a parafollicular or 'C' cell **C** are seen within the follicular epithelium typically located on the basement membrane and not exposed to the follicular lumen. The cytoplasm contains numerous electron-dense secretory granules of the hormone, calcitonin. A fenestrated capillary **Cap** containing an erythrocyte is closely applied to the follicular basement membrane. Part of a mast cell **M** is seen in the interfollicular connective tissue.

Follicular cells concentrate iodide from the blood by means of an iodide pump in the basal plasma membrane. Within the cell, iodide is oxidised to iodine and transported to the follicular plasma membrane where it is released into the follicular lumen. The glycoprotein thyroglobulin is synthesised in the rough endoplasmic reticulum, packaged by the Golgi apparatus, then released into the follicular lumen by exocytosis. Within the follicular lumen (not within the follicular cells), iodine combines with tyrosine residues of the thyroglobulin to form the hormones tri-iodothyronine

(T_3) and tetra-iodothyronine (thyroxine, T_4) which remain bound to the glycoprotein in an inactive form.

Secretion of these hormones involves engulfment of the thyroglobulin-hormone complex to form cytoplasmic vacuoles; the vacuoles then fuse with lysosomes of the follicular cell cytoplasm and hydrolytic enzymes cleave the hormone from the thyroglobulin. The hormones are released in the basal cytoplasm from which they diffuse into the bloodstream. The synthetic and secretory activity of the thyroid gland is dependent on thyroid stimulating hormone (TSH) secreted by the anterior pituitary.

In this micrograph, rough endoplasmic reticulum **rER** is best demonstrated in the basal aspect of a secretory cell of an adjacent follicle. Mitochondria are closely associated with the endoplasmic reticulum and are also scattered throughout the cytoplasm. Golgi complexes **G** are a prominent feature. Small microvilli associated with the exocytosis of thyroglobulin and the endocytosis of thyroglobulin-hormone complex, protrude into the follicular lumen. In one cell a vacuole **V** of thyroglobulin-hormone complex is seen about to fuse with a large lysosome **L**. Electron-dense lysosomes are also seen scattered throughout the cytoplasm.

Parathyroid gland

The parathyroid glands are small, oval endocrine glands closely associated with the thyroid gland. In mammals, there are usually two pairs of glands, one pair situated on the posterior surface of the thyroid gland on each side. The embryological origin of the parathyroid glands are the third and fourth pharyngeal pouches. The parathyroid glands regulate serum calcium and phosphate levels via *parathyroid hormone (parathormone)*.

Parathyroid hormone raises serum calcium levels in three ways:
1. Direct action on bone by increasing the rate of osteoclastic resorption and promoting breakdown of the bone matrix.
2. Direct action on the kidney by increasing the renal tubular reabsorption of calcium ions and inhibiting the reabsorption of phosphate ions from the glomerular filtrate.
3. Promotion of the absorption of calcium from the small intestine; this effect involves vitamin D.

Secretion of parathyroid hormone is stimulated by a decrease in blood calcium levels. In conjunction with calcitonin, secreted by the parafollicular cells of the thyroid gland, blood calcium levels are maintained within narrow limits. Parathyroid hormone is the most important regulator of blood calcium levels and is essential to life, whereas calcitonin may only provide a complementary mechanism for fine adjustment.

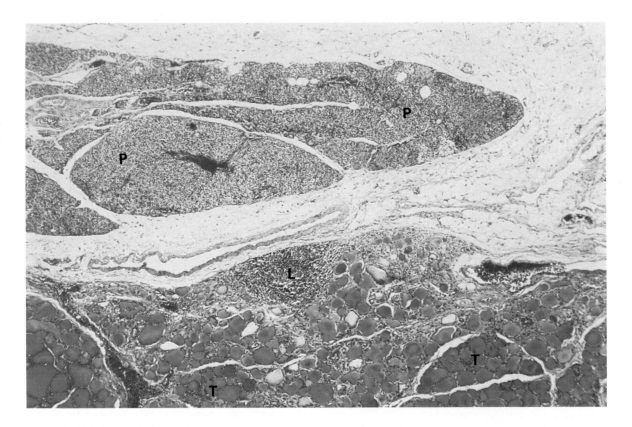

Fig. 17.9 Parathyroid gland
(H & E × 45)

This micrograph shows a parathyroid gland **P** characteristically embedded in the capsule of a thyroid gland **T**. The thin capsule of the parathyroid gland gives rise to delicate connective tissue septa which divide the parenchyma into dense, cord-like masses of secretory cells. The septa carry blood vessels, lymphatics and nerves.

Note that in this specimen, from a 55-year-old woman, there is some infiltration of the thyroid by lymphoid cells **L**; this is a normal feature of the ageing thyroid gland.

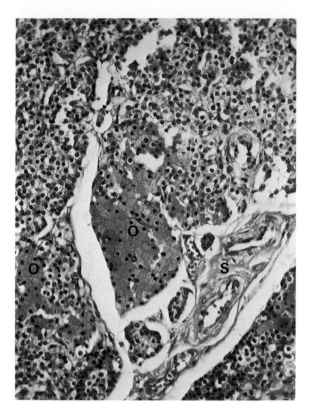

Fig. 17.10 Parathyroid gland
(H & E × 198)

The parathyroid gland contains secretory cells with two types of morphological characteristics:

1. Chief or principal cells: these are the most abundant cells and are responsible for the secretion of parathyroid hormone. Chief cells have a prominent nucleus and relatively little cytoplasm which varies in staining intensity according to the degree of secretory activity of the cell. Actively secreting cells contain much rough endoplasmic reticulum and stain strongly; in contrast, inactive cells contain little rough endoplasmic reticulum and stain poorly.

2. Oxyphil cells: these are larger and much less numerous than chief cells and tend to occur in clumps. They have smaller, densely stained nuclei and strongly eosinophilic (oxyphilic) cytoplasm containing fine granules. Few oxyphil cells are found in the human parathyroid gland until puberty, after which they increase in number with age. Oxyphil cells do not secrete hormones except in certain pathological conditions and their function is poorly understood.

In this micrograph from a young adult, chief cells predominate; note the range of staining intensity from strong to very pale. Oxyphil cells **O** form clumps amongst the chief cells. Note the delicate septa **S** dividing the gland into small lobules and supporting a rich blood supply. With increasing age, adipocytes become characteristically scattered throughout the glandular tissue.

Adrenal gland

The adrenal or supra-renal glands are small, flattened endocrine glands which are closely applied to the upper pole of each kidney. In mammals, the adrenal gland contains two functionally different types of endocrine tissue which have distinctly different embryological origins; in some lower animals, these two components exist as separate endocrine glands. The two components of the adrenal gland are the *adrenal cortex* and *adrenal medulla.*

1. Adrenal cortex: the adrenal cortex has a similar embryological origin to the gonads and like the gonads, secretes a variety of *steroid hormones* all structurally related to their common precursor, *cholesterol.* The adrenal steroids may be divided into three functional classes; *mineralocorticoids, glucocorticoids* and *sex hormones.* The mineralocorticoids are concerned with electrolyte and fluid homeostasis. The glucocorticoids have a wide range of effects on carbohydrate, protein and lipid metabolism. Small quantities of sex hormones secreted by the adrenal cortex supplement gonadal sex hormone secretion.

2. Adrenal medulla: embryologically, the adrenal medulla has a similar origin to that of the sympathetic nervous system and may be considered as a highly specialised adjunct of this system. The adrenal medulla secretes the catecholamine hormones, *adrenaline (epinephrine)* and *noradrenaline (norepinephrine).*

The control of hormone secretion differs markedly between the cortex and medulla. Adrenocortical activity is mainly regulated by the pituitary trophic hormone ACTH, and release of each of the adrenal corticosteroid hormones is controlled by various other circulating hormones and metabolites. In contrast, the secretion of adrenal medullary catecholamines is directly controlled by the sympathetic nervous system. The function of the adrenal medulla is to reinforce the action of the sympathetic nervous system under conditions of stress, the direct nervous control of adrenal medullary secretion permitting a rapid response to stressful stimuli.

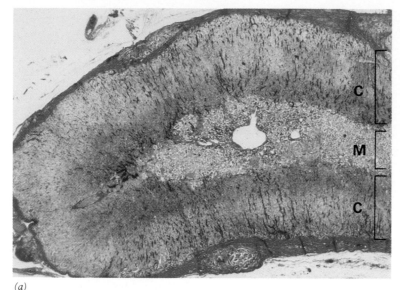

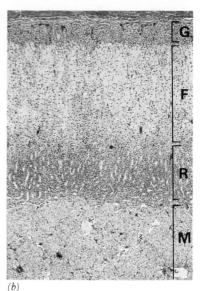

(a)   *(b)*

Fig. 17.11 Adrenal gland

(Azan (a) × 12 (b) × 20)

At low magnification, the adrenal gland is seen to be divided into an outer cortex **C** and a pale-stained inner medulla **M**. A dense fibrous tissue capsule, stained blue in this preparation, invests the gland and provides external support for a delicate collagenous framework supporting the secretory cells. A prominent vein is characteristically located in the centre of the medulla.

At higher magnification in micrograph (b), the adrenal cortex can be seen to consist of three histological zones which are named according to the arrangement of the secretory cells: *zona glomerulosa, zona fasciculata, zona reticularis.*

The zona glomerulosa **G** lying beneath the capsule contains secretory cells arranged in rounded clumps. The intermediate zona fasciculata **F** consists of parallel cords of secretory cells arranged at right angles to the capsule. The zona reticularis **R**, which lies adjacent to the medulla **M**, consists of small, closely-packed, irregularly arranged cells.

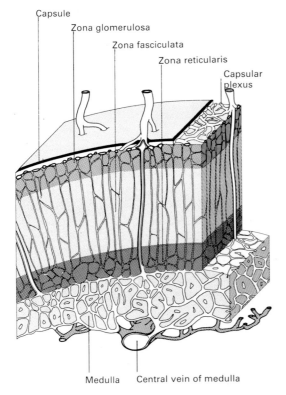

Fig. 17.12 Blood supply of the adrenal

The adrenal gland is supplied by three groups of arteries which form a plexus within the capsule of the gland.

The vascular system of the cortex consists of an anastomosing network of capillary sinusoids supplied by branches of the capsular plexus. The sinusoids descend between the cords of secretory cells in the zona fasciculata into a deep plexus in the zona reticularis before draining into small venules which converge upon the central vein of the medulla. The central medullary veins contain longitudinal bundles of smooth muscle between which the cortical venules enter; contraction of this smooth muscle is thought to dam back cortical blood and thus regulate flow.

The medulla is supplied by small arteries which descend from the capsular plexus through the cortex into the medulla where they ramify into a rich network of dilated capillaries surrounding the medullary secretory cells. The medullary capillaries also drain into the central vein of the medulla. Thus the secretory cells of the medulla are exposed to fresh arterial blood as well as blood rich in adrenocorticosteroids which are believed to have an important influence on the synthesis of adrenaline by the medulla.

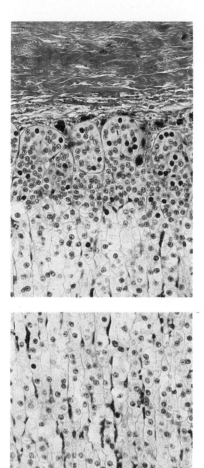

Fig. 17.13 Adrenal cortex: zona glomerulosa

(Azan × 128)

The secretory cells of the zona glomerulosa are arranged in irregular, ovoid clumps separated by delicate connective tissue trabeculae containing capillary sinusoids. The secretory cells have round, strongly stained nuclei and relatively little cytoplasm, thus giving rise to the moderately stained appearance of this zone when seen at lower magnification (see Fig. 17.11). The cytoplasm of the secretory cells contains much smooth endoplasmic reticulum, numerous mitochondria and triglyceride droplets which are the basic substrate for steroid synthesis. The abundance of smooth endoplasmic reticulum and small lipid droplets results in the relatively poor staining properties of the cytoplasm with routine staining methods.

The zona glomerulosa secretes the mineralocorticoid hormones, principally *aldosterone*. The major function of aldosterone is the regulation of body sodium and potassium ion levels by its stimulating action upon the sodium pump of cell membranes particularly in the renal tubules (see Ch. 16). Aldosterone also participates in blood pressure regulation via the renin-angiotensin hormone system controlled by the juxtaglomerular apparatus of the kidney (see Fig. 16.25). Aldosterone secretion is largely independent of ACTH but recent evidence suggests that it may be regulated by a hormone from the pineal gland.

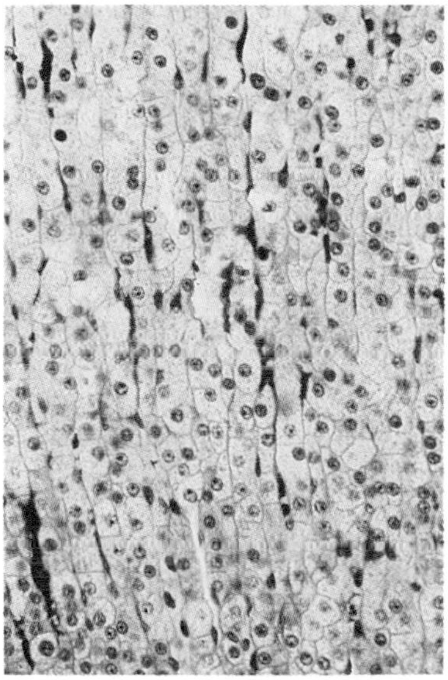

Fig. 17.14 Adrenal cortex: zona fasciculata

(Azan × 128)

The zona fasciculata is the intermediate and broadest of the three zones of the adrenal cortex. It consists of narrow cords of secretory cells, often only one cell thick, separated by connective tissue strands containing capillary sinusoids. The secretory cells are large with an abundant, poorly-stained cytoplasm. The cytoplasm is even richer in smooth endoplasmic reticulum and lipid droplets than the zona glomerulosa and this may confer a foamy appearance to the cells.

The zona fasciculata secretes glucocorticoid hormones, principally *cortisol* which has numerous, wide-ranging metabolic effects. Reflecting the name glucocorticoid, an important metabolic effect is to increase blood glucose levels and the cellular synthesis of glycogen. These effects on carbohydrate metabolism are complemented by increased breakdown of proteins and liberation of lipid from tissue stores.

Control of cortisol secretion is maintained by the hypothalamus via the anterior pituitary hormone ACTH. By this means, many stimuli including stress, promote secretion of glucocorticoids which adjust body metabolism appropriately.

The zona fasciculata is probably also the site of secretion of small amounts of steroid sex hormones.

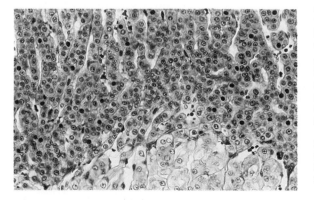

Fig. 17.15 Adrenal cortex: zona reticularis

(Azan × 128)

The zona reticularis is the thin, innermost zone of the adrenal cortex. It consists of an irregular network of branching cords and clumps of glandular cells separated by numerous wide capillary sinusoids. The glandular cells are much smaller than those of the adjacent zona fasciculata, and the cytoplasm, which contains few lipid droplets, stains more strongly.

The zona reticularis may be responsible for the secretion of small quantities of steroid sex hormones or alternatively, it may store, rather than synthesise, the hormones of the zona fasciculata. The two zones may thus constitute a single functional unit.

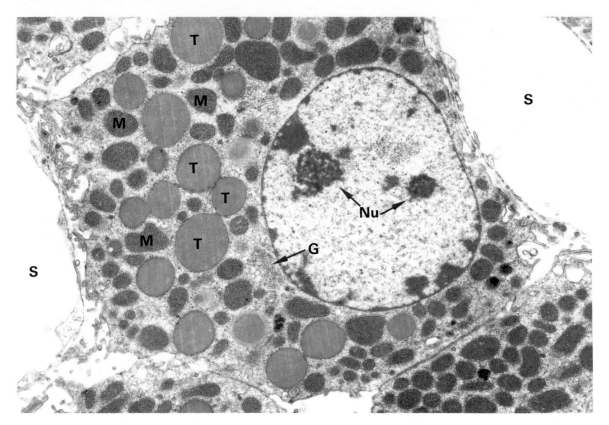

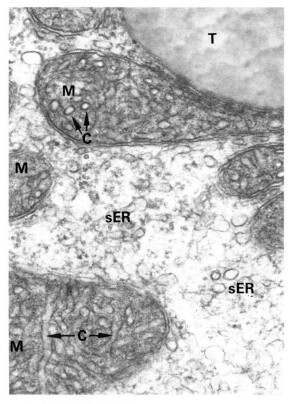

Fig. 17.16 Steroid-secreting cell

(EM (a) × 8500 (b) × 110 500)

These micrographs illustrate the typical ultrastructural features of steroid-secreting cells which are seen not only in the cells of the adrenal cortex but also in the steroid-secreting cells of the ovaries and testes (see Ch.18 and 19). At low magnification, a secretory cell is seen intimately associated with fenestrated capillary sinusoids **S**. Note the numerous irregular projections of the secretory cell plasma membrane subjacent to the sinusoidal endothelium. The rounded secretory cell nucleus is characterised by more than one prominent nucleolus **Nu**.

The abundant cytoplasm contains many large triglyceride droplets **T**. Numerous irregularly shaped mitochondria **M** crowd the cytoplasm; these mitochondria have unusual tubular cristae **C**, clearly seen at high magnification. The cytoplasm contains a prolific system of smooth endoplasmic reticulum **sER** which forms a dense tubular network. A Golgi apparatus **G** is seen close to the nucleus.

Synthesis of steroids begins with the liberation of fatty acids from stored triglycerides. Mitochondrial oxidation of fatty acids provides acetate molecules for synthesis of cholesterol by the smooth endoplasmic reticulum. The basic steroid nucleus, cholesterol, is modified in the smooth endoplasmic reticulum or mitochondria depending on which steroid hormone is being synthesised.

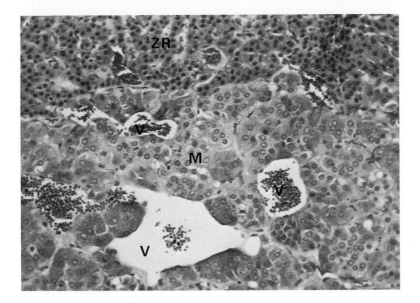

Fig. 17.17 Adrenal medulla

(H & E × 198)

The adrenal medulla **M** is composed of closely packed clumps of secretory cells supported by a fine reticular network containing numerous wide capillaries. Many venous channels **V** draining blood from the sinusoids of the cortex pass through the medulla towards the central medullary vein (see Fig. 17.12).

The secretory cells of the adrenal medulla have large, granular nuclei and extensive strongly basophilic cytoplasm. Note the contrasting eosinophilic cytoplasm of the adjacent zona reticularis **ZR** of the cortex.

The adrenal medulla secretes the catecholamine hormones noradrenaline and adrenaline under the direct control of the sympathetic nervous system. Unlike most of the endocrine glands, adrenal medullary hormones are not secreted continuously but are stored in cytoplasmic granules and released only in response to nervous stimulation in a manner similar to the release of neurotransmitter substances from nerve endings.

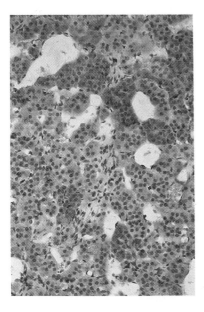

Fig. 17.18 Adrenal medulla

(H & E/Chrome salt fixation × 800)

When fixed in chrome salts, the stored catecholamine granules of some adrenal medullary cells are oxidised to a brown colour; consequently the name *chromaffin cells* is often applied to the secretory cells of the adrenal medulla.

Some adrenal medullary glands synthesise noradrenaline. The majority of the adrenal medullary cells, however, synthesise adrenaline by the addition of a further N-methyl group to noradrenaline, the enzyme responsible being induced by the presence of cortisol percolating down from the cortex. Only those cells containing noradrenaline exhibit a positive chromaffin reaction.

Secretion of catecholamines by the adrenal medulla is controlled by preganglionic neurones of the sympathetic nervous system; thus the secretory cells of the adrenal medulla are functionally equivalent to the post-ganglionic neurones of the sympathetic nervous system. Acute physical and psychological stresses initiate release of adrenal medullary hormones; the released catecholamines act on adrenergic receptors throughout the body particularly in the heart and blood vessels, bronchioles, visceral muscle and skeletal muscle. Adrenaline also has potent metabolic effects such as the promotion of glycogenolysis in liver and skeletal muscle, thus releasing a readily available energy source during stress situations.

Endocrine pancreas

The pancreas is not only a major exocrine gland (see Ch. 15) but it also has important endocrine functions.

The embryonic epithelium of the pancreatic ducts consists of both potential exocrine and endocrine cells. During development, the endocrine cells migrate from the duct system and aggregate around capillaries to form isolated clumps of cells scattered throughout the exocrine glandular tissue. The clumps of endocrine tissue are known as *islets of Langerhans*. The islets vary in size and are most numerous in the tail of the pancreas.

The endocrine pancreas mainly secretes two polypeptide hormones, *insulin* and *glucagon*, both of which play an important role in carbohydrate metabolism. Insulin promotes the uptake of glucose by most cells, particularly those of the liver, skeletal muscle and adipose tissue, thus lowering plasma glucose concentration. In general, glucagon has metabolic effects that oppose the actions of insulin. Apart from their role in carbohydrate metabolism these hormones have a wide variety of other effects on energy metabolism, growth and development.

Release of both insulin and glucagon is primarily controlled by the plasma concentration of glucose. The sympathetic and parasympathetic nervous systems innervate the islets of Langerhans but the significance of their influence is poorly understood.

A third polypeptide, somatostatin, is secreted by cells of the endocrine pancreas. Somatostatin has a wide variety of effects on gastrointestinal function, but it may also inhibit insulin and glucagon secretion.

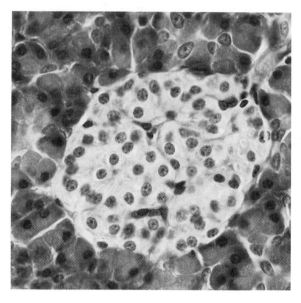

Fig. 17.19 Islets of Langerhans
(H & E × 480)

The islets of Langerhans are composed of clumps of secretory cells supported by a fine reticular network containing numerous fenestrated capillaries. A fine reticular capsule surrounds each islet. The endocrine cells are small with a poorly stained granular cytoplasm; in contrast, the large cells of the surrounding pancreatic acini stain strongly. This difference in staining intensity reflects the relatively greater amount of rough endoplasmic reticulum in the exocrine cells which secrete vast quantities of protein (see Figs. 15.13 to 15.15).

The endocrine pancreas contains secretory cells of three types, *alpha*, *beta* and *delta cells*, which secrete glucagon, insulin and somatostatin respectively. In H & E preparations, these cell types are indistinguishable from one another and special staining methods are required to differentiate between them.

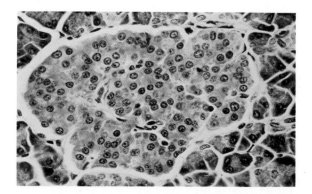

Fig. 17.20 Islet of Langerhans
(Gomori's chrome alum haematoxylin/Phloxine method × 320)

This empirical staining method can be used to distinguish the alpha and beta cells of the endocrine pancreas. The alpha (glucagon-secreting) cells are stained pink and are much less numerous than the blue-stained beta cells (insulin-secreting). Generally, the alpha cells tend to be distributed towards the periphery of the islets. Delta cells (somatostatin-secreting) cannot be differentiated from beta cells with this staining method.

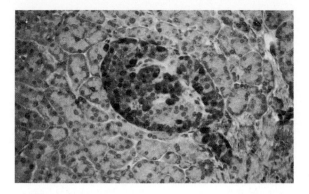

Fig. 17.21 Endocrine pancreas: glucagon cells

(Immunoperoxidase method × 128)

Immunohistochemical techniques may be used to demonstrate the presence of specific molecules within cells; in this preparation, such a method has been used to demonstrate glucagon within the alpha cells of a pancreatic islet. The sites of glucagon localisation within alpha cells appear as brownish deposits; note the characteristic peripheral distribution of alpha cells within the islet.

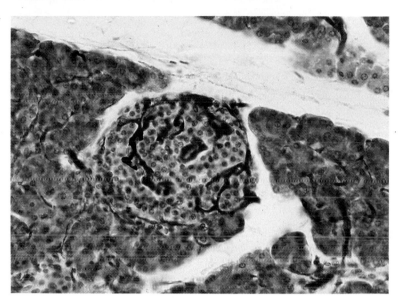

Fig. 17.22 Blood supply of endocrine pancreas

(Carmine perfused/Haematoxylin × 128)

This specimen has been perfused with a red dye before fixation to demonstrate the rich blood supply of the pancreatic islets. Each islet is supplied by as many as three arterioles which ramify into a highly branched network of fenestrated capillaries. The islet is drained by about six venules passing between the exocrine acini to the interlobular veins.

Pineal gland

The pineal gland is a small organ, 6–8 mm long, which represents an evagination from the posterior part of the roof of the third ventricle in the midline. The pineal is connected to the brain via a short stalk containing nerve fibres many of which communicate with the hypothalamus. In reptiles and other lower vertebrates, the pineal lies at, or near, the skin surface where it functions as a photoreceptor organ. In such animals, the pineal secretes a hormone, *melatonin*, which promotes lightening of skin colour by its action on melanophores, pigmented cells analogous to melanocytes in mammals (see Ch. 9). In mammals, the function of the pineal is strongly disputed but at least three important functions may be attributable to it:

1. The pineal may be involved in co-ordinating circadian and diurnal rhythms in many tissues, mediating its effects via the hypothalamus and pituitary gland.

2. There is some evidence that the pineal secretes a hormone which inhibits growth and maturation of the gonads until puberty. After puberty the pineal undergoes partial involution.

3. The pineal may secrete a trophic hormone which regulates the output of aldosterone from the adrenal cortex.

Although the function of the pineal in mammals is poorly understood it has many histological features which suggest that it is an active endocrine gland.

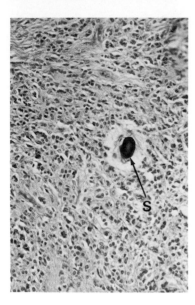

Fig. 17.23 Pineal gland

(H & E × 128)

The pineal consists of two main cell types: *pinealocytes* and *neuroglial cells.* Pinealocytes (pineal chief cells) are highly modified neurones which are arranged in clumps and cords surrounded by a rich network of fenestrated capillaries. In H & E preparations pinealocytes have round, granular nuclei with prominent nucleoli and poorly stained cytoplasm. With special silver impregnation methods, as used in neurohistology (see Ch. 7), pinealocytes appear to have many highly-branched processes, some of which terminate near or upon blood vessels. The cytoplasmic granules of pinealocytes contain a variety of indole compounds, including melatonin, which is not established as a hormone in mammals, and serotonin, which acts as a neurotransmitter substance in parts of the central nervous system. The neuroglial cells, which are similar to the astrocytes of the rest of the CNS (see Fig. 7.22), are dispersed between the clumps of pinealocytes and in association with capillaries. Myelinated sympathetic nerve fibres enter the pineal where they ramify as unmyelinated axons throughout the substance of the gland.

A characteristic feature of the ageing pineal is the presence of basophilic extracellular bodies called *pineal sand* **S** consisting of concentric layers of calcium and magnesium phosphate within an organic matrix. The organic matrix may represent the remnants of carrier proteins for the pineal endocrine secretions.

The gastrointestinal endocrine system

Scattered in the mucosa of the gastrointestinal tract and in the pancreas are a variety of endocrine cells which secrete peptide and amine hormones such as gastrin, secretin, CCK, serotonin and many more recently discovered substances including enteroglucagon, somatostatin, substance P, vasoactive intestinal peptide (VIP), bombesin, gastric inhibitory polypeptide (GIP), motilin and pancreatic polypeptide. These hormones constitute a balanced system of agonists and antagonists which collectively regulate and co-ordinate most aspects of gastrointestinal activity in concert with the autonomic nervous system.

The endocrine cells may be located at any level in the mucosa, from the base of glands to the tips of villi. The cells which are exposed to the tract lumen may be receptive to gastrointestinal contents; these are termed the *open type.* Other endocrine cells are deep to the surface, the *closed type*, and may be receptive to changes in the local tissue environment. The cells responsible for the secretion of a particular hormone tend to be located in a particular anatomical region in the tract but there is considerable overlap in distribution; for example, gastrin-producing cells are located mainly in the pyloric region of the stomach (see Fig. 14.14) although a few gastrin cells are found in the body of the stomach, the duodenum and the pancreas.

The presence of endocrine cells in the gastrointestinal tract has long been demonstrable by staining with silver or chromium salts. Traditionally, the cells were divided into two types, *argentaffin cells* (silver reducing) and *argyrophil cells* (silver absorbing); furthermore, like the catecholamine-secreting 'chromaffin' cells of the adrenal medulla (see Fig. 17.18), both these cell types could be stained specifically with chromium salts and thus the gastrointestinal endocrine cells became collectively known as *enterochromaffin cells.* These classifications were subsequently found to be of little functional significance and currently the term enterochromaffin cell should only be applied to a specific cell type found throughout the tract in large numbers and which is responsible for the secretion of serotonin (5-hydroxytryptamine).

The various gastrointestinal endocrine cells have many ultrastructural features in common but they may be divided into at least 12 different classes according to the shape, size and density of their secretory granules. On the basis of immunohistochemistry and other techniques the various gastrointestinal hormones have been assigned to different ultrastructural cell types. Since gut hormones are a rapidly advancing field of research, there is considerable terminological confusion. It has been the practice for a cell type definitely known to produce a particular hormone to be known by the name of that hormone; for example gastrin-secreting cells are called *gastrin* or *G cells.* Difficulties have arisen where one cell type is found to produce more than one hormone.

Another major problem has been the lack of agreement about which secretory products should be classified as hormones since some of the known secretory products have only local activity. An example is serotonin, a potent local smooth muscle constrictor, which is not generally recognised as a hormone since it does not normally have more distant effects. For such substances which appear to act principally on adjacent or nearby cells and tissues, the term *paracrine* may be applied.

A further problem has arisen with the discovery that some of the gastrointestinal endocrine secretory products such as gastrin, CCK, VIP, substance P, bombesin and serotonin are also found in the brain where they appear to act as neurotransmitters; indeed, this may be the mode of action of some of these substances in the gastrointestinal tract.

In summary, there is a mass of peptide and amine-secreting cells scattered throughout the gastrointestinal tract which may be considered as a diffuse endocrine organ. The substances produced by this organ have specific and overlapping activities which regulate and co-ordinate the function of the gastrointestinal system.

The APUD cell concept and diffuse neuroendocrine system

From comparative ultrastructural studies of endocrine tissues it became evident that the diverse group of peptide or amine secreting cells have certain ultrastructural features in common. These cells have little rough endoplasmic reticulum, much smooth endoplasmic reticulum, numerous free ribosomes and small membrane-bound secretory granules. Subsequent histochemical investigation revealed that many of these cells share some common metabolic processes related to hormone synthesis. Amongst others, these processes include a high uptake of amine precursors and the ability to decarboxylate; on this basis, the descriptive term *APUD cell* (amine precursor uptake and decarboxylation) was applied and this group is now known to include at least the following diverse cells: adrenal medullary chromaffin cells, thyroid 'C' cells, all pancreatic endocrine cells, all gastrointestinal hormone cells including enterochromaffin (serotonin) cells, ACTH and MSH cells of the pituitary, chemoreceptors of the carotid body and mast cells.

Further research has suggested that the APUD cells include an even more diverse group of cells which are derived embryologically from neural crest tissue and therefore may be considered as highly modified neurones. For this reason, the term *diffuse neuroendocrine system* has been applied to encompass all these cell types and the term *paraneurone* has been proposed to describe the cells.

In summary, the principal features of the diffuse neuroendocrine system are as follows:

1. The cells produce amines or peptides with hormone-like activity and/or produce substances identical with, or related to, known or suspected neurotransmitters.
2. The cells should possess synaptic vesicle-like structures or neurosecretory-like granules;
3. The cells should exhibit both receptor and secretory functions;
4. The cells should be of neuroectodermal origin.

At present, few cells have been shown to meet all these criteria; nevertheless, if further substantiated, the concept of a *paraneuronal system* may provide a more functional basis for understanding the often interrelated activities of a highly diverse group of cells.

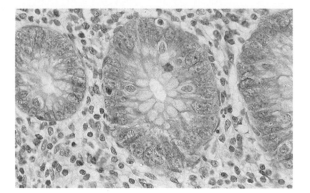

Fig. 17.24 APUD cells in the large intestinal mucosa

(Alkaline diazo method × 320)

This specimen of colonic mucosa has been stained by a histochemical method which demonstrates the presence of APUD cells, the secretory granules of which are stained orange-brown. The endocrine cells are typically small and in this example are of the 'closed type' as they lie deep to the mucosal surface.

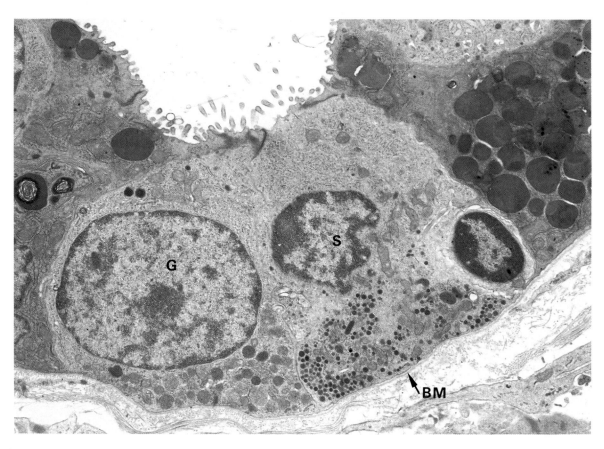

Fig. 17.25 Gastrointestinal endocrine cells

(EM × 8300)

This micrograph shows two endocrine cells from the human pylorus, both of which exhibit the typical characteristics of open-type gastrointestinal APUD cells. The endocrine cell **G** is a gastrin-secreting cell recognised on the basis of its large, moderately dense secretory granules. The adjacent endocrine cell **S** contains much smaller and more dense granules of the secretory product *somatostatin* which appears to have a broad range of actions including the inhibition of insulin and glucagon secretion and inhibition of the secretion of many gastrointestinal hormones. The open-type APUD cells are usually pyramidal in shape, the apex extending to the tract lumen and the base resting on the basement membrane **BM**. The apical surface forms a few microvilli which may receive stimuli from the tract lumen. Secretory granules are aggregated in the basal cytoplasm from which they are released into the capillaries of the lamina propria. Typically, the cytoplasm contains only a few short profiles of rough endoplasmic reticulum and numerous free ribosomes. The closed-type of APUD cells are usually rounded and lack the polarity of the open-type but otherwise have similar ultrastructural features.

18. Male reproductive system

Introduction

The male reproductive system may be divided into four major functional components:

1. The *testes* or male gonads, paired organs lying in the scrotal sac, are responsible for production of the male gametes, *spermatozoa*, and secretion of male sex hormones.

2. A paired system of ducts, each consisting of *ductuli efferentes, epididymis, ductus deferens* and *ejaculatory duct*, collect, store and conduct spermatozoa from each testis. The ejaculatory ducts converge on the *urethra* from which spermatozoa are expelled into the female reproductive tract during copulation.

3. Two exocrine glands, the paired *seminal vesicles* and the single *prostate gland*, secrete a nutritive and lubricating fluid medium called *seminal fluid* in which spermatozoa are conveyed to the female reproductive tract. Seminal fluid, spermatozoa and cells desquamated from the lining of the duct system comprise *semen*.

4. The *penis* is the organ of copulation. A pair of small accessory glands, the *bulbo-urethral glands of Cowper*, secrete a fluid which prepares the urethra for the passage of semen during ejaculation.

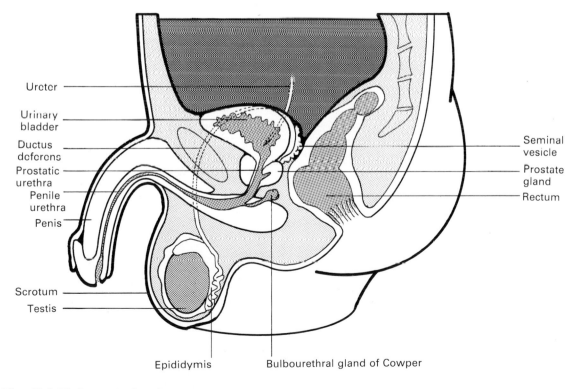

Ureter
Urinary bladder
Ductus deferens
Prostatic urethra
Penile urethra
Penis
Scrotum
Testis
Epididymis
Bulbourethral gland of Cowper
Seminal vesicle
Prostate gland
Rectum

Fig. 18.1 Male reproductive system

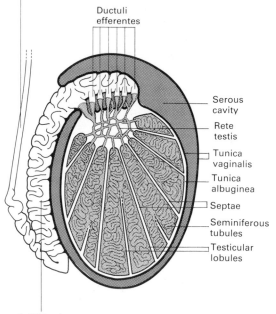

Ductus deferens

Ductuli efferentes

Serous cavity

Rete testis

Tunica vaginalis

Tunica albuginea

Septae

Seminiferous tubules

Testicular lobules

Epididymis

Fig. 18.2 Testis

During development, each testis with the first part of its duct system, blood vessels, lymphatics and nerves, descends along a tortuous path from the posterior wall of the peritoneal cavity to the scrotum. During migration, the testis carries with it an investing layer of peritoneum so that in the scrotum the testis is almost completely surrounded by a serous cavity which is an extension of the peritoneal cavity. This serous cavity protects the testis by allowing it to move freely in the scrotal sac; the lining of the cavity is known as the *tunica vaginalis*.

The testis is encapsulated by a dense, fibrous, connective tissue layer, the *tunica albuginea*, from which, at the posterior aspect, numerous ill-defined connective tissue septa divide the testis into about 250 *testicular lobules*. Within each lobule are from one to four highly convoluted loops, the *seminiferous tubules*, in which spermatozoa are produced. The seminiferous tubules converge upon a plexus of spaces, the *rete testis*. From the rete testis, about twelve small ducts, called the *ductuli efferentes*, conduct spermatozoa to the extremely tortuous first part of the *ductus deferens* which is known as the *epididymis*.

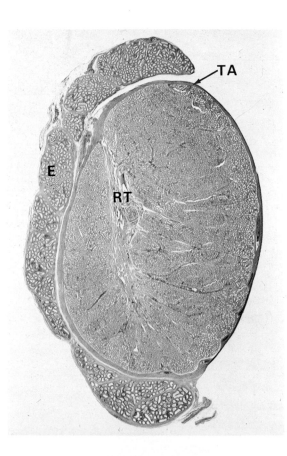

Fig. 18.3 Testis

(Monkey: H & E × 3)

This micrograph illustrates the gross morphological features of a testis cut in the sagittal plane so as to show the relationship of the epididymis **E** which lies on its posterior aspect. The testis is packed with numerous, coiled, seminiferous tubules which can just be seen in various planes of section at this magnification. Groups of about four seminiferous tubules are segregated into testicular lobules; the connective tissue septa are so delicate as to be barely seen at this magnification. The dense fibrous capsule which invests the testis, and which is continuous with many of the interlobular septa, is called the tunica albuginea **TA** since it appears white on gross examination. Spermatozoa pass from the seminiferous tubules into the rete testis **RT** which is connected to the epididymis via the ductuli efferentes at the upper posterior pole of the testis; the ductuli are not seen in this plane of section. The epididymis is a tightly coiled tube which forms a compact mass extending down the whole length of the posterior aspect of the testis. The epididymis is the major site of storage of newly formed spermatozoa. At the lower pole of the testis, the epididymal tube becomes continuous with the relatively straight ductus (vas) deferens which is not seen in this section.

Gametogenesis

In all somatic cells, cell division (mitosis) results in the formation of two daughter cells each one genetically identical to the mother cell. Somatic cells contain a full complement of chromosomes (the diploid number) which function as homologous pairs (see Ch. 2). The process of sexual reproduction involves the fusion of specialised male and female cells called *gametes* to form a *zygote* which has the diploid number of chromosomes. Each gamete contains only half the diploid number of chromosomes; this half complement of chromosomes is known as the *haploid number*.

The production of haploid cells involves a unique form of cell division called *meiosis* which occurs only in the germ cells of the gonads during the formation of gametes; meiotic cell division is thus also called *gametogenesis*. Meiosis involves two cell division processes of which only the first is preceded by duplication of chromosomes (see Ch. 2). Thus, meiotic cell division of a single diploid germ cell gives rise to four haploid gametes. In the male, each of the four gametes undergoes morphological development into a mature spermatozoon whereas in the female, unequal distribution of the cytoplasm during meiosis results in one gamete gaining almost all the cytoplasm from the mother cell, whilst the other three acquire almost no cytoplasm; the large gamete matures to form an *ovum* and the other three, the so-called *polar bodies*, degenerate.

The primitive germ cells of the male, the *spermatogonia*, are present only in small numbers in the male gonads before sexual maturity. After sexual maturity, spermatogonia multiply continuously by mitosis to provide a supply of cells which then undergo meiosis to form male gametes. In contrast, the germ cells of the female, called *oogonia*, multiply by mitosis only during early fetal development thereby producing a fixed complement of cells with the potential to undergo gametogenesis. Gametogenesis in the female is discussed more fully in Chapter 19. The production of male gametes is called *spermatogenesis* and the subsequent development of the male gamete into a motile spermatozoon is called *spermiogenesis*; both these processes occur within the testes.

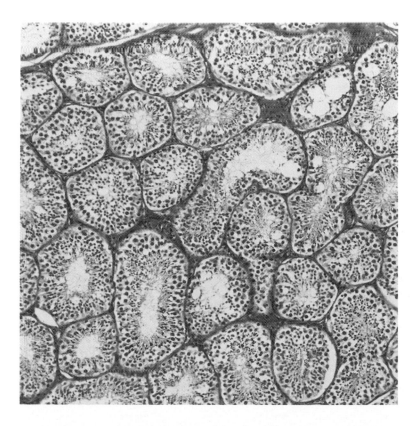

Fig. 18.4 Seminiferous tubules
(H & E × 100)

This micrograph illustrates seminiferous tubules cut in various planes of section. The seminiferous tubules are highly convoluted tubules lined by a stratified epithelium which consists of two distinct populations of cells:

1. Cells in various stages of spermatogenesis and spermiogenesis, collectively referred to as the *spermatogenic series*;

2. Non-spermatogenic cells, called *Sertoli cells*, which support and nourish the developing spermatozoa.

In the interstitial spaces between the tubules, cells with an endocrine function, called *Leydig cells*, are found either singly or in clumps in the supporting connective tissue.

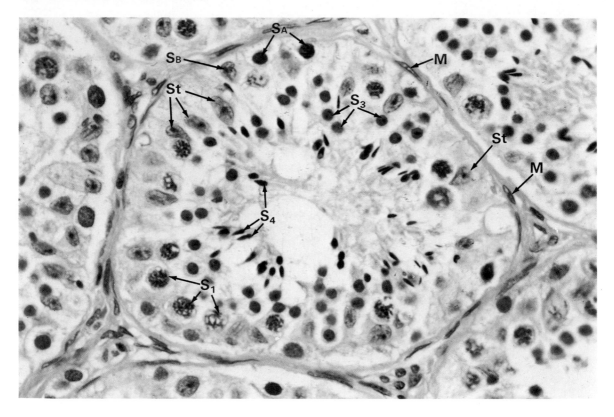

Fig. 18.5 Seminiferous tubule

(H & E × 640)

This micrograph illustrates an active seminiferous tubule cut in transverse section. The processes of spermatogenesis and spermiogenesis occur in waves along the length of the tubule, taking about 9 weeks to complete in man; thus in any one histological section all development phases are seldom represented.

Spermatogonia, the germ cells, are found in the basal layer of the seminiferous epithelium where they divide by mitosis giving rise to further spermatogonia (designated as Type A), and to spermatogonia which will proceed through meiosis to become spermatozoa (designated as Type B). Spermatogonia Type A S_A are characterised by a large, spheroidal or elliptical nucleus with fine, moderately condensed chromatin; nucleoli, which are associated with the nuclear envelope, and a nuclear vacuole may be prominent. Spermatogonia Type B S_B have a paler-stained nucleus, centrally located nucleoli, and no nuclear vacuole. Both types of spermatogonia have relatively little cytoplasm and this is poorly stained.

Spermatogonia Type B enter the first stages of meiotic division when they become known as *primary spermatocytes*. Primary spermatocytes S_1 are readily recognised by their extensive cytoplasm and large nuclei containing either coarse clumps or thin threads of chromatin; cells may be seen in chromosomal division. In man, the first meiotic cell division cycle takes approximately 3 weeks to complete, after which time the daughter cells become known as *secondary spermatocytes*. The smaller, secondary spermatocytes rapidly undergo the second meiotic division and are therefore much less commonly seen.

The gametes thus produced by meiosis, called *spermatids* S_3, then proceed through the long metamorphosis known as spermiogenesis to become recognisable as spermatozoa. As spermiogenesis proceeds, the nuclei of spermatids become smaller, more condensed and less granular until they assume the small pointed form of spermatozoa S_4 (see Fig. 18.7).

Throughout the entire developmental process from spermatogonia to spermatozoa, the daughter cells of each division remain connected to one another by narrow cytoplasmic bridges which only break down upon release of spermatozoa into the lumen of the tubule. This phenomenon has been used to explain the observation that synchronous develoment of spermatozoa occurs in waves throughout the seminiferous tubules.

During the developmental process, the cells of the spermatogenic series are supported by Sertoli cells St, the nuclei of which are usually found towards the basement membrane of the seminiferous tubule. The characteristic Sertoli cell nucleus is often triangular or ovoid in shape with a very prominent nucleolus and relatively homogeneous chromatin. Although not evident with light microscopy, Sertoli cells have an extensive cytoplasm which ramifies throughout the whole germinal epithelium enclosing all the cells of the spermatogenic series.

The basal layer of germinal cells is supported by a basement membrane beneath which are a variable number of layers of cells structurally similar to smooth muscle cells M. These cells have a contractile function in some mammalian species but their function in man is unknown.

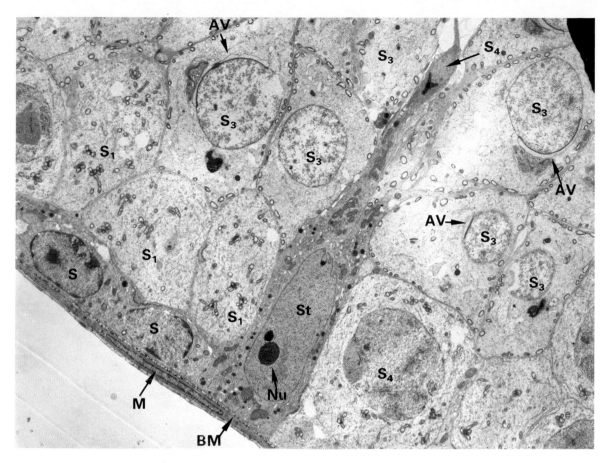

Fig. 18.6 Sertoli cell

(EM × 3400)

The intimate relationship of a Sertoli cell **St** to cells of the spermatogenic series is demonstrated in this electron micrograph.

The Sertoli cell rests on the basement membrane **BM** of the seminiferous tubule and its cytoplasm extends to the lumen of the tubule, thereby filling all the narrow spaces between the cells of the spermatogenic series. The cytoplasmic outline of the Sertoli cell is thus highly irregular and constantly changing to permit the progressive movement of developing spermatozoa towards the luminal surface. The ovoid nucleus of the Sertoli cell is characteristically orientated at right angles to the basement membrane and often exhibits a deep indentation; a large, dense nucleolus **Nu** is a constant feature and dense chromatin bodies are often associated with the nucleolus. The cytoplasm contains a moderate number of mitochondria, many lipid droplets, and relatively little rough endoplasmic reticulum. The presence of a highly ordered smooth endoplasmic reticulum suggests that Sertoli cells are, for some unknown reason, highly active in lipid biosynthesis.

Sertoli cells are postulated to act as 'nurse' cells, in some way providing structural and metabolic support for the developing spermatogenic cells. During spermiogenesis, Sertoli cells phagocytise excess cytoplasm cast off by spermatids.

Note in this micrograph the variety of cells of the spermatogenic series. Spermatogonia **S** rest upon the basement membrane beneath which is a slender smooth muscle-like (myoid) cell **M**. Above the germ cell layer, primary spermatocytes S_1 are seen; secondary spermatocytes are short-lived and therefore rarely seen. Spermatids S_3 in different phases of spermiogenesis are seen in the upper layers; these cells have developing acrosomal vesicles **AV** (see Fig. 18.7). At the luminal surface, the Sertoli cell envelops an almost fully formed spermatozoon S_4.

The control of spermatogenesis and spermiogenesis remains the subject of intense investigation; it is believed that Sertoli cells mediate some important regulatory mechanisms. It is well established that high concentrations of androgen hormones secreted by Leydig cells of the testicular interstitium (see Fig. 18.9) are essential for production and maturation of spermatogenic cells. Recent evidence suggests that Sertoli cells secrete an androgen-binding protein which concentrates androgens in seminiferous epithelium; production of this binding protein is believed to be dependent on the pituitary gonadotrophin, follicle-stimulating hormone.

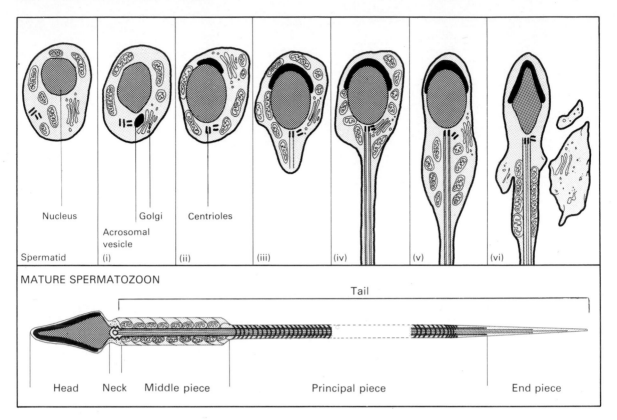

Nucleus Golgi Centrioles

Acrosomal
vesicle

Spermatid (i) (ii) (iii) (iv) (v) (vi)

MATURE SPERMATOZOON

Tail

Head Neck Middle piece Principal piece End piece

Fig. 18.7 Spermiogenesis

Spermiogenesis is the process by which spermatids, the gametes produced by meiotic division, are transformed into the potentially motile forms, the mature spermatozoa. This involves the following major stages:

1. The Golgi apparatus elaborates a large vesicle, the *acrosomal vesicle*, which accumulates carbohydrates and hydrolytic enzymes.

2. The acrosomal vesicle becomes applied to one pole of the progressively elongating nucleus to form a structure known as the *acrosomal head cap*.

3. Both centrioles migrate to the end of the cell opposite to the acrosomal head cap and the centriole aligned parallel to the long axis of the nucleus elongates to form a flagellum which has a basic structure similar to that of a cilium (see Fig. 5.21).

4. As the flagellum elongates, nine coarse fibrils, which may contain contractile proteins, become arranged

longitudinally around the core of the flagellum. Further rib-like fibrils then become disposed circumferentially around the whole flagellum.

5. The cytoplasm migrates to surround the first part of the flagellum with the remainder of the flagellum appearing to project from the cell but in fact remaining surrounded by plasma membrane. This migration of cytoplasm thus concentrates mitochondria in the flagellar region.

6. As the flagellum elongates, excess cytoplasm is cast off and phagocytised by the enveloping Sertoli cell. The mitochondria become arranged in a condensed, helical manner around the fibrils which surround the first part of the flagellum.

The structure of fully formed spermatozoa varies in detail from species to species, but conforms to the basic structure seen in this diagram of a human spermatozoon.

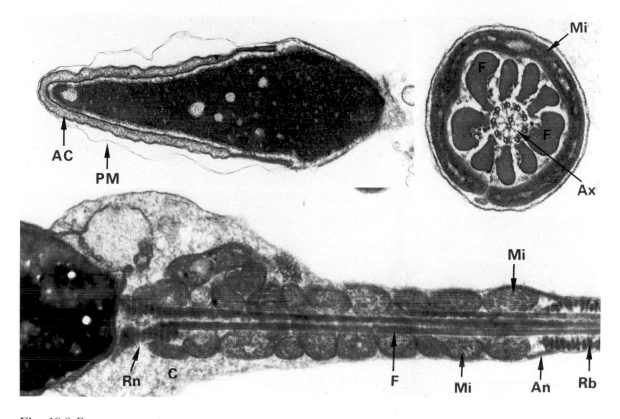

Fig. 18.8 Spermatozoon

(EM (a) Head; LS × 14 000 (b) Neck, middle piece and principal piece; LS × 17 000 (c) Middle piece; TS × 48 000)

The ultrastructural features of human spermatozoa are shown in these micrographs. The spermatozoon is an extremely elongated cell (about 65 μm long) consisting of three main components, the *head, neck* and *tail*. The tail is subdivided into three segments, the so-called *middle piece, principal piece* and *end piece* (see Fig. 18.7). The head is the most variable structure between different mammalian species. In man, the head is about 7 μm long and has a flattened pear-shape. The nucleus, which occupies most of the head, is composed of extremely condensed chromatin; in man, the nucleus is characterised by a variable number of clear spaces called *nuclear vacuoles* which are areas of dispersed chromatin. Surrounding the anterior two-thirds of the nucleus is the acrosomal cap **AC**, a flattened, membrane-bound vesicle containing a range of glycoproteins and a variety of hydrolytic enzymes, principally *hyaluronidase*; these enzymes disaggregate the cells of the corona radiata and dissolve the zona pellucida during penetration of the ovum at fertilisation (see Ch. 19.). Note the plasma membrane **PM** which has become partially separated during preparation.

The neck is a very short segment which connects the head with the tail. It contains vestiges of the centrioles, one of which gives rise to the axoneme **Ax** of the flagellum. The axoneme has the standard 'nine plus two' arrangement of microtubule doublets seen in cilia (see Fig. 5.21). The axoneme of the neck is surrounded by several condensed fibrous rings **Rn**. In human spermatozoa, a significant amount of cytoplasm **C** often remains in the neck region.

The middle piece, the first part of the tail, is about the same length as the head and consists of the flagellar axoneme surrounded by nine coarse outer fibrils **F** arranged longitudinally. External to this core, elongated mitochondria **Mi** are arranged in a tightly packed helix; the mitochondria are thought to generate the energy required for flagellar movement. A fibrous thickening beneath the plasma membrane, called the anulus **An**, prevents mitochondria from slipping into the principal piece.

The principal piece, which constitutes most of the tail length, consists of a central core, comprising the axoneme and the nine longitudinal fibrils continuing from the middle piece. Surrounding this core are numerous fibrous ribs **Rb** arranged in a circular manner. Two of the longitudinal fibrils of the core are fused with the surrounding ribs so as to form anterior and posterior columns extending throughout the length of the principal piece. This arrangement divides the principal piece longitudinally into two functional compartments, one containing three coarse fibrils and the other containing four. Although little is known of the mechanism of flagellar motion, it had been suggested that this asymmetry accounts for the more powerful stroke of the tail in one direction, the so-called 'power stroke'; this can easily be observed in fresh, live preparations of spermatozoa viewed with the light microscope. The end piece, not shown in these micrographs, is merely a short tapering portion of the tail containing the axoneme only.

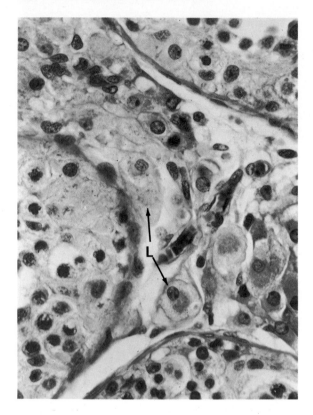

Fig. 18.9 Interstitial cells of the testis (Leydig cells)

(H & E × 480)

Leydig cells, responsible for secretion of the male sex hormones, are the principal cell type found in the connective tissue between seminiferous tubules. Leydig cells **L** occur singly or in clumps and are intimately associated with rich plexuses of blood and lymph capillaries which surround the seminiferous tubules. These large cells have an extensive, eosinophilic cytoplasm containing variable numbers of lipid vacuoles; the ultrastructural features closely resemble those of the steroid-secreting cells of the adrenal cortex (see Fig. 17.16). In man, but no other species, Leydig cells also contain elongated cytoplasmic crystals, called *crystals of Reinke*, which are large enough to be seen with light microscopy when suitably stained; these crystals become more numerous with age but their function is completely unknown.

Testosterone is the principal hormone secreted by Leydig cells. Testosterone is not only responsible for the development of male secondary sexual characteristics at puberty but is also essential for the continued function of the seminiferous epithelium. The secretory activity of Leydig cells is controlled by the pituitary gonadotrophic hormone, luteinising hormone, often referred to as *interstitial cell stimulating hormone (ICSH)* in the male.

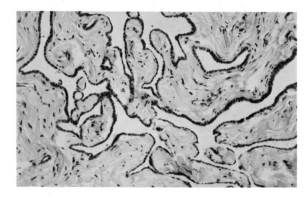

Fig. 18.10 Rete testis

(H & E × 128)

The seminiferous tubules converge upon the so-called *mediastinum testis* which consists of a plexiform arrangement of spaces, the *rete testis*, spported by highly vascular, collagenous connective tissue. The rete testis is lined by a single layer of cuboidal epithelial cells some of which may possess a flagellum. Flagellar activity is presumed to aid the progress of spermatozoa which do not become motile until after maturation is completed in the epididymis.

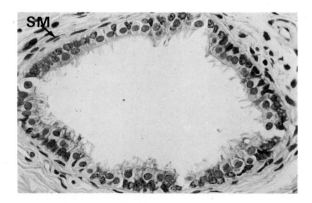

Fig. 18.11 Ductulus efferens

(H & E × 320)

The rete testis drains into the head of the epididymis via approximately 12 convoluted ducts, the *ductuli efferentes*. The ductuli are lined by a single layer of epithelial cells some of which are tall, columnar and ciliated and others which are short and non-ciliated; both cell types often contain a brown pigment of unknown composition. Ciliary action in the ductuli propels spermatozoa towards the epididymis. A thin band of circularly arranged smooth muscle **SM** surrounds each ductulus.

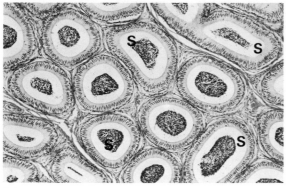

(a)

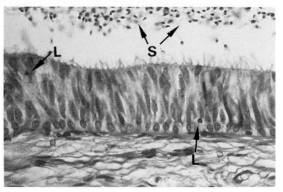

(b)

Fig. 18.12 Epididymis

(H & E (a) × 50 (b) × 320)

The epididymis is a long, extremely convoluted duct extending down the posterior aspect of the testis to the lower pole where it becomes the ductus deferens. The major function of the epididymis is thought to be the accumulation and storage of spermatozoa **S** during which time the spermatozoa develop motility. The epididymis is a tube of smooth muscle lined by a pseudostratified epithelium. From the proximal to the distal end of the epididymis, the muscular wall increases from a single, circular layer as in these micrographs to three layers organised in the same manner as in the ductus deferens (see Fig. 18.13). The smooth muscle at the proximal end exhibits slow, rhythmic contractility; this activity gently moves spermatozoa towards the ductus deferens. Distally, the smooth muscle is richly innervated by the sympathetic

nervous system which produces intense contractions of the lower part of the epididymis during ejaculation.

The epithelial lining of the epididymis shows a gradual transition from a tall, pseudostratified columnar form proximally as seen in micrograph (b) to a shorter pseudostratified form distally. The principal cells of the epididymal epithelium bear tufts of very long microvilli, inappropriately called stereocilia (see Fig. 5.23); stereocilia are thought to be involved in absorption of a vast excess of fluid accompanying the spermatozoa from the testis. The ultrastructure of the cells strongly suggests an additional secretory function but the nature of epididymal secretory products, if any, remains unknown. Occasional lymphocytes **L** may be seen within the epithelium

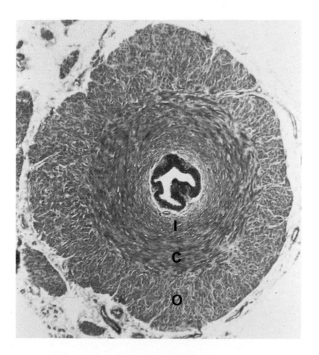

Fig. 18.13 Ductus deferens

(H & E × 30)

The ductus (or vas) deferens, which conducts spermatozoa from the epididymis to the urethra, is a thick-walled muscular tube consisting of inner **I** and outer **O** longitudinal layers and a thick intermediate circular layer **C**. Like the distal part of the epididymis, the ductus deferens is innervated by the sympathetic nervous system and contracts strongly to expel its contents into the urethra during ejaculation.

The ductus deferens is lined by a pseudostratified epithelium similar to that of the epididymis (see Fig. 18.12); the epithelial lining and its supporting lamina propria are thrown into longitudinal folds which permit expansion of the duct during ejaculation. The dilated distal portion of each ductus deferens, known as the *ampulla*, receives a short duct draining the seminal vesicle, thus forming the short ejaculatory duct; the ejaculatory ducts from each side converge to join the urethra as it passes through the prostate gland.

This specimen was obtained during male sterilisation (*vasectomy*).

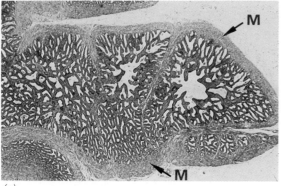

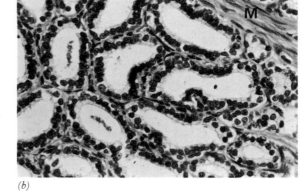

(a)

(b)

Fig. 18.14 Seminal vesicle

(H & E (a) × 10 (b) × 320)

Each seminal vesicle is a highly convoluted, glandular outpocketing of the associated ductus deferens. The central lumen of each seminal vesicle is highly irregular and recessed giving a honeycomb appearance at low magnification. The prominent muscular wall **M** is arranged into inner circular and outer longitudinal layers. The epithelial lining is simple, usually pseudostratified in man, and consists of secretory cells which produce a yellowish, viscid, alkaline fluid containing fructose, fibrinogen and vitamin C; this secretion contributes to the nutritive and supporting fluid of semen. Although not thought to store spermatozoa, seminal vesicles are often seen to contain spermatozoa which have probably entered by reflux from the ampulla. The smooth muscle of the seminal vesicles is supplied by the sympathetic nervous system; during ejaculation, muscle contraction forces secretions from the seminal vesicles into the urethra via the ampullae.

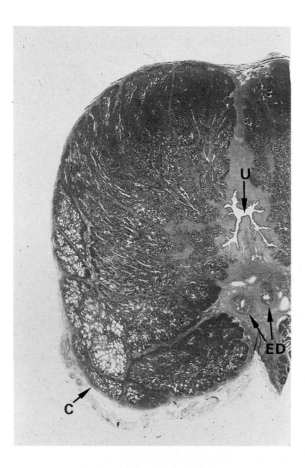

Fig. 18.15 Prostate gland

(Dog: H & E × 5)

The prostate is a large gland which surrounds the bladder neck and the first part of the urethra in the midline; the wall of the prostatic urethra is formed by the substance of the prostate gland. As seen in this micrograph, the prostate gland consists of glandular lobules, up to 50 in all, which converge to open via about 20 separate ducts into irregular outpockets of the prostatic urethra **U** throughout its length. In addition to prostatic glandular tissue proper, numerous, small *paraurethral glands* (not seen in this micrograph) open into the prostatic urethra throughout its length, and it is these glands and their supporting connective tissue which increase greatly in size as a normal part of the ageing process of human males; this process, known as *benign prostatic hypertrophy*, may cause obstruction of urinary outflow by occluding the prostatic urethra. Note in this micrograph, the ejaculatory ducts **ED** which join the prostatic urethra just before its exit from the prostate gland.

The secretory product of the prostate, which makes up about 75% of the seminal fluid, is thin and milky; it is rich in citric acid and hydrolytic enzymes, notably fibrinolysin, which liquefies coagulated semen after it has been deposited within the female genital tract.

The supporting stroma and capsule **C** of the prostate gland consists of dense fibro-elastic connective tissue which contains numerous smooth muscle fibres. The smooth muscle of the prostate, like that of the seminal vesicles and the rest of the tract, is innervated by the sympathetic nervous system which stimulates powerful contractions during ejaculation.

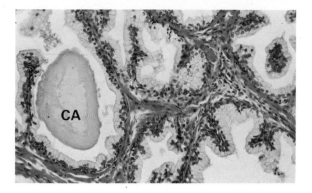

Fig. 18.16 Prostate gland
(H & E × 128)

The prostatic glandular epithelium varies from inactive, low cuboidal to active, pseudostratified columnar depending on the degree of stimulation by androgens from the testis. The histological appearance seen in this micrograph is that of highly active secretory cells. The secretory product is stored temporarily within the gland and often forms amorphous masses called *corpora amylacea* **CA**, one of which is seen in this section from a young man. With increasing age, these bodies become progressively calcified to form lamellated deposits called *prostatic concretions* or *prostatic salt*.

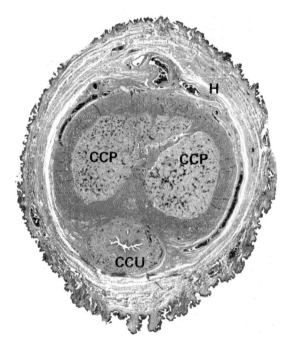

Fig. 18.17 Penis
(TS: H & E × 3)

This transverse section through the penis of an adult human male demonstrates the general arrangement of the penile tissues. The penis consists of three cylindrical masses of erectile tissue: the paired *corpora cavernosa penis* **CCP** in the dorsal aspect, and the midline *corpus cavernosum urethrae* **CCU** (formerly called the *corpus spongiosum*) which surrounds and supports the penile urethra. Condensed fibro-elastic tissue invests the cavernous bodies, being thickest around the corpora cavernosa penis which are incompletely separated by a midline septum. This dense connective tissue is continuous with the very loose hypodermis **H** which allows the thin penile skin to move freely over the underlying structures. Note the prominent blood vessels of the hypodermis.

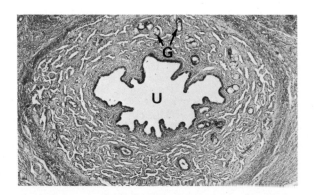

Fig. 18.18 Corpus cavernosum urethrae
(TS: H & E × 20)

The erectile tissue of the penis consists of broad vascular lacunae or cavernous sinuses supported by trabeculae of fibro-elastic connective tissue containing smooth muscle fibres. The lacunae are lined by the usual vascular endothelium. The penile urethra **U** has an irregular outline due to the presence of deep outpocketings which are continuous with the ducts of simple acinar glands, the *paraurethral glands* **G**.

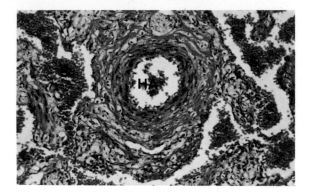

Fig. 18.19 Penile erectile tissue
(H & E × 128)

The vascular sinuses **S** of the cavernous bodies of the penis are directly supplied by numerous anastomosing thick-walled arteries and arterioles called *helicine arteries* **HA** since they follow a spiral course in the flaccid state. Blood drains from the sinuses via veins which lie immediately beneath the dense fibro-elastic tissue investing the cavernous bodies. During erection, dilatation of the helicine arteries, mediated by the parasympathetic nervous system, results in engorgement of the vascular sinuses which enlarge, compressing and restricting venous outflow. Engorgement of the corpus cavernosum urethrae tends to collapse the penile urethra, but this is overcome by the extremely forceful contractions of the seminal tract during ejaculation.

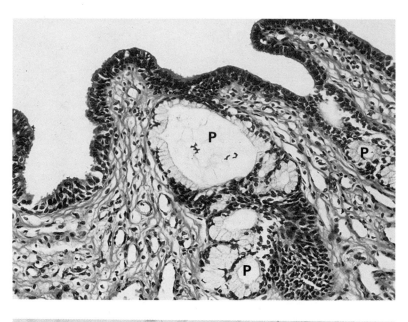

Fig. 18.20 Penile urethra
(H & E × 200)

Apart from the prostatic urethra which is lined by urinary epithelium, the male urethra is lined by stratified or pseudostratified columnar epithelium although small areas of stratified squamous epithelium may be found along the length of the penile urethra in human adult males. The external opening (*urethral meatus*) is always lined by stratified squamous epithelium.

The urethra is lubricated by mucous secretions from the paraurethral glands **P** and the bulbo-urethral glands of Cowper which have a similar, but more discrete, organisation.

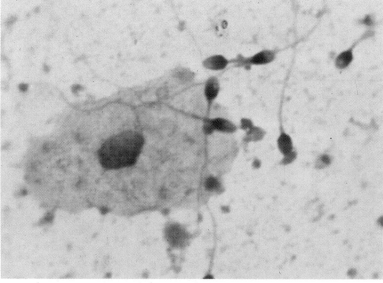

Fig. 18.21 Semen
(H & E × 1200)

Semen, the product of ejaculation, consists of spermatozoa and seminal fluid which is derived principally from the seminal vesicles and prostate gland. The volume of each human ejaculate is about 3.5 ml, containing from 50–150 million spermatozoa per ml. In normal fertile human males, up to 25% of the ejaculated spermatozoa are abnormal or degenerate forms. By the time of ejaculation, spermatozoa have matured and acquired the property of motility; they remain incapable of fertilising an ovum until after undergoing an incompletely understood process called *capacitation*, within the female genital tract. Metabolites for motility are provided in the form of fructose and citrate in the seminal fluid. Note that desquamated cells, prostatic concretions and other tract debris are normal constituents of semen.

19. Female reproductive system

Introduction

The female reproductive system has the following major functions:

1. The production of female gametes, the *ova*, by a process called *oogenesis*;
2. The reception of male gametes, the spermatozoa;
3. The provision of a suitable environment for the fertilisation of ova by spermatozoa;
4. The provision of an environment for the development of the fetus;
5. A means for the expulsion of the developed fetus to the external environment;
6. Nutrition of the newborn.

These functions are all integrated by hormonal and nervous mechanisms.

The female reproductive system may be divided into three structural units on the basis of function: the ovaries, the genital tract and the breasts.

The *ovaries*, paired organs lying in the pelvic cavity, are the sites of oogenesis. In sexually mature mammals, ova are released by the process of *ovulation* in a cyclical manner either seasonally or at regular intervals throughout the year. The cyclical ovulations are suspended during pregnancy. The process of ovulation is controlled by the cyclical release of gonadotrophic hormones from the anterior pituitary. The ovaries themselves have an endocrine function; they secrete the hormones *oestrogen* and *progesterone* which co-ordinate the activities of the genital tract and breasts with the ovulatory cycle.

The *genital tract* extends from near the ovaries to open at the external surface and provides an environment for reception of male gametes, fertilisation of ova, development of the fetus, and expulsion of the fetus at birth. The genital tract begins with a pair of *uterine tubes*, also called *oviducts* or *Fallopian tubes*, which conduct ova from the ovaries to the *uterus* where fetal development occurs. Fertilisation of ova by spermatozoa occurs within the uterine tubes. The uterus is a muscular organ, the mucosal lining of which undergoes cyclical proliferation under the influence of ovarian hormones. This provides a suitable environment for implantation of the fertilised ovum. At birth, or *parturition*, strong contractions of the muscular uterine wall expel the fetus through the *cervix* into the birth canal or *vagina*. The vagina is an expansile muscular tube specialised for the passage of the fetus to the external environment and the reception of the penis during coitus. At the external opening of the vagina are thick folds of skin which constitute the *vulva*.

The breasts are highly modified apocrine sweat glands which, in the female, develop at puberty and regress at menopause. During pregnancy, the breasts undergo structural changes in preparation for milk production or *lactation*.

In the non-pregnant state, the female reproductive system undergoes continuous cyclical changes from puberty to menopause. When ovulation is not followed by the implantation of a fertilised ovum, the proliferated mucosal lining regresses and a new ovulation cycle commences. In humans, the proliferated uterine mucosa is shed in a period of bleeding known as *menstruation*; the first day of bleeding marks the beginning of a new cycle of proliferation of the uterine mucosa which is known as the *menstrual cycle*. In humans, the menstrual cycle is usually of 28 days duration and ovulation usually occurs at the midpoint of the cycle. The ovulatory and menstrual cycles are integrated by hormones secreted by the ovaries; these hormones also promote cyclical changes in all other parts of the female reproductive system.

In other animals, the proliferated uterine mucosa is absorbed rather than shed and the female is receptive to the male only during the period of ovulation which is known as *oestrus* (or heat). The remaining part of the cycle is called the *dioestrus* and the whole cycle is known as the *oestrus cycle*.

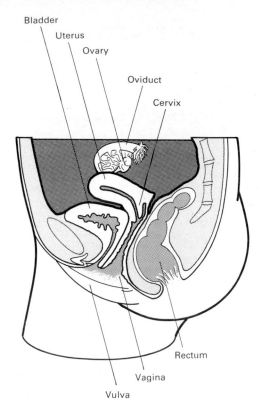

Fig. 19.1 Human female reproductive system

(sagittal section)

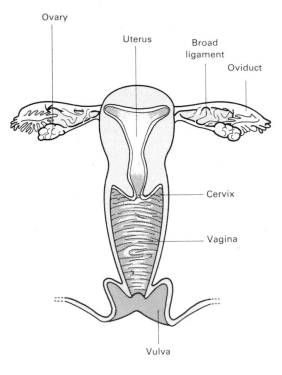

Fig. 19.2 Human female reproductive system

(coronal view)

Fig. 19.3 Ovary *(illustrations opposite)*

(a) Monkey: Azan × 18 (b) Human: H & E × 8

The ovaries of all mammals have a similar basic structure. However, their overall appearance varies considerably in accordance with the species differences in the pattern of the ovarian cycle and the state in the cycle at which the ovary is examined. These micrographs compare the ovarian appearance of the monkey with that of the human.

The ovaries are flattened, oval organs encapsulated in a fibrous connective tissue layer called the *tunica albuginea*, named for its white appearance on gross examination.

The body of the ovary consists of spindle-shaped cells, reticular fibres and ground substance which together constitute the *ovarian stroma*. In the peripheral zone of the stroma, known as the *cortex*, are numerous *follicles* which contain female gametes in various stages of development. In addition, there may also be post-ovulatory follicles of various kinds, i.e. corpora lutea (see Fig. 19.7) or degenerative

follicles i.e. corpora albicantes (see Fig. 19.9) and atretic follicles (see Fig. 19.10).

In the monkey ovary, note the numerous follicles **F** of various sizes and states of development. In contrast, developing follicles are difficult to see in the human ovary at this magnification; this human ovary is dominated by an active corpus luteum **CL** and several degenerating corpora lutea and corpora albicantes.

The central zone of the ovarian stroma, the medulla **M** is highly vascular, the arteries being coiled giving rise to the term *helicine arteries*; these are well-demonstrated in micrograph (a). The blood vessels of the ovary, together with autonomic nerves and lymphatics, pass in the broad ligament **L** into the ovary at the hilum. Note in micrograph (b), the nearby oviduct **O** included in the plane of section.

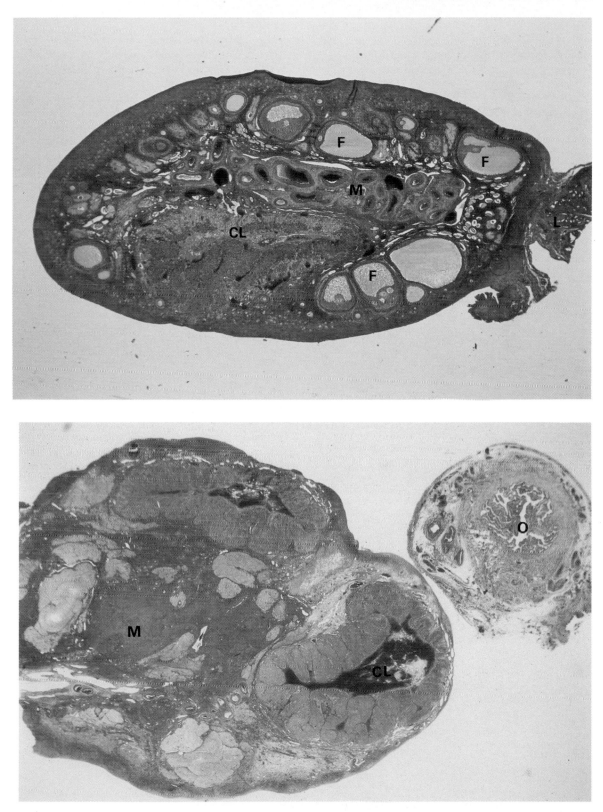

Follicular development

During early fetal development, primordial germ cells called *oogonia* migrate into the ovarian cortex where they multiply by mitosis. By the fourth and fifth months of fetal development in the human, some oogonia enlarge and assume the potential for development into mature gametes. At this stage they become known as *primary oocytes* and commence the first stage of meiotic division (see Ch. 2). By the seventh month of fetal development, the primary oocytes become encapsulated by a single layer of flattened *follicular cells*, of epithelial origin, to form *primordial follicles*. This encapsulation arrests the first meiotic division and no further development of the primordial follicle then occurs until after the female reaches sexual maturity. The remaining phases of meiotic division occur during a final phase of follicular maturation leading to ovulation and fertilisation. Thus all the female germ cells are present at birth and the process of meiotic division is completed between 15 and 50 years later. In contrast, in males, meiotic division of germ cells commences only after sexual maturity and sperm formation is accomplished within about 2 months (see Ch. 18). Female germ cells may undergo degeneration (*atresia*) at any stage of follicular maturation.

During each ovarian cycle, up to 20 primordial follicles are in some way activated to undergo the maturation process; nevertheless, usually only one follicle reaches full maturity and is ovulated whilst the remainder undergo atresia before the point of ovulation. The reason for this apparent wastage is unclear; during maturation, however, the follicles have an endocrine function which may be far beyond the capacity of a single follicle and the primary purpose of the other follicles may be to act as an endocrine gland.

Follicular maturation involves changes in the oocyte, the follicular cells and the surrounding stromal tissue. Follicular maturation is stimulated by the gonadotrophic hormone FSH secreted by the anterior pituitary.

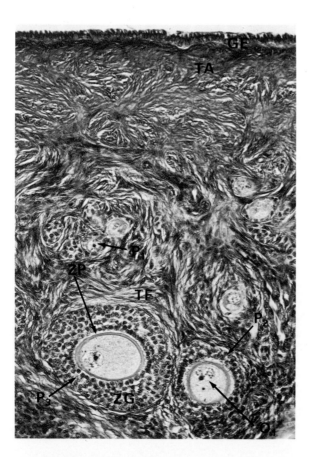

Fig. 19.4 Ovarian cortex

(Azan × 120)

This micrograph, taken from a monkey, shows the typical appearance of follicles in the ovarian cortex and illustrates several stages in early follicular development.

In the mature ovary, undeveloped follicles exist as *primordial follicles* P_1 which are composed of a *primary oocyte* surrounded by a single layer of flattened follicular cells. The primary oocyte has a large nucleus, a prominent nucleolus and little cytoplasm. When stimulated to develop, the primordial follicle enlarges to form a *primary follicle* P_2 in which the oocyte O_1 has greatly enlarged and the follicular cells have become cuboidal. A homogeneous glycoprotein layer, the *zona pellucida* ZP, develops between the oocyte and the surrounding follicular cells. During this stage of follicular maturation the surrounding connective tissue stroma begins to form an organised layer around the follicle called the *theca folliculi* TF. With further development, the primary follicle P_3 continues to enlarge and the follicular cells proliferate to form a layer several cells thick called the *zona granulosa* ZG. The external connective tissue layer, the theca, begins to differentiate into two layers, the *theca interna* and *theca externa*.

Note also in this micrograph, the fibrous tunica albuginea TA and the single layer of cuboidal epithelial cells on the surface of the ovary. This epithelial layer is continuous with the mesothelial lining of the peritoneal cavity and is known as the *germinal epithelium* GE from the mistaken belief that these cells were the origin of the female germ cells.

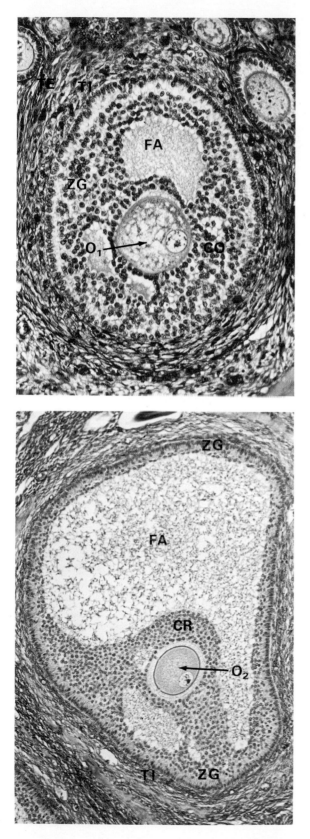

Fig. 19.5 Secondary follicle
(Azan × 120)

Primary follicles continue to develop until the stage at which they become known as *secondary follicles*. Secondary follicles are usually situated deeper in the ovarian cortex and are recognised by the following features. The zona granulosa **ZG** has proliferated greatly and a space, called the *follicular antrum* **FA**, appears in which follicular fluid accumulates. At this stage, the oocyte O_1 has almost reached its mature size and becomes situated eccentrically in a thickened area of the granulosa called the *cumulus oophorus* **CO**. The theca interna **TI** and the theca externa **TE** are now well defined.

By this stage, the cells of the theca interna have differentiated into typical steroid secreting cells (see Fig. 17.16) and have commenced the secretion of oestrogen hormones. Oestrogens promote proliferation of the uterine mucosa in readiness for the implantation of a fertilised ovum. The theca externa is merely composed of connective tissue and has no endocrine function.

Fig. 19.6 Graafian follicle
(Azan × 75)

Approaching maturity, further growth of the oocyte ceases and the first meiotic division is completed just before ovulation. At this stage the oocyte becomes known as the *secondary oocyte* and commences the second meiotic division. The first polar body, containing very little cytoplasm, remains inconspicuously within the zona pellucida (see Ch. 2). The follicular antrum **FA** enlarges markedly and the zona granulosa **ZG** forms a layer of even thickness around the periphery of the follicle. The cumulus oophorus diminishes leaving the oocyte O_2 surrounded by a layer several cells thick, the *corona radiata* **CR**, which remains attached to the zona granulosa by thin bridges of cells. Before ovulation these bridges break down and the oocyte, surrounded by the corona radiata, floats free inside the follicle.

At ovulation, the mature follicle ruptures and the ovum, comprising the secondary oocyte, zona pellucida and corona radiata, is expelled into the peritoneal cavity near the entrance to the uterine tube. The second meiotic division of the oocyte is not completed until after penetration of the ovum by a spermatozoon.

During the process of follicular maturation the amount of oestrogen-secreting tissue, the theca interna **TI**, increases progressively and there is a corresponding rise in the level of circulating oestrogens. Atresia of all but the follicle destined to ovulate probably accounts for the fall in circulating oestrogens which occurs just prior to ovulation (see Fig. 19.19).

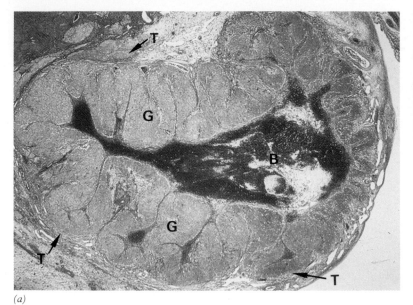

(a)

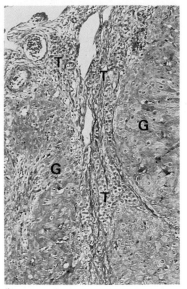

(b)

Fig. 19.7 Corpus luteum

(H & E (a) × 42 (b) × 128)

Following ovulation the ruptured follicle collapses and fills
with a blood clot and the three layers of the follicular wall
become re-organised to form a temporary endocrine gland,
the *corpus luteum*. Under the influence of luteinising
hormone (LH) secreted by the anterior pituitary, the cells of
the former zona granulosa increase greatly in size and begin
secretion of the steroid hormone progesterone. The
cytoplasm of these cells contains a bright yellow pigment
which gives rise to the name *granulosa luteal cells* and the
name corpus luteum to the whole structure. Progesterone
promotes exocrine secretion by glands in the mucosal lining
of the uterus, which are now greatly proliferated under the
influence of the oestrogens secreted by the theca interna
cells of the follicle before ovulation. This provides a suitable
environment for the implantation of a fertilised ovum.

The cells of the former theca interna also increase in size
but to a lesser extent. Although interrupted by ovulation,
these cells continue to secrete oestrogens, which are
necessary to maintain the proliferated uterine mucosa. These
cells become known as *theca luteal cells* or *paraluteal cells*.

The blood clot, granulosa luteal and theca luteal layers are
invaded by capillaries from the former theca externa to form
a rich vascular network characteristic of endocrine glands.

The corpus luteum is dependent on the secretion of LH
from the anterior pituitary; however, rising levels of
progesterone inhibit LH secretion. Without the continuing
stimulus of LH, the corpus luteum cannot be maintained
and 12–14 days after ovulation it regresses to form the
functionless *corpus albicans* (see Fig. 19.9). Once the corpus
luteum regresses, secretion of both oestrogens and
progesterone ceases. Without these hormones the mucosal
lining of the uterus collapses with the onset of menstruation.

Implantation of a fertilised ovum in the uterine wall

interrupts the integrated ovarian and menstrual cycles. After
implantation, a hormone called *human chorionic
gonadotrophin* (HCG) is secreted into the maternal
circulation by the developing placenta. HCG, which has an
analogous function to that of LH, maintains the function of
the corpus luteum in secreting oestrogens and progesterone
until about the twelfth week of pregnancy. After this time,
the corpus luteum of pregnancy slowly regresses to form the
functionless corpus albicans and the placenta takes over the
major role of oestrogen and progesterone secretion until
parturition.

At low magnification, the remnant of the blood clot **B** is
seen in the centre of the corpus luteum, surrounded by a
broad zone of granulosa luteal cells **G**. Peripherally, a thin
zone of theca luteal (paraluteal) cells **T** can be seen. The
corpus luteum is bounded by a connective tissue zone
representing the theca externa of the antecedent Graafian
follicle.

At higher magnification, granulosa luteal cells **G** may be
compared with theca luteal (paraluteal) cells **T**. Granulosa
luteal cells have a relatively large amount of pale-stained
cytoplasm containing numerous lipid droplets which give
rise to the vacuolated appearance seen in this preparation;
lipid is utilised in the synthesis of the steroid hormone,
progesterone.

Theca luteal (paraluteal) cells form a thin zone around the
periphery of the granulosa luteal layer with finger-like
extensions of the theca luteal layer extending into the
granulosa luteal layer. Theca luteal cells are smaller, with a
more densely staining, less vacuolated cytoplasm; these cells
are responsible for the secretion of oestrogens.

The ultrastructure of the endocrine cells of the corpus
luteum is characteristic of all steroid secretory cells (see
Fig. 17.16).

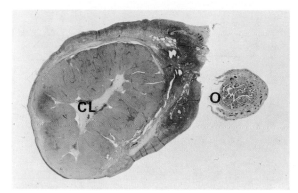

Fig. 19.8 Corpus luteum of pregnancy

(H & E × 3)

The corpus luteum of pregnancy is a much larger structure than the corpus luteum of the ovarian cycle but has a similar basic organisation; the corpus luteum of pregnancy produces oestrogens and progesterone for approximately the first trimester of pregnancy and then slowly regresses, its function being taken over by the placenta.

This micrograph shows a human ovary during the first trimester. The corpus luteum **CL** is greatly enlarged compared with that of the second half of the menstrual cycle and the corpus luteum occupies most of the ovary. Note the adjacent oviduct **O**.

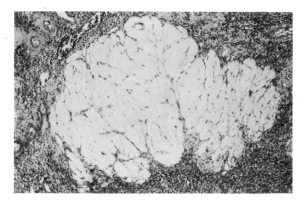

Fig. 19.9 Corpus albicans

(H & E × 20)

The corpus albicans is the inactive fibrous tissue mass which forms following the involution of a corpus luteum. The secretory cells of the degenerate corpus luteum autolyse and are phagocytised by macrophages. The vascular supporting tissue regresses to form a relatively acellular scar which eventually merges with the surrounding ovarian stroma.

In the human ovary, corpora albicantes are a dominant feature, increasing in number with age and often appearing to occupy almost the whole ovarian stroma.

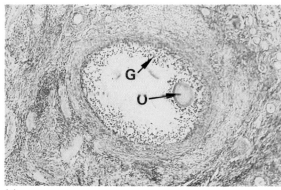
(a)

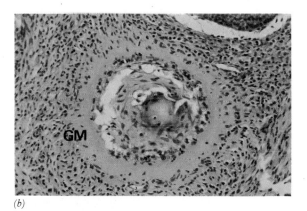
(b)

Fig. 19.10 Atretic follicles

(H & E (a) × 128 (b) × 128)

The process of follicular atresia (degeneration) may occur at any stage in the development of the ovum. By the sixth month of development the fetal ovary contains approximately 6 million primordial follicles, four million of which undergo atresia by the time of birth. Atresia continues until puberty when less than half a million follicles remain and thereafter follicular atresia continues at a slow rate amongst primordial follicles.

In addition, with each ovarian cycle approximately 20 follicles begin to mature, usually all but one becoming atretic at some stage before complete maturity.

The histological appearance of *atretic follicles* varies enormously, depending on the stage of development reached and the progress of atresia. The atretic follicle seen in micrograph (a) is a secondary follicle in early atresia; the oocyte **O** has degenerated and the granulosa cells **G** have begun to disorganise. Advanced atresia, as seen in micrograph (b), is characterised by gross thickening of the basement membrane between the granulosa cells and the theca interna forming the so-called *glassy membrane* **GM**. Atretic follicles are ultimately replaced completely by fibrous connective tissue.

DEVELOPMENT OF HUMAN OVA

DEVELOPMENTAL EVENTS

DEVELOPMENTAL STAGE

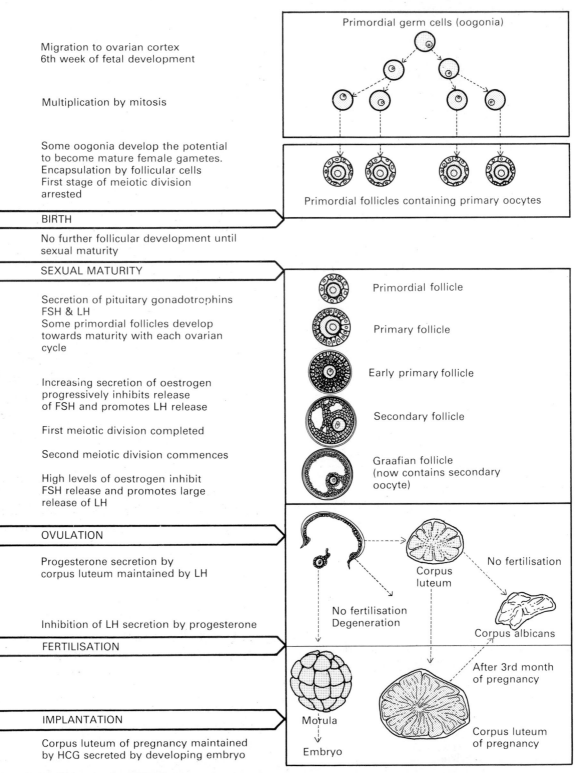

Migration to ovarian cortex
6th week of fetal development

Multiplication by mitosis

Some oogonia develop the potential
to become mature female gametes.
Encapsulation by follicular cells
First stage of meiotic division
arrested

Primordial germ cells (oogonia)

Primordial follicles containing primary oocytes

BIRTH

No further follicular development until
sexual maturity

SEXUAL MATURITY

Secretion of pituitary gonadotrophins
FSH & LH
Some primordial follicles develop
towards maturity with each ovarian
cycle

Increasing secretion of oestrogen
progressively inhibits release
of FSH and promotes LH release

First meiotic division completed

Second meiotic division commences

High levels of oestrogen inhibit
FSH release and promotes large
release of LH

Primordial follicle

Primary follicle

Early primary follicle

Secondary follicle

Graafian follicle
(now contains secondary
oocyte)

OVULATION

Progesterone secretion by
corpus luteum maintained by LH

Inhibition of LH secretion by progesterone

FERTILISATION

Corpus
luteum

No fertilisation

No fertilisation
Degeneration

Corpus albicans

IMPLANTATION

Corpus luteum of pregnancy maintained
by HCG secreted by developing embryo

Morula

Embryo

After 3rd month
of pregnancy

Corpus luteum
of pregnancy

Fig. 19.11 Summary of follicular development

The genital tract

The genital tract comprises the oviducts, uterus and the vagina, all of which have the same basic structure; a wall of smooth muscle, an inner mucosal lining and an outer layer of loose connective tissue. The mucosal and muscular components vary greatly according to their location and functional requirements; the whole tract undergoes cyclical changes under the influence of ovarian hormones released during the ovarian cycle.

The cyclical changes in the genital tract facilitate the entry of ova into the oviduct, the passage of spermatozoa into the oviduct, the passage of the fertilised ovum into the uterus and the implantation and development of the fertilised ovum in the mucosal lining of the uterine wall. Implantation of a fertilised ovum results in the secretion of hormones which inhibit the ovarian cycle and produce the gross changes in the genital tract necessary for fetal development and parturition.

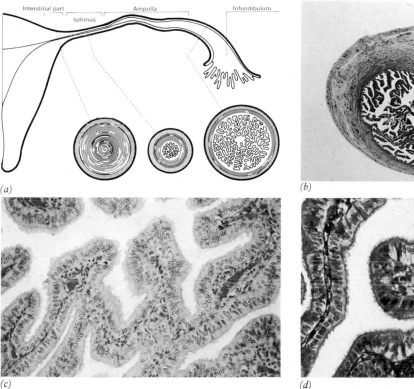

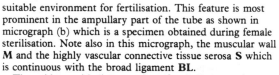

Fig. 19.12 Oviduct

(a) Parts of oviduct (b) H & E × 10 (c) H & E × 128 (d) Azan × 128

The oviducts (also called uterine tubes or Fallopian tubes) conduct ova from the surface of the ovaries to the uterine cavity and are also the site of fertilisation by spermatozoa.

The oviduct is shaped like an elongated funnel and is divided anatomically into four parts as shown diagrammatically in (a).

The *infundibulum* moves so as to overlie the site of rupture of the Graafian follicle at ovulation; finger-like projections called *fimbriae*, extending from the end of the tube, envelop the ovulation site and direct the ovum into the tube.

Movement of the ovum down the tube is mediated by gentle peristaltic action of the longitudinal and circular smooth muscle layers of the oviduct wall and is aided by a current of fluid propelled by the action of the ciliated epithelium lining the tube.

The mucosal lining of the oviduct is thrown into a labyrinth of branching, epithelial-lined folds which provide a suitable environment for fertilisation. This feature is most prominent in the ampullary part of the tube as shown in micrograph (b) which is a specimen obtained during female sterilisation. Note also in this micrograph, the muscular wall **M** and the highly vascular connective tissue serosa **S** which is continuous with the broad ligament **BL**.

The oviduct epithelium consists of a single layer of columnar cells which are of two types: ciliated and non-ciliated. The non-ciliated cells, which are stained blue in micrograph (d), produce a secretion which is propelled towards the uterus by the ciliated cells. This secretion may have a role in the nutrition and protection of the ovum. The ratio of ciliated to non-ciliated cells and the height of the cells undergo cyclical variations under the influence of ovarian hormones. The epithelial folds are supported by a highly vascular connective tissue core, the collagen of which is stained blue in micrograph (d).

The human menstrual cycle

The uterus is a flattened pear-shaped organ approximately 7 cm long in the non-pregnant state. Its mucosal lining, the *endometrium*, provides the environment for fetal development and the thick muscular wall, the *myometrium*, which expands greatly during pregnancy, provides protection for the fetus and a mechanism for the expulsion of the fetus at parturition.

The endometrial lining of the uterine cavity, consists of a simple columnar ciliated epithelium supported by a broad, highly cellular, connective tissue stroma containing many simple tubular glands. Under the influence of the hormones oestrogen and progesterone, secreted by the ovary during the ovarian cycle, the endometrium undergoes regular cyclical changes so as to offer a suitable environment for implantation of a fertilised ovum. For successful implantation, the fertilised ovum requires an easily penetrable, highly vascular tissue and an abundant supply of glycogen for nutrition until vascular connections are established with the maternal environment.

The cycle of changes in the endometrium proceeds through two distinct phases, proliferation and secretion, which involve both the epithelium and supporting connective tissue stroma.

1. The proliferative phase: the endometrial stroma proliferates to form a deep, richly vascularised stroma resembling primitive mesenchyme (see Fig. 4.2). The simple tubular glands proliferate to form numerous glands which begin secretion coincident with ovulation. The proliferative phase is initiated and sustained until ovulation by the increasing production of oestrogens from developing ovarian follicles.

2. The secretory phase: release of progesterone from the corpus luteum after ovulation promotes production of copious, thick, glycogen-rich secretion by the proliferated endometrial glands.

Unless implantation of a fertilised ovum occurs, the continuing production of progesterone is inhibited by negative feedback via the anterior pituitary, thus suppressing LH release leading to involution of the corpus luteum. In the absence of progesterone, the endometrium is unable to be maintained and most of it is shed during the period of bleeding known as menstruation. Activation of FSH secretion initiates a new cycle of follicular development and oestrogen secretion; this, in turn, initiates a new cycle of proliferation of the uterine mucosa from the remnants of the endometrium of the previous cycle. Although the process of menstruation represents the end-point of the cycle of endometrial changes, the first day of menstruation is the most easily recognisable point and is usually taken to mark the first day of the 28-day menstrual cycle. Menstruation is usually completed by the fifth day, after which the proliferative phase continues until about the fourteenth day. Ovulation, which usually occurs at the fifteenth day, marks the beginning of the secretory phase which culminates in menstruation about the twenty-eighth day.

The endometrium is divided into three histologically and functionally distinct layers; the deepest or basal layer, the *stratum basalis*, adjacent to the myometrium, undergoes the least dramatic changes during the menstrual cycle and is not shed during menstruation. The broad, intermediate layer is characterised by a stroma with a spongy appearance and is called the *stratum spongiosum*. The thinner, superficial layer which has a compact stromal appearance is known as the *stratum compactum*. The compact and spongy layers exhibit dramatic changes throughout the cycle and are both shed during menstruation; hence they are jointly referred to as the *stratum functionalis*.

The arrangement of the arterial supply of the endometrium has important influences on the menstrual cycle. Branches of the uterine arteries pass through the myometrium and immediately divide into two different types of arteries: *straight arteries* and *spiral arteries*. Straight arteries are short and pass a small distance into the endometrium then bifurcate to form a rich plexus supplying the stratum basalis. Spiral arteries are long, coiled, and thick walled and pass to the surface of the endometrium giving off numerous branches which give rise to a rich capillary plexus around the glands and in the stratum compactum. Unlike the straight arteries, the spiral arteries are highly responsive to the hormonal changes of the menstrual cycle. The withdrawal of progesterone secretion at the end of the cycle causes the spiral arteries to constrict and this precipitates an *ischaemic phase* which immediately precedes menstruation.

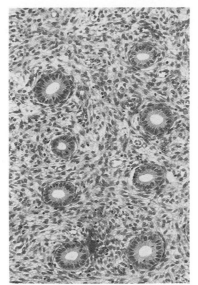

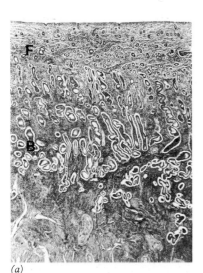

(a)

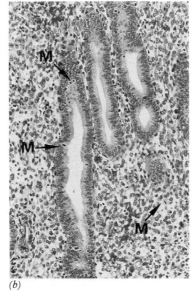

(b)

(a)

(b)

Fig. 19.13 Endometrium: early proliferative phase

(H & E (a) × 8 (b) × 128)

The low-magnification micrograph illustrates the myometrium **M** and the relatively thin endometrium consisting of the stratum basalis **B**, stratum spongiosum **S** and stratum compactum **C**. At this early proliferative stage, the stroma of the stratum functionalis (spongiosum plus compactum) has proliferated but the simple tubular glands have as yet barely proliferated into the stratum compactum.

At high magnification the proliferating glandular epithelium is seen to consist of low columnar cells. Occasional mitotic figures can be seen. Note the highly cellular connective tissue stroma almost devoid of collagen fibres which resembles primitive mesenchyme.

Fig. 19.14 Endometrium: late proliferative phase

(H & E (a) × 8 (b) × 128)

By the late proliferative stage the glands have extended to open on to the endometrial surface and the endometrium has doubled in thickness. Note that in contrast to the stratum functionalis **F**, the appearance of the stratum basalis **B** is little changed when compared with the early proliferative phase.

At high magnification many mitotic figures **M** are evident in both the glandular epithelium and the connective tissue stroma. At this stage the glandular epithelium may have a pseudostratified appearance.

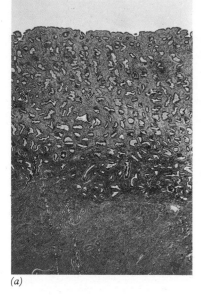

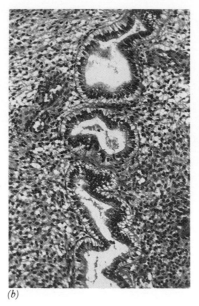

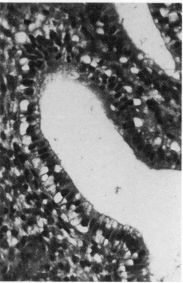

(a)   *(b)*   *(c)*

Fig. 19.15 Endometrium: early secretory phase

(H & E (a) × 8 (b) × 128 (c) × 320)

Ovulation marks the onset of the secretory phase although endometrial proliferation continues for several days. At low magnification, the glands are seen to have developed an irregular corkscrew configuration and the endometrium approaches its maximum thickness.

Under the influence of progesterone, the glandular epithelium is stimulated to synthesise glycogen. Initially the glycogen accumulates to form vacuoles in the basal aspect of the cells, thus displacing the nuclei towards the centre of the now tall columnar cells. This *basal vacuolation* of the cells is the characteristic feature of early secretory endometrium as seen at high magnification.

Glycogen is an important source of nutrition for the fertilised ovum.

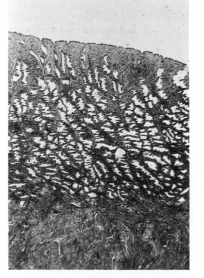

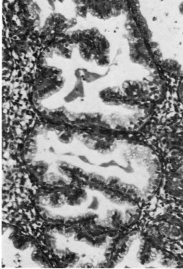

Fig. 19.16 Endometrium: late secretory phase

(H & E (a) × 8 (b) × 128)

At low magnification, the late secretory phase is characterised by a saw-tooth appearance of the glands which contain copious, thick, glycogen-rich secretions.

At high magnification, basal vacuolation is not now evident in the glandular epithelium since active secretion is taking place. Mitotic figures are rarely seen. Note the highly vascular connective tissue stroma which has become infiltrated with leucocytes.

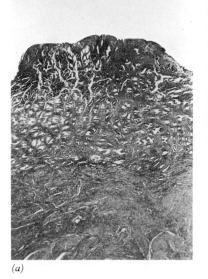

(a)

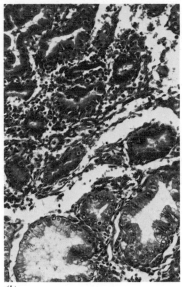

(b)

Fig. 19.17 Endometrium: onset of menstruation

(H & E (a) × 8 (b) × 128)

In the absence of implantation of a fertilised ovum, degeneration of the corpus luteum results in cessation of oestrogen and progesterone secretion which initiates phases of spasmodic constriction in the spiral arterioles. The resulting ischaemia is initially manifest by degeneration of the superficial layers of the endometrium and leakage of blood into the stroma, as seen at low magnification in micrograph (a).

Further ischaemia leads to degeneration of the whole stratum functionalis which is progressively shed as *menses*. Menses is thus composed of blood, glandular epithelium and stromal elements. Normally menses is unable to clot due to the local release of inhibitory (anticoagulant) factors. At high magnification the degenerating endometrium is seen to be heavily infiltrated by leucocytes.

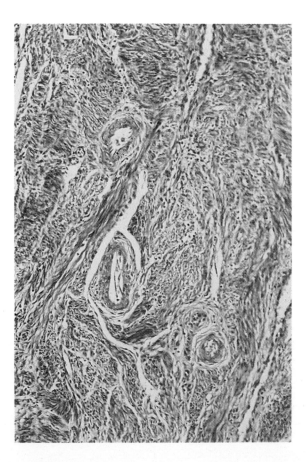

Fig. 19.18 Myometrium

(H & E × 198)

The main bulk of the uterus consists of smooth muscle, the myometrium, which is composed of interlacing bundles of long, slender fibres arranged in ill-defined layers; within the muscle is a rich network of arteries and veins supported by dense connective tissue. During pregnancy, under the influence of oestrogen, the myometrium increases greatly in size by both cell division and cell growth.

At parturition, strong contractions of the myometrium are reinforced by the action of the hormone oxytocin secreted by the posterior pituitary. These contractions expel the fetus from the uterus into the vagina and also constrict the blood supply to the placenta, thus precipitating its detachment from the uterine wall.

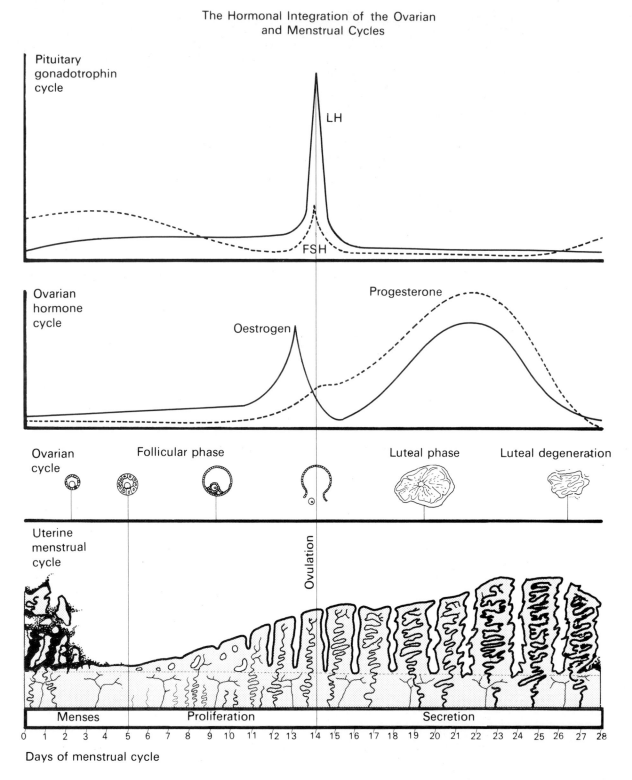

Days of menstrual cycle

Fig. 19.19 The hormonal integration of the ovarian and menstrual cycles

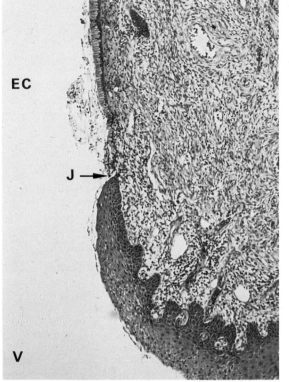

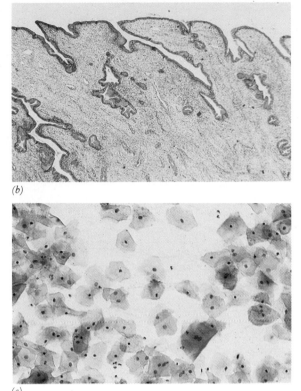

(a)

(b)

(c)

Fig. 19.20 Uterine cervix

(a) H & E × 200 (b) H & E × 28 (c) Papanicolou method × 400

The uterine cervix protrudes into the upper vagina and contains the *endocervical canal* linking the uterine cavity with the vagina. The function of the cervix is to admit spermatozoa to the genital tract at the time when fertilisation is opportune i.e. around the time of ovulation, but at other times, including pregnancy, to protect the uterus and upper tract from bacterial invasion. In addition, the cervix must be capable of great dilatation to permit the passage of the fetal head during parturition.

As seen in micrograph (a), the endocervical canal **EC** is lined by a single layer of tall, columnar, mucus-secreting cells similar to the surface epithelium of the endometrium. Where the cervix is exposed to the more hostile environment of the vagina **V** it is lined by thick stratified squamous epithelium identical to that of the rest of the vagina. The junction **J** between the vaginal and endocervical epithelium is quite abrupt and is normally located at the external os, the point at which the endocervical canal opens into the vagina.

The main bulk of the cervix is composed of tough, collagenous connective tissue containing relatively little smooth muscle. Beneath the region of the squamo-columnar junction, the cervical stroma is often infiltrated with leucocytes, as seen in micrograph (a), forming part of the defence against ingress of micro-organisms.

As seen in micrograph (b), the mucus-secreting epithelial lining of the endocervical canal is thrown into deep furrows and tunnels giving the appearance of branched tubular glands and giving rise to the rather inaccurate term 'endocervical glands'.

During the menstrual cycle, the 'endocervical glands' undergo cyclical changes in secretory activity. In the proliferative phase, rising levels of oestrogen promote secretion of thin watery mucus which permits the passage of

spermatozoa into the uterus around the period of ovulation. Following ovulation, the cervical mucus becomes highly viscid forming a plug which inhibits the entry of microorganisms from the vagina; this is particularly important should pregnancy occur. These changes in the quality of the cervical mucus form the basis for one of the 'natural' methods of contraception.

The cervical stroma is also influenced by the ovarian hormones, particularly oestrogens, which cause softening of the tissue by reducing collagenous cross-linkages and increasing uptake of water by the ground substance. At its most extreme, this provides the means by which the cervix stretches, thins and dilates in late pregnancy and during parturition. To a much smaller extent, similar changes occur during the normal menstrual cycle. One such effect is that the volume of the cervical stroma varies during each cycle causing eversion of the columnar epithelium near the squamo-columnar junction and exposing it to the vaginal environment. This induces the growth of stratified squamous epithelium over the exposed area accounting for the red, inappropriately named 'erosions' of the cervix often seen in normal women of reproductive age. The importance of this *transformation zone* is that it may undergo malignant change causing cancer of the cervix.

This area can be studied by scraping cells from the surface with a wooden spatula, smearing them on a glass slide, and staining them by the Papanicolou method; this is known as *exfoliative cytology* and is demonstrated in micrograph (c) on a specimen from a normal, healthy cervix. The surface cells of the stratified squamous epithelium have small degenerative nuclei and are stained pink due to a small content of keratin; the deeper cells have plump nuclei of normal appearance and the cytoplasm is stained blue.

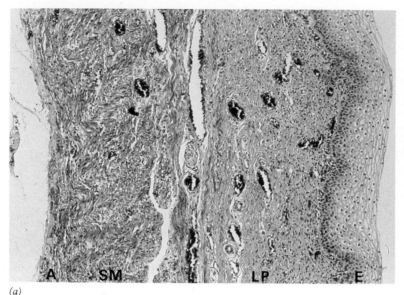

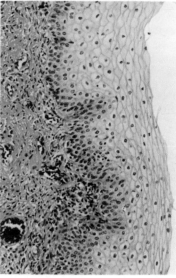

(a) *(b)*

Fig. 19.21 Vagina

(Masson's trichrome (a) × 75 (b) × 128)

The vagina is a fibromuscular canal and, as seen in micrograph (a), the wall consists of a mucosal layer lined by stratified squamous epithelium **E**, a layer of smooth muscle **SM** and an outer connective tissue adventitia **A**. In the relaxed state, the vaginal wall collapses to obliterate the lumen and the vaginal epithelium is thrown up into folds. The dense lamina propria **LP** contains many elastic fibres, has a rich plexus of small veins and is devoid of glands. The vagina is lubricated by cervical mucus, a fluid transudate from the rich vascular network of the lamina propria and mucus secreted by glands of the labia minora. The smooth muscle bundles of the muscular layer are arranged in ill-defined circular and longitudinal layers; the longitudinal layers predominate especially in the outer region.

The combination of a muscular layer and a highly elastic

lamina propria permits the gross distension which occurs during parturition. Conversely after coitus, involuntary contraction of the smooth muscle layer ensures that a pool of semen remains in the cervical region. Thick elastic fibres in the outer adventitial layer also facilitate these functions.

Micrograph (b) illustrates the stratified squamous epithelium which lines the vagina. During the menstrual cycle, this epithelium undergoes cyclical changes which includes slight keratinisation of the superficial cells; histological examination of cells scraped from the surface provides a useful means for estimation of the time of the last ovulation. Throughout the cycle, the superficial cells produce glycogen which is anaerobically metabolised by commensal bacteria in the vagina to form lactic acid which inhibits the growth of pathogenic micro-organisms.

The breasts

The breasts, or mammary glands, are highly modified apocrine sweat glands (see Fig. 9.13) which develop embryologically along two lines, the *milk lines*, extending from the axillae to the groin. In humans, only one gland develops on each side of the thorax although accessory breast tissue may be found anywhere along the milk lines.

The breasts of both sexes follow an identical course of development until puberty, after which the female breasts develop under the influence of pituitary, ovarian and other hormones. Until the menopause, the breasts undergo cyclical changes in activity which are controlled by the hormones of the ovarian cycle. After menopause, the breasts, like the other female reproductive tissues, undergo progressive atrophy and involution.

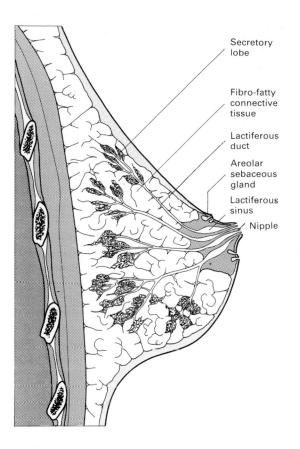

Secretory
lobe

Fibro-fatty
connective
tissue

Lactiferous
duct

Areolar
sebaceous
gland

Lactiferous
sinus

Nipple

Fig. 19.22 Structure of the breast

This highly schematic diagram illustrates the general
organisation of the breast. Each breast consists of 15–25
independent glandular units called *breast lobes*, each
consisting of a compound tubulo-acinar gland (see Fig.
5.25). The lobes are arranged radially at different depths
around the *nipple* or *mammary papilla*. A single large duct,
the *lactiferous duct*, drains each lobe via a separate opening
on the surface of the nipple. Just before each duct opens on
to the surface, the duct forms a dilatation called the
lactiferous sinus. The nipple contains bands of smooth muscle
orientated parallel to the lactiferous ducts and circularly near
the base; contraction of this muscle causes erection of the
nipple.

Each breast lobe is divided into a variable number of
lobules; the lobules consist of a system of ducts, *the alveolar
ducts*, from which large numbers of secretory alveoli develop
during pregnancy. The lobules are separated from each other
by loose connective tissue whereas each lobe is separated by
dense connective tissue often containing a large amount of
adipose tissue.

The skin surrounding the nipple, the *areola*, is pigmented
and contains sebaceous glands which are not associated with
hair follicles. The secretions of these glands probably help to
protect the nipple and areola during suckling.

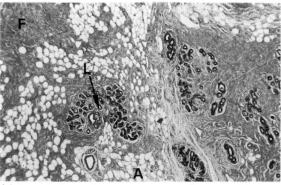

(a)

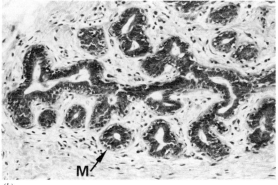

(b)

Fig. 19.23 Breast

(H & E (a) × 20 (b) × 128)

These micrographs show breast tissue from a non-pregnant
woman of reproductive age. At low magnification, the
lobules **L** of the breast are seen to form islands of glandular
tissue within an extensive mass of dense fibrous **F** and
adipose **A** connective tissue. At higher magnification, the
lobules are seen to consist of alveolar ducts lined by a
cuboidal epithelium supported by a prominent basement
membrane. Like sweat glands, a discontinuous layer of
myoepithelial cells **M** lies between the duct-lining cells and
the basement membrane. During the reproductive years, the
duct epithelium undergoes cyclical changes under the
influence of ovarian hormones. Early in the cycle, the duct
lumina are not clearly evident but later in the cycle the
lumina become more prominent and may contain an
eosinophilic secretion.

The interlobular connective tissue is usually dense and
fibrous whereas the connective tissue within the lobule is
loose, highly cellular, rarely contains fat, and has a rich
capillary network; these features can be seen in micrograph
(b). This loose intralobular connective tissue may facilitate
proliferation and expansion of breast alveoli during
pregnancy.

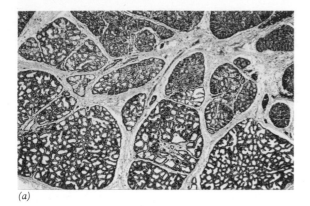

(a)

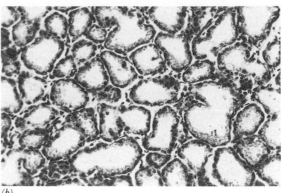

(b)

Fig. 19.24 Breast during pregnancy

(H & E (a) × 20 (b) × 128)

These micrographs demonstrate the histological changes which occur in the breast during pregnancy. Under the influence of oestrogens and progesterone produced by the corpus luteum, and later by the placenta, the alveolar duct epithelium proliferates to form numerous secretory alveoli. Breast proliferation also depends on prolactin, a prolactin-like hormone produced by the placenta called human placental lactogen (HPL), thyroid hormone and corticosteroids. At low magnification, the breast lobules are seen to have expanded greatly at the expense of the intralobular connective tissue and interlobular adipose tissue.

As pregnancy progresses the alveoli begin to secrete a protein-rich fluid called *colostrum*, the accumulation of which dilates the alveolar and duct lumina. Colostrum is the form of breast secretion available during the first few days of suckling; it contains a laxative substance and maternal antibodies which are thought to confer upon the newborn passive immunity to some diseases. Unlike milk, colostrum contains little lipid. Breast secretion is controlled by the hormone prolactin secreted by the anterior pituitary. During pregnancy, prolactin secretion progressively increases but its activity is suppressed by high levels of circulating oestrogens and progesterone.

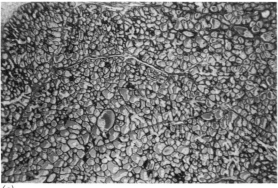

(a)

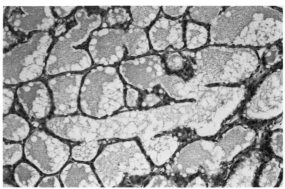

(b)

Fig. 19.25 Lactating breast

(H & E (a) × 20 (b) × 128)

After parturition the levels of circulating progesterone and oestrogens fall, thus promoting prolactin activity. Prolactin stimulates milk production (lactation) in conjunction with several other hormones.

As seen in micrograph (a) the lactating breast is composed almost entirely of alveoli greatly distended with milk; the interlobular connective tissue is reduced to thin septa between the lobules. At higher magnification in (b), the alveoli are seen to be filled with an eosinophilic material containing clear vacuoles representing lipid droplets dissolved out during tissue preparation. Some individual alveoli have an appearance reminiscent of thyroid follicles; however, in most cases the irregular branching pattern of the alveoli is clear evidence of an exocrine gland.

Milk production proceeds for as long as suckling continues and may even occur for some years after childbirth. This process is mediated by a neuro-hormonal reflex involving nipple stimulation by suckling and release of prolactin from the anterior pituitary. A different neuro-hormonal reflex promotes milk expulsion from the breasts; this reflex, also initiated by suckling, causes the release of the hormone oxytocin from the posterior pituitary. Oxytocin causes contraction of the myoepithelial cells which embrance the secretory alveoli and ducts, thus propelling milk into the lactiferous sinuses. Withdrawal of the suckling stimulus, and hence the release of pituitary hormones at weaning, results in regression of the lactating breast and resumption of the ovarian cycle.

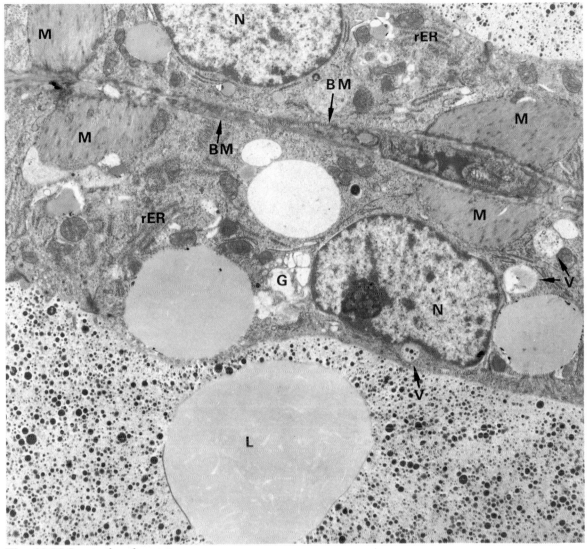

Fig. 19.26 Lactating breast

(EM × 9000)

This micrograph shows two secretory cells of adjacent alvcoli in a lactating breast. Their nuclei **N** are large with prominent nucleoli. Each alveolus is bounded by a basement membrane **BM**, the basement membranes in this example being separated by only a shred of connective tissue. Within the basement membrane of each alveolus in intimate association with the secretory cells are the cytoplasmic processes of myoepithelial cells **M**, contraction of which expels milk from the gland; the nuclei of the myoepithelial cells are not shown in this field.

The compositon of milk varies somewhat during the period of lactation and even during the period of each suckling episode but its main constituents are as follows: water (88%), ions (particularly sodium, potassium, chloride, calcium and phosphate), protein (1.5%, mainly lactalbumin and casein), carbohydrate (7%, mainly lactose), lipids (3.5%, mainly triglyceride), vitamins and antibodies (of the IgA class).

The water, ions and protein are secreted in a manner common to other serous glands, the proteins being synthesised on the rough endoplasmic reticulum **rER**, packaged in the Golgi apparatus **G** and secreted in secretory vacuoles **V** by exocytosis; note that the protein in the milk is represented by extremely electron-dense granules. The Golgi apparatus is extensive and the protein-containing secretory vacuoles also contain a considerable amount of other less electron-dense material so it appears likely that these organelles are also involved in synthesis and secretion of lactose.

The cytoplasm of the secretory cells contains lipid droplets **L** of various sizes not bounded by a membrane; these contain triglyceride though whether this is derived directly from blood or synthesised in the secretory cells is uncertain. The lipid is discharged by the process called apocrine secretion which involves the lipid droplet, surrounding cytoplasm and plasma membrane being cast off into the lumen. A large lipid droplet with thin overlying rim of cytoplasm can be seen in the lower alveolus just prior to secretion; a large droplet surrounded by a shred of cytoplasm and plasma membrane is seen in the lumen close by.

Vitamins and IgA are probably transported across the cell from the bloodstream in small membranous vesicles.

20. Central nervous system

Introduction

The central nervous system, comprising the brain and spinal cord, is composed entirely of neurones, their axons and dendrites, and the supporting cells of the CNS, the neuroglial cells; the histology of these and the meninges which invest the CNS are described in Chapter 7.

On gross examination, sections of any part of the CNS are made up of grey matter and white matter, the grey matter mainly containing the neurone cell bodies and the white matter the axons; lipid in the myelin sheaths of the axons accounts for the white appearance of white matter. The distribution of grey matter and white matter differs greatly from one part of the brain to the other as does the morphology and arrangement of the neurones. This chapter provides an outline of the histological features of the main regions of the brain and spinal cord.

The histological methods used in the study of the CNS can be divided into three broad groups. Firstly, there are techniques which demonstrate nuclei and cell bodies, and their cytoplasmic constituents; such methods include routine stains such as H & E and more specific methods for demonstrating particular cytoplasmic constituents such as the Nissl method for RNA. These methods show minimal detail of axons and dendrites. Moreover, since myelin (lipid) is dissolved out during preparation, white matter remains almost unstained by such methods. In contrast, there is a second group of stains which specifically demonstrates lipid; these so-called myelin methods, e.g. Weigart-Pal, are particularly useful for studying the arrangement of grey matter (nuclei) and white matter in the brain stem and spinal cord (see Figs. 20.1–20.3), as well as abnormalities of myelination. With myelin methods, the white matter stains strongly, the grey matter remaining unstained. Heavy metal impregnation methods applied to thick tissue sections, make up the third group of histological techniques. These methods (see Fig. 20.7) demonstrate overall cell morphology and, apart from showing the distinctive shapes of the neurone cell bodies in various parts of the CNS, they also outline axons and dendrites permitting study of neuronal interconnections. Such methods, which are extremely protracted and technically exacting, were widely used around the turn of the 20th century by the great pioneers of neuroanatomy such as Cajal and Golgi from whom they take their names.

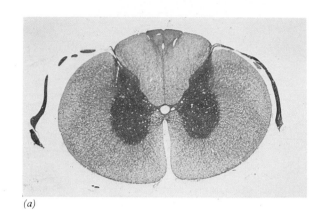

(a)

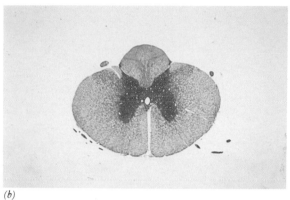

(b)

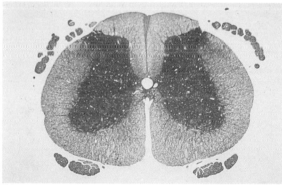

(c)

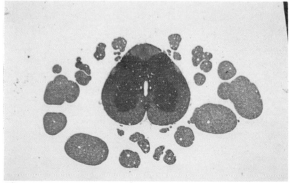

(d)

Fig. 20.1 Spinal cord

(Cat: Weigart-Pal × 10 (a) Cervical (b) Thoracic (c) Lumbar (d) Sacral)

The structure of the spinal cord is basically similar over its whole length. However, the functional differences at the four main levels are reflected in corresponding characteristic features which are demonstrated in this series of micrographs. In transverse section, the central mass of grey matter has the shape of a butterfly, the ventral horns being most prominent and containing the cell bodies of the large lower motor neurones. The dorsal horns are much less prominent and contain the cell bodies of small second order sensory neurones which relay sensory information to the brain from primary afferent neurones for the modalities of temperature and pain whose cell bodies lie in the dorsal root ganglia. Small lateral horns, which contain the cell bodies of preganglionic, sympathetic efferent neurones, are found in the thoracic and upper lumbar regions corresponding to the level of the sympathetic outflow from the cord. The volume of grey matter is much more extensive in the cervical and lumbar regions corresponding to the great sensory and motor innervation of the limbs and this is reflected in the much greater diameter of the spinal cord in these areas. The central canal containing CSF and lined with ependymal cells lies in the central commissure of grey matter.

The white matter of the spinal cord consists of ascending tracts of sensory fibres and descending motor tracts; passing up the spinal cord towards the brain, more and more fibres enter and leave the cord so that the volume of white matter increases progressively from the sacral to cervical regions.

Externally, the spinal cord has a deep ventral median fissure but dorsally there is only a shallow dorsal midline sulcus. On each side, a dorso-lateral sulcus marks the line of entry of the dorsal nerve roots. The roughly triangular area of white matter between the dorsal horns represents the ascending dorsal columns which convey fibres for the senses of vibration, proprioception and discriminatory touch to the medulla where they synapse with second order sensory neurones in the gracile and cuneate nuclei. In the cervical region, each dorsal column is subdivided into two fascicles, the medial fasciculus gracilis conveying fibres from the lower limbs, and the lateral fasciculus cuneatus conveying fibres from the upper limbs.

Ventrolateral sulci may be discernible on each side (see micrograph (c)) marking the sites of exit of the ventral nerve roots.

The ventrolateral white matter on each side is made up of various ascending and descending tracts most notably the lateral spinothalamic tract (pain and temperature), ventral spinothalamic tract (light touch), spinocerebellar tracts and corticospinal tract (motor).

Like the brain, the spinal cord is invested by meninges, the outer surface of the dura mater being loosely connected by fibrous strands to the periosteum of the vertebral canal and the intervening epidural space being filled with loose adipose tissue and an extensive venous plexus. During development, the vertebral column lengthens to a greater degree than the enclosed spinal cord and the segmental levels of the lower part of the cord therefore lie above the corresponding intervertebral foramina. Consequently, below the cervical region, the nerve roots have an increasingly oblique course in the subarachnoid space before passing through the intervertebral foramina and thus can be seen adjacent to the cord particularly in the lumbar and sacral regions.

Fig. 20.2 Medulla

*(Weigart-Pal × 4 (a) Upper-mid level
(b) Lower level)*

The medulla, the most distal part of the
brain stem, can be roughly divided into
two parts, the characteristic features of
which are seen in these micrographs;
this myelin staining method leaves grey
matter relatively unstained.

The most obvious feature of the
upper half of the medulla is the inferior
olivary nucleus **O** with its peculiar
convoluted appearance in transverse
section; adjacent are the smaller dorsal
and medial accessory olivary nuclei
which complete the inferior olivary
complex. The neurones of the inferior
olivary complex relay central and spinal
afferent stimuli to the cerebellar cortex.
Also, at the upper mid medullary level
shown in micrograph (a), the fourth
ventricle **IV** closes to become a narrow
central canal which continues down into
the spinal cord. Thus the medulla is
often divided into an upper, open part
and a lower, closed part.

All of the ascending (sensory) and
descending (motor) pathways found in
the spinal cord pass through the
medulla, although their arrangement in
the medulla differs considerably from
that in the spinal cord. The most easily
recognisable features of these pathways
in the medulla are the gracile and
cuneate nuclei and fasciculi, and the
pyramids.

The dorsal white matter columns of
the spinal cord convey ascending
proprioceptive, vibration and
discriminatory touch fibres from the
lower limbs and upper limbs in the
fasciculus gracilis **FG** and fasciculus
cuneatus **FC** respectively. In the
similarly situated nucleus gracilis and
nucleus cuneatus in the dorsum of the
medulla, these fibres synapse with cell
bodies of second order neurones which
then pass upwards to the thalamus via
the medial lemniscus which lies medial
to the olivary complex.

Axons originating in the motor cortex
descend through the internal capsule,
break up into small bundles in the
pons, then converge again in the
medulla to form a prominent ventral
pyramid **P** on each side of the medulla;
in the pyramids, about 85% of fibres
cross to the other side in the
decussation of the pyramids.

The medulla also contains the various
tracts and nuclei of the 8th to the 12th
cranial nerves as well as the spinal
nucleus and tract of the trigeminal
nerve which extends from the pons
down into the upper cervical cord. The
spinal nucleus of the trigeminal tract

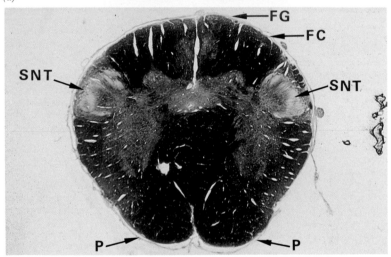

(a)

(b)

SNT is easily recognisable
dorsolaterally throughout the medulla
with its tract of white matter lying
superficially. The hypoglossal nucleus
HN can also be identified in
micrograph (a). In the centre of the
lower medulla, grey matter can be seen,
still roughly resembling the
characteristic butterfly shape seen in
sections of the spinal cord; the ventral
grey matter horns contain cell bodies of
lower motor neurones running in the
spinal accessory and first cervical
nerves.

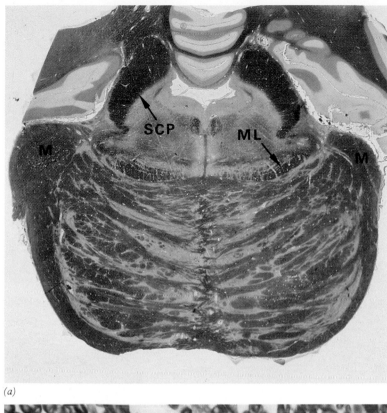

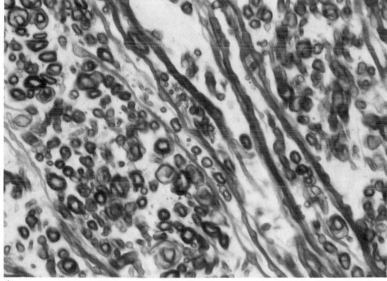

(a)

(b)

Fig. 20.3 Pons

(Weigart-Pal (a) Mid level × 3 (b) Basal pons × 480)

The pons is the middle portion of the brain stem, lying between midbrain proximally and medulla distally. In transverse section, it comprises two parts, a bulky ventral region (the *basal pons*) and a smaller dorsal (*tegmental*) region.

The basal pons consists of crisscrossed bundles of longitudinal and transverse fibres between which lie collections of neurone cell bodies known as pontine nuclei. Micrograph (b) shows a small area of this region at higher magnification, the myelin investing the axons being stained blue; neurone cell bodies are not stained and are therefore not identifiable. The longitudinal fibres of the basal pons consist of descending fibres of two main types. Firstly, there are axons from the motor cortex passing down to synapse with lower motor neurones of the ventral horns of the spinal cord; on leaving the pons, these axons converge to form the characteristic pyramids (pyramidal tracts) in the medulla. The second group of descending fibres have widespread cortical origins and synapse in the pontine nuclei from which fibres then pass in the transverse bundles, crossing the mid-line, to enter the cerebellum via the middle peduncles **M**.

The dorsal tegmentum contains the ascending spinothalamic (sensory) tracts and the nuclei of the fifth, sixth and seventh cranial nerves. On each side, the medial lemniscus **ML** is readily identifiable; this represents the upward continuation of proprioceptive, vibration and fine touch pathways from the gracile and cuneate nuclei of the medulla. The cerebellar peduncles are a readily recognisable feature of the pons, the middle peduncle being still present in sections through the mid pontine level as in micrograph (a) at which level the superior peduncles **SCP** are very prominent. The main bulk of the superior cerebellar peduncles is made up of fibres from the central nuclei of the cerebellum passing upwards to the thalamus and then projecting to the motor cortex.

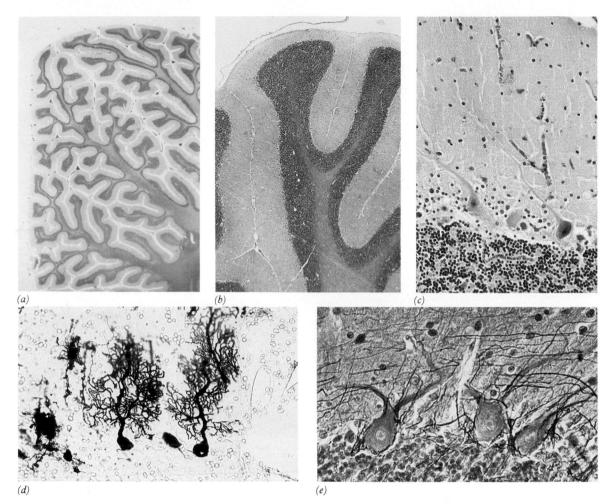

(a) (b) (c)

(d) (e)

Fig. 20.4 Cerebellum

(H & E (a) × 4 (b) × 64 (c) × 320 (d) Golgi-Cox × 320 (e) Bielschowsky/neutral red × 600)

The cerebellum, which co-ordinates muscular activity and maintains posture and equilibrium, consists of a cortex of grey matter with a central core of white matter containing four pairs of nuclei. Afferent and efferent fibres pass to and from the brain stem via inferior, middle and superior cerebellar peduncles linking medulla, pons and midbrain respectively.

As seen in micrograph (a), the cerebellar cortex forms a series of deeply convoluted folds or *folia* supported by a branching central medulla of white matter. At higher magnification in micrograph (b), the cortex is seen to consist of three layers, an outer layer containing relatively few cells (the so-called *molecular layer*), an extremely cellular inner layer (the so-called *granule cell layer*) and a single intervening layer of huge neurones called *Purkinje cells*. The Purkinje cells, seen at further magnification in micrograph (c), have huge cell bodies, a relatively fine axon extending down through the granule cell layer, and an extensively branching dendritic system which arborises into the outer molecular layer; this extraordinary dendritic system is best demonstrated by heavy metal methods as in micrograph (d).

The deep granule cell layer of the cortex contains numerous small neurones, the non-myelinated axons of which pass outwards to the molecular layer where they bifurcate to run parallel to the surface to synapse with the dendrites of Purkinje cells; each granule cell synapses with several hundred Purkinje cells. Micrograph (e) demonstrates the course of granule cell axons in the molecular layer. The axons are stained black with silver and the cell bodies are counter-stained with neutral red. In addition to the Purkinje and granule cells already described, there are three other types of small neurones in the cerebellar cortex, namely, *stellate cells* and *basket cells* scattered in the outer molecular layer and *Golgi cells* scattered in the superficial part of the granule cell layer.

In simple terms, afferent fibres enter the cerebellum from the brain stem and then pass via the white matter core to make complex connections with granule cells, Purkinje dendrites and other neurones of the cerebellar cortex; these cortical cells also make numerous interconnections with each other within the molecular layer. The only efferent fibres from the cerebellar cortex are the Purkinje cell axons which pass down through the granule cell layer into the white matter where they synapse in the central nuclei of the cerebellum.

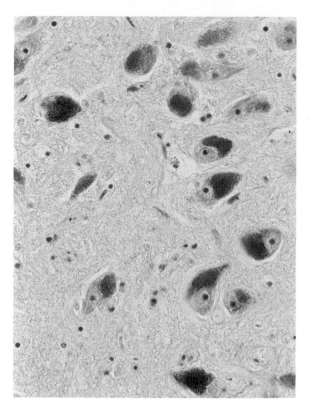

Fig. 20.5 Substantia nigra

(H & E × 480)

The *substantia nigra* is a large mass of grey matter extending throughout the midbrain; on each side it divides the cerebral peduncles into dorsal and ventral parts and in sections of the midbrain it is easily recognised by the black pigment from which its name derives.

The substantia nigra has extensive connections with the cortex, spinal cord, corpus striatum and reticular formation and appears to play an important part in the fine control of motor function. The neurones of the substantia nigra are multipolar in form and in adults the cytoplasm contains numerous granules of melanin pigment as seen in this micrograph. The pigmented neurones of the substantia nigra contain dopamine which appears to act as a neurotransmitter causing inhibitory effects particularly on neurones in the corpus striatum.

DOPA (dihydroxyphenylalanine) is a precursor of dopamine and also of melanin, and the melanin of substantia nigra neurones may merely represent a residual product of normal metabolic activity; this is supported by the fact that very little melanin is present at birth with the amount increasing considerably during childhood and thereafter rising at a slower rate into old age.

Parkinson's disease, a debilitating disorder characterised by tremor, muscular rigidity and impaired speed and precision of motor functions, is associated with degeneration of neurones in the substantia nigra and a marked reduction in dopamine synthesis. Symptoms can be alleviated by the drug L-dopa, a dopamine precursor which crosses the blood-brain barrier (see Fig. 7.25).

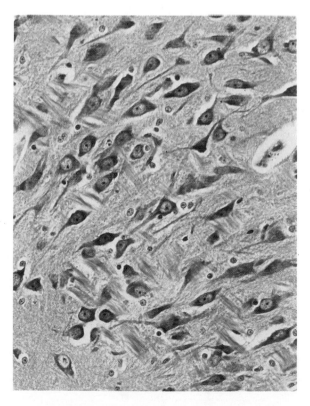

Fig. 20.6 Thalamus

(H & E × 480)

The thalami are large masses of grey matter lying on each side of the third ventricle and comprising the main bulk of the diencephalon, the central core of the cerebrum. Functionally, the thalamus is subdivided into a large number of nuclei including reticular and motor nuclei as well as specific sensory nuclei containing the cell bodies of neurones with axons projecting to the cerebral cortex. The thalamus constitutes an extremely complex relay and integration centre for information from almost all parts of the CNS.

This micrograph shows the histological appearance of a typical thalamic nucleus consisting of a dense aggregation of neurone cell bodies criss-crossed by tracts of afferent and efferent nerve fibres.

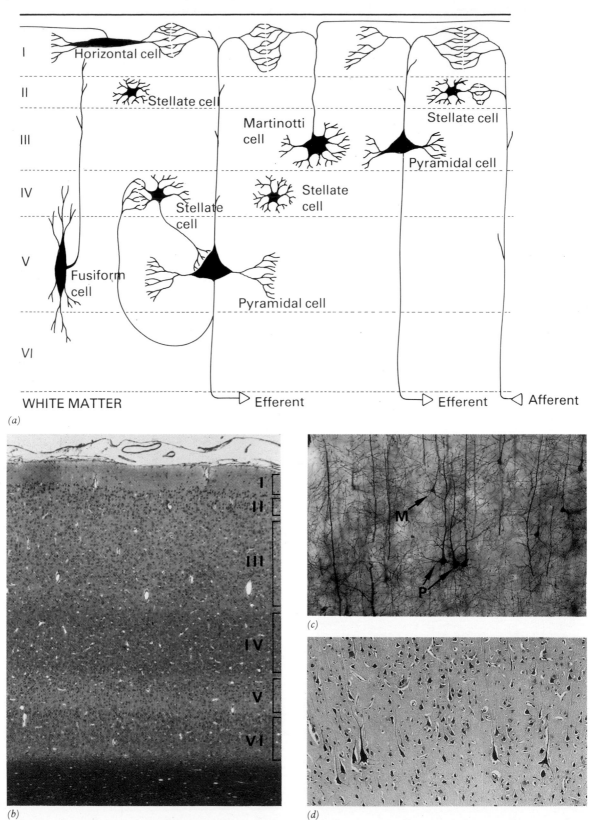

(a)

I Horizontal cell

II Stellate cell

III Martinotti cell — Stellate cell — Pyramidal cell

IV Stellate cell — Stellate cell

V Fusiform cell — Pyramidal cell

VI

WHITE MATTER — Efferent — Efferent — Afferent

(b)

I
II
III
IV
V
VI

(c)

M

P

(d)

Fig. 20.7 Cerebral cortex *(illustrations opposite)*

(a) Neurone cell types (b) Methyline blue × 42 (c) Golgi method × 320 (d) Nissl method × 320

The cerebral hemispheres consist of a convoluted cortex of grey matter overlying the central medullary mass of white matter which conveys fibres between different parts of the cortex and to and from other parts of the CNS.

Histologically, the neurones of the cerebral cortex are divided into five different morphological types which are arranged in several layers. In submammalian species, the major function of the cortex concerns the sense of olfaction (smell) and the neurones are arranged into three layers. In mammals, there has evolved the so-called *neocortex* consisting of six layers of neurones. The neocortex comprises the sensory and motor areas of the cortex as well as the vast association cortex and in all, constitutes about 90% of the cerebral cortex in humans. The primitive three-layered pattern persists only in the olfactory cortex and cortical part of the limbic system in the temporal lobe.

Neurone types in the cerebral cortex

The five characteristic types of cortical neurone are shown diagrammatically in (a), the pyramidal and stellate cells being by far the most common type.

1. Pyramidal cells, as their name implies, have pyramid-shaped cell bodies, the apex being directed towards the cortical surface. A thin axon arises from the base of the cell and passes into the underlying white matter, though in the case of small superficially located cells, the axon may synapse in the deep layers of the cortex. From the apex, a thick branching dendrite passes towards the surface where it has a prolific array of fine dendritic branches. In addition, short dendrites arise from the edges of the base and ramify laterally. The size of the pyramidal cells varies from small to large, the smallest tending to lie more superficially. The huge upper motor neurones of the motor cortex, known as *Betz cells*, are the largest of the pyramidal cells in the cortex.

2. Stellate (granule) cells are small neurones with a short vertical axon and several short branching dendrites giving the cell body the shape of a star; basket and neurogliaform subtypes are also described. With routine histological methods the cells look like small granules giving rise to their alternative name.

3. Cells of Martinotti are small polygonal cells with a few short dendrites and the axon extending toward the surface and bifurcating to run horizontally, most commonly in the most superficial layer.

4. Fusiform cells are spindle-shaped cells oriented at right angles to the surface. The axon arises from the side of the cell body and passes superficially. Dendrites extend from each end of the cell body branching so as to pass vertically into deeper and more superficial layers.

5. Horizontal cells of Cajal are small and spindle-shaped but oriented parallel to the surface. They are the least common cell type and are only found in the most superficial layer where their axons pass laterally to synapse with the dendrites of pyramidal cells.

In addition to neurones, the cortex contains supporting neuroglial cells i.e. astrocytes, oligodendroglia and microglia.

Layers of the neocortex

As previously stated, the neurones in the neocortex are arranged into six layers, the layers differing in characteristic neurone morphology, size and population density. The layers merge with one another rather than being highly demarcated and vary somewhat from one region of the cortex to another depending on cortical thickness and function.

Micrograph (b) illustrates the typical layered appearance of the cerebral cortex, the more detailed characteristics of each layer being as follows:

I. *Plexiform (molecular) layer*. This most superficial layer mainly contains dendrites and axons of cortical neurones making synapses with one another; the sparse nuclei are those of neuroglia and occasional horizontal cells of Cajal.

II. *Outer granular layer*. A dense population of small pyramidal cells and stellate cells make up this thin layer which also contains various axons and dendritic connections from deeper layers.

III. *Pyramidal cell layer*. Pyramidal cells of moderate size predominate in this broad layer, the cells increasing in size deeper in the layer.

IV. *Inner granular layer*. This narrow layer consists mainly of densely packed stellate cells.

V. *Ganglionic layer*. Large pyramidal cells and smaller numbers of stellate cells and cells of Martinotti make up this layer, the name of the layer originating from the huge pyramidal (ganglion) Betz cells of the motor cortex.

VI. *Multiform cell layer*. So named on account of the wide variety of differing morphological forms found in this layer, the layer contains numerous small pyramidal cells and cells of Martinotti, as well as stellate cells especially superficially, and fusiform cells in the deeper part.

Micrograph (c) shows part of layer V using a thick section stained with a heavy metal impregnation technique which demonstrates considerable morphological detail. Several pyramidal cells P are easily identifiable, the principal dendrite of each (but not the axon) being included in the plane of section. A cell of Martinotti M can also be identified by its polygonal shape.

Micrograph (d) also shows layer V but in this case the section is thinner and stained by a routine histological method; in this example there is little morphological detail, nevertheless most of the cells are identifiable as pyramidal cells, increasing in size in the deeper part and including several huge cells.

The synaptic inter-connections within the cortex are exceedingly complex with any one cell synapsing with several hundred other neurones. However, there are several basic principals of cortical organisation and function. Firstly, the functional units are disposed vertically, corresponding to the general orientation of axons and major dendrites. Secondly, afferent fibres (their cell bodies lying elsewhere in the CNS) generally synapse high in the cortex with dendrites of efferent neurones, the cell bodies of which lie in deeper layers of the cortex. Thirdly, efferent pathways, typically the axons of pyramidal cells, tend to give off branches which pass back into more superficial layers to communicate with their own dendrites via interneuronal connections involving other cortical cell types.

21. Special sense organs

Introduction

The organs of special sense are highly sophisticated sensory receptors in which the specific neural receptors are incorporated in a non-neural structure which enhances and refines the reception of incoming stimuli. The eye and audio-vestibular apparatus of the ear are the main special sense organs but the gustatory (taste) and olfactory (smell) receptors are usually also included in this category.

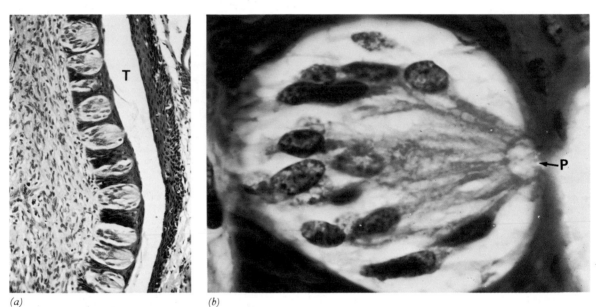

(a)   *(b)*

Fig. 21.1 Taste buds

(H & E (a) × 128 (b) × 1200)

Taste buds, the chemoreceptors for the sense of taste or *gustation*, are in man mainly located in the epithelium of the circumvallate papillae of the tongue (see Fig. 13.12), although they are also found scattered in other parts of the tongue, palate, pharynx and epiglottis. In the circumvallate papillae, taste buds face into the deep troughs **T** surrounding the papillae as shown in micrograph (a). Serous glands, called the glands of von Ebner, drain into the troughs where the serous secretion is thought to act as a solvent for taste-provoking substances.

The taste bud is a barrel-shaped organ extending the full thickness of the epithelium and opening at the surface via a pore known as the *taste pore* **P**. Each taste bud contains from twenty to thirty long, spindle-shaped cells which extend from the basement membrane to the taste pore. Classically, two types of cell are described in the taste bud: light *gustatory cells* and dark *supporting* or *sustentacular cells*. A third cell type, the *basal cell*, is now generally recognised and may constitute the precursor of one or both of the other cell types. Both gustatory and sustentacular cells have long

microvilli which extend into the taste pore which contains a glycoprotein substance thought to be secreted by the sustentacular cells.

Ultrastructural studies have shown non-myelinated nerve fibres to be associated with both cell types, but there appears to be a more intimate, synapse-like relationship between the nerve fibres and the gustatory cells. Although the so-called gustatory cells are thought to be the taste receptors, the sustentacular cells may also serve some receptor function. Like the oral epithelium, all the cells of the taste bud, which represent highly specialised epithelial cells, are renewed continuously though the gustatory and sustentacular cells are replaced at different rates.

Four taste modalities are recognised: sweet, bitter, acid and salt. Each modality tends to be principally perceived in a specific region of the tongue; however, no structural differences have been demonstrated between taste buds from different areas. The sensations of taste and smell are closely associated and loss of olfactory sense is accompanied by diminished gustatory perception.

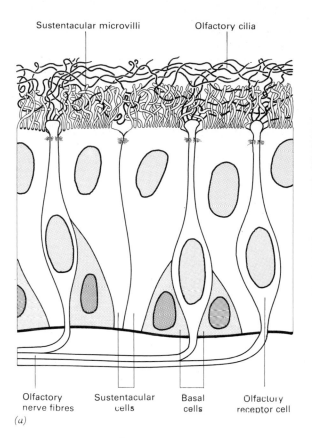

Sustentacular microvilli   Olfactory cilia

Olfactory nerve fibres   Sustentacular cells   Basal cells   Olfactory receptor cell

(a)

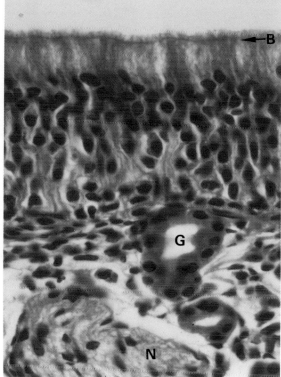

(b)

Fig. 21.2 Olfactory receptors

(a) Schematic diagram (b) H & E × 720

The receptors for the sense of smell are located in a modified form of respiratory epithelium called *olfactory epithelium* in the nasal cavity; although extensive in some mammals such as the dog, the olfactory epithelium is restricted to a small area in the roof of the nasal cavity in man. The olfactory epithelium is extremely tall, pseudostratified columnar in form and contains cells of three types: olfactory receptor cells, supporting epithelial (*sustentacular*) cells and basal epithelial cells.

The *olfactory receptor cells* are true bipolar neurones (see Fig. 7.2), the cell bodies of which are located in the middle stratum of the olfactory epithelium. A single dendritic process extends from the cell body to the free surface where it terminates as a small swelling which gives rise to about a dozen extremely long, modified cilia. These cilia, which contain the usual '9 plus 2' arrangement of microtubules, are nonmotile and lie flattened against the epithelial surface. The cilia are thought to be the sites of interaction between odiferous substances and the receptor cells. At the basal aspect, each receptor cell gives rise to a single fine, non-myelinated axon which penetrates the basement membrane to join the axons of other receptor cells. The bundles of axons pass via about 20 small holes on each side of the cribriform plate of the ethmoid bone to reach the olfactory bulbs of the forebrain where they synapse with second order sensory neurones.

The supporting or sustentacular cells are elongated cells with their tapered bases resting on the basement membrane. Many long microvilli extend from their luminal surfaces to form a tangled mat with the cilia of the receptor cells. At the luminal surface, the plasma membranes of the sustentacular and receptor cells are bound by typical junctional complexes. The functions of the sustentacular cells are poorly understood but they probably provide mechanical and physiological support for the receptor cells. The basal cells are small, conical cells which may represent epithelial stem cells although recent evidence suggests that some may represent immature receptor cells.

In histological section, it is difficult to distinguish individual cell types within the olfactory epithelium; however, the nuclei of sustentacular cells occupy the uppermost stratum, those of the receptor cells the middle stratum, and the basal cells lie close to the basement membrane. Note the terminal bar **B** at the luminal surface representing junctional complexes; note also the tangled meshwork of microvilli and cilia on the surface.

The olfactory epithelium is supported by vascular, loose connective tissue containing bundles of afferent nerve fibres **N** and numerous serous glands called *Bowman's glands* **G** which produce the watery surface secretions in which odiferous substances are dissolved.

The Eye

The eye is a highly specialised organ of photoreception, a process which involves the conversion of different quanta of light energy into nerve action potentials.

The photoreceptors are modified dendrites of two types of nerve cells, *rod cells* and *cone cells*. The rods are integrated into a system which is receptive to light of differing intensity; this is perceived in a form analogous to a black and white photographic image. The cones are of three functional types receptive to the colours blue, green and red and constitute a system by which coloured images may be perceived. The rod and cone receptors and a system of integrating neurones are located in the inner layer of the eye, the *retina*. The remaining structures of the eye serve to support the retina or to focus images of the visual world upon the retina.

In addition, several accessory structures namely the *eyelids*, *lacrimal gland* and *conjunctiva* protect the eye from external damage.

Fig. 21.3 The eye *(illustration opposite)*

The eye is made up of three basic layers: the outer *corneo-scleral layer*, the intermediate *uveal layer (uveal tract)* and the inner *retinal layer*.

1. Corneo-scleral layer: The corneo-scleral layer forms a tough, fibro-elastic capsule which supports the eye. The posterior five-sixths, the *sclera*, is opaque and provides insertion for the extra-ocular muscles.

The anterior one-sixth, the *cornea*, is transparent and has a smaller radius of curvature than the sclera. The cornea is the principal refracting medium of the eye and roughly focuses an image on to the retina; the focusing power of the cornea depends mainly on the radius of curvature of its external surface. The corneo-scleral junction is known as the *limbus* and is marked internally and externally by a shallow depression.

2. Uveal layer: The middle layer, the uvea or uveal tract, is a highly vascular layer which is made up of three components: the *choroid*, *ciliary body* and the *iris*. The choroid lies between the sclera and retina in the posterior five-sixths of the eye. It provides nutritive support for the retina and is heavily pigmented, thus absorbing light which has passed through the retina. Anteriorly, the choroid merges with the ciliary body which is a circumferential thickening of the uvea lying beneath the limbus.

The ciliary body surrounds the coronal equator of the *lens* and is attached to it by the *suspensory ligament* or *zonule*. The lens is a biconvex transparent structure, the shape of which can be varied to provide fine focus of the corneal image upon the retina. The ciliary body contains smooth muscle, the tone of which controls the shape of the lens via the suspensory ligament. The lens, suspensory ligament and ciliary body partition the eye into a large posterior compartment and a smaller anterior compartment.

The iris, the third component of the uvea, forms a diaphragm extending in front of the lens from the ciliary body so as to incompletely divide the anterior compartment into two chambers; these are known by the terms *anterior* and *posterior chamber* (not to be confused with the anterior and posterior compartments mentioned above). The highly pigmented iris acts as an adjustable diaphragm which regulates the amount of light reaching the retina. The aperture of the iris is called the *pupil*.

The anterior and posterior chambers contain a watery fluid, the *aqueous humor*, which is secreted into the posterior chamber by the ciliary body and circulated through the pupil to drain into a canal at the angle of the anterior chamber, the *canal of Schlemm*. The aqueous humor is a source of nutrients for the non-vascular lens and cornea, and acts as an optical medium which is non-refractive with respect to the cornea. The pressure of aqueous humor maintains the shape of the cornea.

The large, posterior compartment of the eye contains a gelatinous mass known as the *vitreous body* consisting of transparent *vitreous humor*. The vitreous body supports the lens and retina from within as well as providing an optical medium which is non-refractive with respect to the lens. In life, the vitreous body contains a canal which extends from the exit of the optic nerve to the posterior surface of the lens; this *hyaloid canal* represents the course of the hyaloid artery which supplies the vitreous body during embryological development. The vitreous body and hyaloid canal are rarely preserved in histological preparations.

3. Retinal layer: The photosensitive retina forms the inner lining of most of the posterior compartment of the eye and terminates along a scalloped line, the *ora serrata*, behind the ciliary body. Anterior to the ora serrata, the retinal layer continues as a non-photosensitive epithelial layer which lines the ciliary body and the posterior surface of the iris.

The visual axis of the eye passes through a depression in the retina called the *fovea* which is surrounded by a yellow pigmented zone, the *macula lutea*. The fovea is the area of greatest visual acuity.

Afferent nerve fibres from the retina converge to form the *optic nerve* which leaves the eye through a part of the sclera known as the *lamina cribrosa*. The retina overlying the lamina cribrosa, the *optic papilla (optic disc)* is devoid of photoreceptors and thus represents a blind spot.

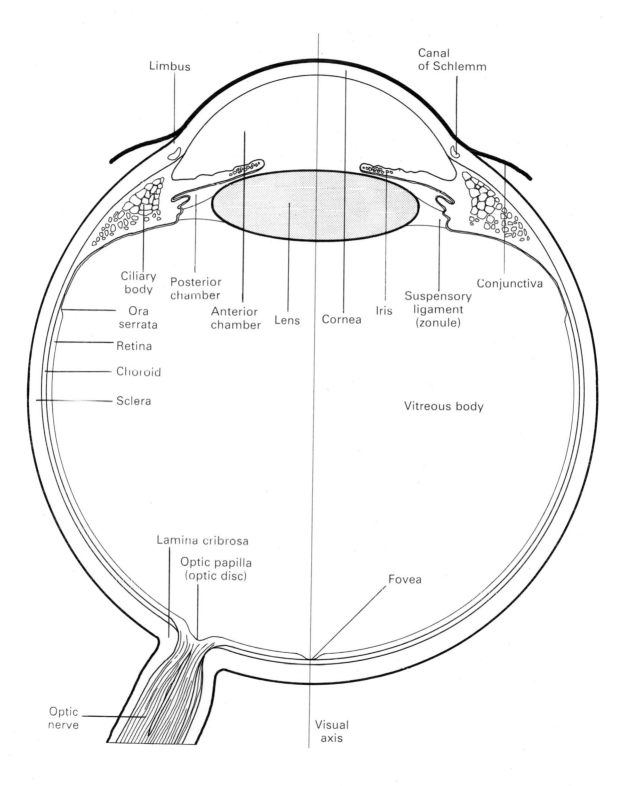

Limbus

Canal
of Schlemm

Ciliary
body

Posterior
chamber

Conjunctiva

Ora
serrata

Anterior
chamber

Lens   Cornea   Iris

Suspensory
ligament
(zonule)

Retina

Choroid

Sclera

Vitreous body

Lamina cribrosa

Optic papilla
(optic disc)

Fovea

Optic
nerve

Visual
axis

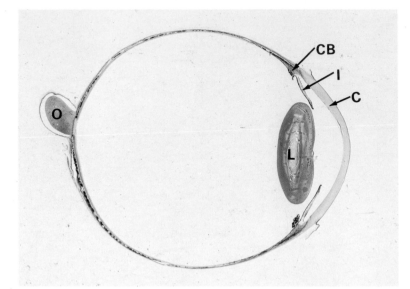

Fig. 21.4 Eye

(Monkey: H & E × 5)

This horizontal section shows the relative sizes of the components of the eye. At this magnification, the three layers comprising the wall of the globe are not readily distinguishable although in the wall of the posterior compartment, the middle layer of choroid is recognisable by its high content of pigment.

The other uveal structures, the ciliary body **CB** and iris **I** are readily visible. The lens **L** has been artefactually distorted during preparation and the suspensory ligament by which it is attached to the ciliary body is not preserved. Note the relative thickness of the cornea **C**.

The optic nerve **O** is seen to penetrate the sclera medial to the visual axis; the fovea is not present in this plane of section.

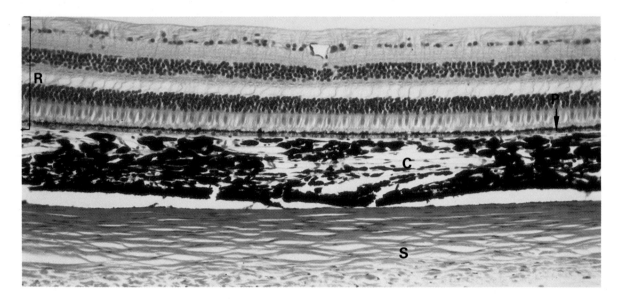

Fig. 21.5 Wall of the eye

(H & E × 300)

The three layers of the wall of the eye are illustrated in this micrograph.

The inner photosensitive retina is a multi-layered structure, the outermost limit of which is defined by a layer of *pigmented epithelial cells* **P**.

The choroid **C** is a layer of loose, highly vascular connective tissue lying between the sclera **S** externally and the retina **R** internally. The choroid and retina are separated by a thin membrane known as *Bruch's membrane* which probably represents the basement membrane of the pigmented epithelium. The blood supply of the uveal layer of the eye is provided by branches of the ophthalmic artery which penetrate via the sclera. Larger vessels predominate in the superficial aspect of the choroid with a rich capillary plexus in the deeper aspect providing nourishment for the outer layers of the retina by diffusion across Bruch's membrane. The choroid contains numerous large, heavily pigmented melanocytes which confer the dense pigmentation characteristic of the choroid. The pigment absorbs light rays passing through the retina and prevents interference due to light reflection.

The sclera consists of dense fibro-elastic connective tissue, the fibres of which are arranged in bundles parallel to the surface. This layer contains little ground substance and few fibroblasts. The sclera varies in thickness, being thickest posteriorly and thinnest at the coronal equator of the globe.

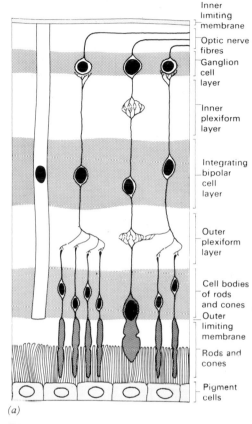

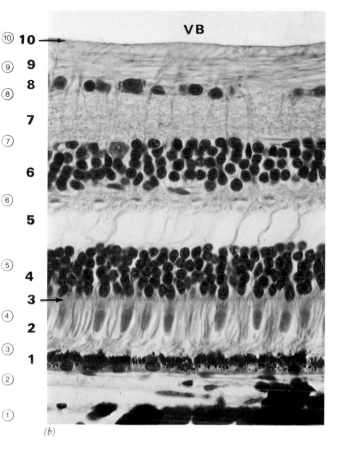

Fig. 21.6 Retina

(a) Schematic diagram (b) H & E × 640

The retina is made up of three basic cell types, neurones, pigmented epithelial cells and neurone support cells. The neurones are divided into three functional groups namely photoreceptor cells (rod cells and cone cells), the cells of afferent fibres passing in the optic nerve and a group of neurones interposed between the first two types which integrate sensory input from the photoreceptors before transmission to the cerebral cortex. The integrating neurones are further subdivided into three basic types, *bipolar cells*, *horizontal cells* and *amacrine cells*.

Histologically, the retina is traditionally divided into 10 distinct histological layers as shown in the micrograph, the distribution of the different cell types being illustrated in a highly schematic manner in the diagram.

The outermost layer (1) consists of the *pigmented epithelial cells* forming a single layer resting on Bruch's membrane which separates them from the choroid superficially. *Rod and cone processes* of the photoreceptor cells comprise the next layer (2) with a thin eosinophilic structure known as the *outer limiting membrane* (3) separating them from a layer of densely packed nuclei described as the *outer nuclear layer* (4). The outer nuclear layer contains the cell bodies of the rod and cone photoreceptors. The almost featureless layer deep to this is known as the *outer plexiform layer* (5) and contains synaptic connections between the short axons of the photoreceptor cells and integrating neurones, the cell bodies of which lie in the *inner nuclear layer* (6). In the *inner plexiform layer* (7), the integrating neurones make synaptic

connections with dendrites of neurones whose axons form the optic tract. The cell bodies of the optic tract neurones (sometimes called *ganglion cells*) comprise the *ganglion cell layer* (8). Deep to this is the layer of *afferent fibres* (9) passing towards the optic disc to form the optic nerve. Finally, the *inner limiting membrane* (10) demarcates the innermost aspect of the retina from the *vitreous body* **VB**. Note in the diagram that only bipolar cells are represented in the integrating cell layer; this layer also contains the cell bodies of the horizontal and amacrine cells as illustrated in Figure 21.8.

Towards the left of the diagram is represented an extremely elongated support cell extending between inner and outer limiting membranes and with its nucleus in the same layer as the integrating neurones. These cells, known as *Muller cells*, are analogous to the neuroglia of the CNS and have long cytoplasmic processes which embrace and sometimes even encircle the retinal neurones filling all the intervening spaces. Muller cells provide structural support and may also mediate the transfer of essential metabolites such as glucose to the retinal neurones.

The outer limiting membrane is not a true membrane but merely represents the line of intercellular junctions between Muller cells and the photoreceptor cells (shown diagrammatically in Fig. 21.7). In contrast, the inner limiting membrane represents the basement membrane of the Muller cells resting on the vitreous body.

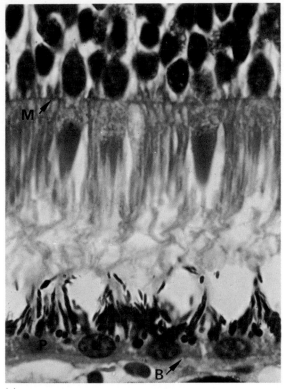

(a)

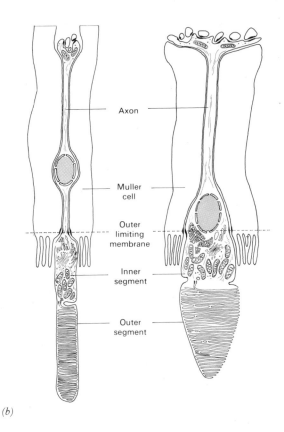

(b)

Fig. 21.7 Retinal photoreceptors

(a) H & E × 1200 (b) Schematic diagram

The rod and cone photoreceptor layer of the retina is shown at very high magnification in this micrograph, the cell bodies of the rod and cone cells lying deep to the outer limiting membrane **M**. Peripherally, the rods and cones mingle with long microvilli extending from the pigment epithelial cells **P**.

As shown in the diagram, the rod photoreceptors are long slender bipolar cells, the single dendrite of each cell extending beyond the outer limiting membrane as the rod proper. The rod proper consists of *inner* and *outer segments* connected by a thin eccentric strand of cytoplasm containing nine microtubule doublets similar to those of a cilium but without the inner pair of microtubules. The inner segment contains a prominent Golgi apparatus and many mitochondria. The outer segment has a regular cylindrical shape and contains a stack of flattened membranous discs which incorporate the pigment *rhodopsin* (visual purple). The membranous discs are continuously shed from the end of each rod and phagocytised by the pigmented epithelial cells, the discs being continuously replaced from the inner segment. In essence, the transduction process involves the interaction of light with rhodopsin molecules which promotes a configurational change within the membrane, thus initiating an action potential. The action potential then passes inwards along the dendrite and axon to the layer of integrating neurones.

Cones are similar in basic structure to the rods but they differ in several details. The outer segment of the cone is a long conical structure about two-thirds the length of a rod and containing a similar number of even more flattened membranous discs. Unlike the situation in the rods however, the disc membrane is continuous with the plasma membrane

so that, on one side, the spaces between the discs are continuous with the extracellular environment (see diagram). The discs are not shed although the tips of the cones are invested by processes of pigmented epithelial cells. The cones contain pigments similar to rhodopsin, receptive to blue, green and red light, and the mechanism of transduction is probably similar. The bodies of the cone cells are generally continuous with the inner segment of the cone proper without an intervening dendritic process and the nuclei of cone cells thus form a row of nuclei immediately deep to the outer limiting membrane.

As seen in the micrograph, the pigmented epithelial cells are cuboidal in shape with the nuclei located basally towards Bruch's membrane **B**. Apically, the cells are crammed with melanin granules, numerous mitochondria and lipofuscin, a residual product of phagocytosis (see Fig. 1.3). The pigment cell microvilli which are from 5–7 μm long, extend between the photoreceptors and, with electron microscopy, are seen to contain membranous lamellae similar to those in the rod outer segments; these appear to disintegrate as they pass deeper into the pigment cells. In addition to phagocytosis, the pigment epithelial cells provide structural and metabolic support for the rods and cones and in addition absorb light thus preventing back reflection.

During histological preparation, the retina frequently becomes detached from the wall of the eye and the plane of cleavage is usually between the rods and cones and the layer of pigmented epithelial cells corresponding to the cavity of the embryonic optic vesicle. This is also the plane along which the retina cleaves in the living eye in the pathological condition known as *retinal detachment*.

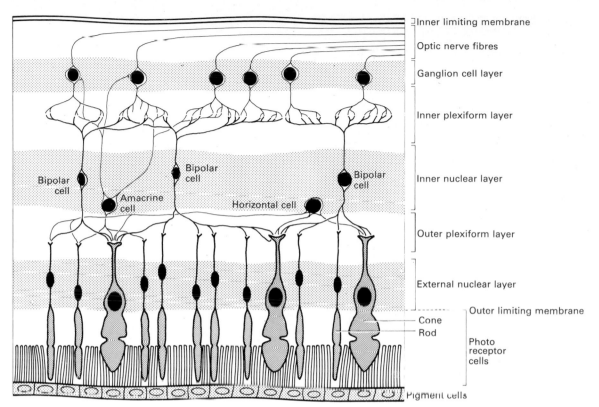

Inner limiting membrane

Optic nerve fibres

Ganglion cell layer

Inner plexiform layer

Inner nuclear layer

Outer plexiform layer

External nuclear layer

Outer limiting membrane

Cone
Rod

Photo receptor cells

Pigment cells

Bipolar cell

Bipolar cell

Bipolar cell

Amacrine cell

Horizontal cell

Fig. 21.8 Neuronal interconnections in the retina

This diagram demonstrates the basic pattern of neuronal interconnections between the photoreceptor cells and the afferent neurones of the optic tract. The interneurones consist of three basic cell types, bipolar cells, horizontal cells and amacrine cells, their cell bodies all being located in the inner nuclear layer (along with those of the supporting Muller cells).

Bipolar cells, the most numerous of the integrating neurones, in general make direct connections between one or more photoreceptors and one or more optic tract neurones. Horizontal cells have several short processes and one long process, the terminal branches of each making lateral connections between adjacent and more distant rods and cones in the outer plexiform layer. The amacrine cells have one or two short dendritic trunks giving rise to numerous branches which make connections with bipolar and optic tract neurones in the inner plexiform layer as well as making occasional feedback connections with photoreceptors in the outer plexiform layer.

As seen in the Figure 21.7 (b) opposite, the axons of the rod photoreceptors terminate in spherical processes into which are invaginated their small number of synaptic connections. In contrast, the cone photoreceptors have a flattened pedicle which accommodates hundreds of intercellular contacts.

In all, there are more than 100 million rods and 6 million cones. The cones are particularly dense in the macula and the immediately surrounding area and, in the fovea itself, the photoreceptors are almost exclusively cones. The density of both rods and cones diminishes towards the retinal periphery. The foveal cones have an almost one to one relationship with the optic tract neurones giving maximal visual discrimination. There are only about 1 million optic tract neurones and the more peripheral the photoreceptors, the larger is their ratio to the optic tract neurones. This is consistent with the main function of the more peripheral receptors (predominantly rods) which is for determination of light and dark rather than fine two-point discrimination.

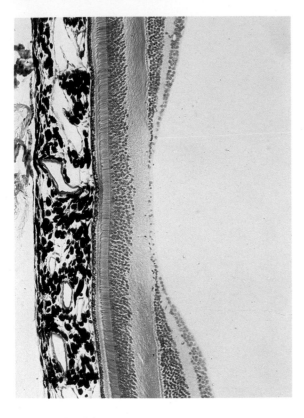

Fig. 21.9 Fovea

(Masson's trichrome × 320)

The fovea is a conical depression in the retina corresponding to the point where the visual axis of the cornea and lens meets the retina and lying about 4 mm lateral and slightly inferior to the exit of the optic nerve fibres via the optic disc. Consequently, the fovea is the area subject to the least refractory distortion. To complement this, the foveal retina is modified to obtain the maximum photoreceptor sensitivity and is thus the area of the retina with the greatest visual discrimination; however, its function is poor in conditions of low light intensity. Surrounding the fovea is an ovoid yellow area about 1 mm wide called the *macula lutea*.

As seen in this micrograph, at the fovea the inner layers of the retina are flattened laterally so as to present the least barrier to light reaching the photoreceptors. Retinal blood vessels are absent at the fovea, as can be readily seen with the ophthalmoscope, and the brownish colour of the choroidal melanin shows through the much attenuated retina. At the fovea, the photoreceptors are almost exclusively cones which are elongated and closely packed (approximately 100 000 cones are contained in the fovea). Neuronal interconnections in the bipolar cell layer provide for a one-to-one ratio of these cones to optic nerve fibres which means that each foveal photoreceptor is individually represented at the visual cortex.

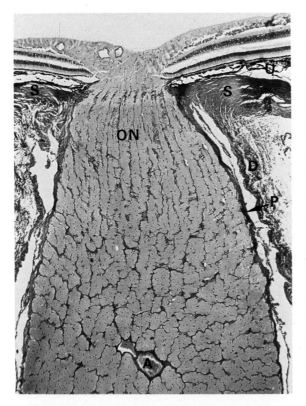

Fig. 21.10 Optic nerve

(Haematoxylin/van Gieson × 30)

The afferent fibres from the retina converge at a point medial to the fovea, the optic papilla or optic disc, fibres from the lateral quadrants sweeping above and below the macula to avoid the fovea. The fibres then penetrate the sclera **S** through the lamina cribrosa to form the optic nerve **ON**. Note the thickness of the optic tract layer overlying the disc and the absence of photoreceptor cells from the optic papilla which is thus a blind spot on the retina.

In their course across the retina, the afferent fibres are not myelinated as this would obstruct light passing to the photoreceptors. Myelination commences at the optic disc which imparts the white colour seen with the ophthalmoscope.

The optic nerve and retina develop embryologically as an outgrowth of the primitive forebrain, thus the optic nerve is invested by meninges. The dura mater **D** becomes continuous with its developmental equivalent, the sclera, while the pia-arachnoid **P** continues into the eye as the uveal tract **U**.

The main blood supply of the retina is provided by the central artery of the retina **A**, a branch of the ophthalmic artery. This divides at the optic disc into four branches supplying the quadrants of the retina. These vessels course within the optic fibre layer breaking up into a rich capillary network which drains back into a venous system closely following the course of the arterial supply. The vessels are confined to the optic tract layer and more superficial layers are dependent on diffusion, the most peripheral retinal layers also being supplied likewise from the choroid.

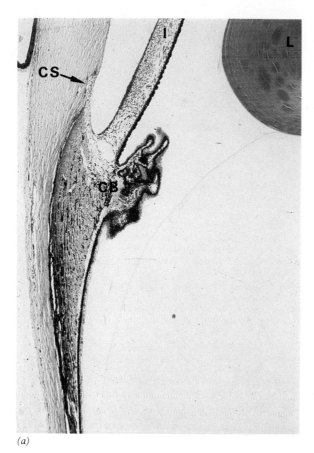

(a)

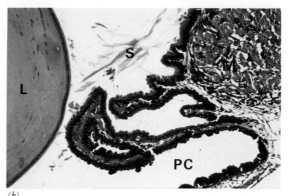

(b)

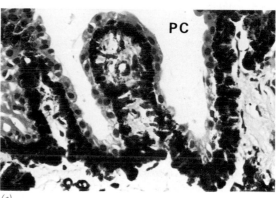

(c)

Fig. 21.11 Ciliary body

(H & E (a) × 30 (b) × 128 (c) × 320)

The ciliary body is a circumferential structure which bulges into the eye between the ora serrata and the limbus (see Fig. 21.3). As seen in micrograph (a), the ciliary body **CB** represents the forward continuation of the choroid layer **C** (uveal tract) of the posterior five-sixths of the wall of the eye and, like it, it is highly vascular and contains a considerable amount of melanin pigment. Anteriorly, it is continuous with the third component of the uveal tract, the iris **I**, passing in front of the lens **L**.

As can be seen in each of these micrographs, the ciliary body is lined with a double layer of cuboidal epithelium. The deep layer is highly pigmented and represents a forward continuation of the pigmented epithelial layer of the retina whilst the surface layer, which is not pigmented, is a non-photosensitive forward extension of the receptor layer of the retina.

The ciliary body is attached to the coronal equator of the lens **L** by the suspensory ligament which consists of extremely fine collagenous strands which seldom remain intact after histological preparation; a few aggregated shreds of the suspensory ligament **S** are seen in micrograph (b). Tension in the suspensory ligament tends to flatten the lens which, in the relaxed state, assumes a more globular shape. The bulk of the ciliary body consists of smooth muscle **M** arranged in such a manner that, when it contracts, tension

upon the suspensory ligament is reduced thus permitting the lens to assume a more convex shape. This mechanism permits fine focusing of images already roughly focused upon the retina by the cornea. The ciliary muscle is innervated by parasympathetic nerve fibres.

From that part of the ciliary body exposed to the angle of the posterior chamber **PC**, there project a number of branching epithelial folds called *ciliary processes* containing a connective tissue core rich in fenestrated capillaries. The ciliary processes are responsible for the continuous production of aqueous humor which then circulates into the anterior chamber via the pupil. Aqueous humor is continuously reabsorbed into the canal of Schlemm **CS** seen at the angle of the anterior chamber in micrograph (a).

Aqueous humor is a clear, watery fluid somewhat similar in composition to CSF and hypotonic with respect to plasma. The production of aqueous humor is presumed to be an active process mediated by the two epithelial layers lining the ciliary processes. Balanced rates of secretion and reabsorption of aqueous humor result in the maintenance of a constant intra-ocular pressure of about 15 mm of mercury which stabilises the lens and cornea. The flow of aqueous humor also provides for a continuous exchange of metabolites with the cells of the avascular cornea and lens.

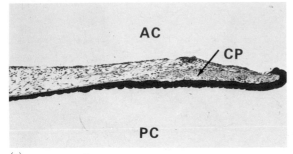

(a)

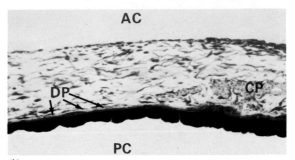

(b)

Fig. 21.12 Iris

(H & E (a) × 20 (b) × 80)

The iris is the most anterior part of the uveal layer of the eye. It arises from the ciliary body and forms a diaphragm in front of the lens so dividing the anterior compartment of the eye into posterior **PC** and anterior chambers **AC** which communicate via the pupil. The pupillary edge of the iris rests on the anterior edge of the lens in life.

The main mass of the iris consists of loose, highly vascular connective tissue which is pigmented due to the presence of numerous melanocytes scattered in the stroma. The anterior surface of the iris is irregular and consists of a discontinuous layer of fibroblasts and melanocytes; in the fetus the surface is lined by endothelial cells but these become absent during early childhood. In contrast, the posterior surface is relatively smooth and is lined by epithelium which is derived embryologically as a continuation of the two layers which line the surface of the ciliary body. The surface layer, nonpigmented in the ciliary body, becomes heavily pigmented in the iris such that the individual cells are completely obscured. The deep layer, pigmented in the ciliary body, is transformed in the iris into lightly pigmented myoepithelial cells which constitute the radially orientated *dilator pupillae* **DP** muscle of the iris. Even at high magnification, these myoepithelial cells are difficult to distinguish.

The *constrictor muscle of the pupil (constrictor pupillae)* **CP** consists of a band of circumferentially oriented smooth muscle fibres in the pupillary aspect of the stroma. Like the smooth muscle of the ciliary body, the constrictor pupillae is innervated by the parasympathetic nervous system whereas the myoepithelial cells of the dilator pupillae are innervated by the sympathetic nervous system.

The colour of the iris depends on the amount of pigment in the connective tissue stroma, the amount of pigment in the posterior epithelial layer being relatively constant between individuals. Blue eyes contain little stromal pigment whereas brown eyes have much stromal pigment.

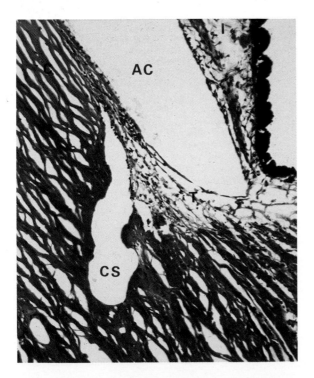

Fig. 21.13 Canal of Schlemm

(H & E × 75)

The canal of Schlemm **CS** is a circumferential canal lined by endothelium which is situated in the inner aspect of the corneal margin **C** immediately adjacent to the angle of the anterior chamber **AC**. At the angle of the anterior chamber there is a meshwork of fine connective tissue trabeculae **T** lined by endothelium; aqueous humor percolates through the spaces between the trabeculae before reaching the canal of Schlemm. There is no direct communication between the trabecular spaces and the canal of Schlemm thus reabsorption of aqueous humor involves passage across two layers of endothelium and intervening connective tissue. The mechanism of transport is not understood; disruption of this process leads to increased intraocular pressure as in the disease known as *glaucoma*. The canal of Schlemm drains via minute channels through the sclera into the episcleral venous system, a pressure gradient being maintained to prevent reflux of blood. Note the close relationship of the root of the iris **I** with the canal of Schlemm.

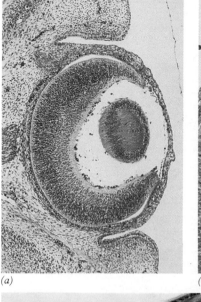

(a)

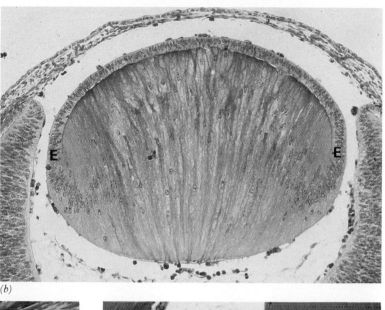

(b)

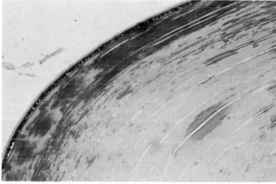

(c)

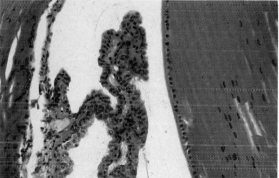

(d)

Fig. 21.14 The lens and its development

(H & E (a) × 64 (b) × 150 (c) × 50 (d) × 50)

The lens is an elastic biconvex structure which, although transparent and apparently amorphous, is almost entirely composed of living cells. The lens cells are highly modified epithelial cells derived embryologically from ectoderm which forms a depression, the *lens pit*, overlying the embryonic optic vesicle.

With further development, the lens pit becomes deeper, its margins fusing to form the *lens vesicle* which becomes detached from the surface and sinks deeper to become enveloped by the growing optic vesicle; at this stage the lens vesicle merely consists of a single layer of epithelial cells.

The posterior cells of the lens vesicle now become greatly elongated antero-posteriorly filling the central cavity of the vesicle as seen in micrograph (a). The lens cells in the central antero-posterior axis then undergo maturation as seen in micrograph (b) losing their nuclei to become known as *lens fibres*. Proliferation of the cells at the lens equator **E** adds further fibres to the central mass, the growth process continuing at a slow rate even into old age.

When fully developed, the lens substance consists of two to three thousand anucleate fibres, each stretching between anterior and posterior poles of the lens. The fibres have the shape of extremely elongated, six-sided prisms, the more peripheral fibres curving to follow the antero-posterior surface contour of the lens. The fibres contain a crystalline protein and the cell membranes of adjacent fibres are fused, leaving little intervening extracellular substance.

The anterior surface is covered by a single layer of cuboidal cells which retain their nuclei, this layer merging with the residual proliferative cells at the equatorial margin of the lens. The whole lens is enveloped by a thick epithelial basement membrane forming the *lens capsule* which is connected via the suspensory ligament to the ciliary body.

Micrograph (c) shows part of a mature lens including the anterior cuboidal epithelium and lens capsule. The cellular nature of the lens substance is not readily apparent and the lens substance is particularly prone to artefactual distortion during histological preparation. Micrograph (d) shows the equatorial region of the lens and nearby ciliary processes. Note the anterior epithelial layer and the presence of nuclei in the more recently formed peripheral fibres.

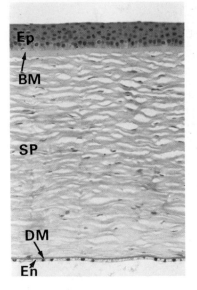

Fig. 21.15 Cornea

(H & E × 80)

The cornea is the thick, transparent portion of the corneo-scleral layer enclosing the anterior one-sixth of the eye. The relatively fixed convexity of the external surface provides the principal mechanism for focusing images upon the retina.

The cornea is an avascular structure consisting of five layers. The outer surface is lined by stratified squamous epithelium **Ep** about five cells thick which is not normally keratinised. This epithelium is supported by a specialised basement membrane known as *Bowman's membrane* **BM** which is particularly prominent in man. The bulk of the cornea, the *substantia propria* **SP**, consists of a highly regular form of dense collagenous connective tissue forming thin lamellae. Fibroblasts and occasional leucocytes are scattered in the ground substance between the lamellae. The inner surface of the cornea is lined by a layer of flattened endothelial cells **En** which are supported by a very thick elastic basement membrane known as *Descemet's membrane* **DM**.

The cornea is sustained by diffusion of metabolites from the aqueous humor and the blood vessels of the limbus; some oxygen is derived directly from the external environment.

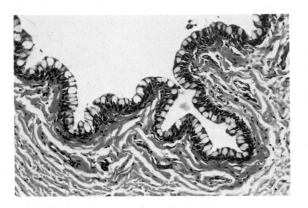

Fig. 21.16 Conjunctiva

(Haematoxylin/van Gieson × 128)

The conjunctiva is the epithelium which covers the exposed part of the sclera and inner surface of the eyelids. It is stratified columnar in form and for a stratified epithelium is unusual in that it contains goblet cells in the surface layers. The conjunctival mucous secretions contribute to the protective layer on the exposed surface of the eye.

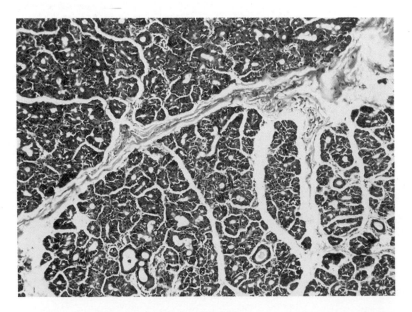

Fig. 21.17 Lacrimal gland

(H & E × 150)

The lacrimal gland is responsible for the secretion of tears, a watery fluid containing the antibacterial enzyme *lysozyme* and electrolytes of similar concentration to that of plasma.

Histologically, the lacrimal glands are similar to the salivary glands in lobular structure and compound tubulo-acinar form of the secretory units. The secretory cells have the typical appearance of serous (protein-secreting) cells with basally located nuclei and strongly stained granular cytoplasm.

Each gland drains via a dozen or more small ducts into the superior fornix. Tears drain to the inner aspect of the eye and then into the nasal cavity via the nasolacrimal duct.

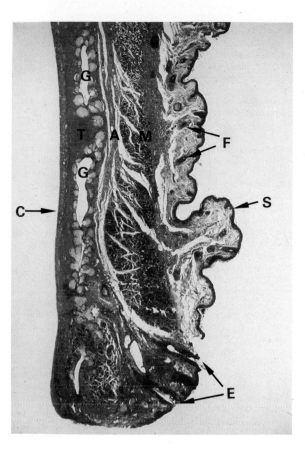

Fig. 21.18 Eyelid
(H & E × 16)

Each eyelid consists of a dense fibro-elastic plate, the *tarsus* **T**, covered externally by thin, highly-folded skin **S** and on the internal aspect by smooth conjunctiva **C**. The skin contains scattered fine hair follicles **F** and the underlying connective tissue is extremely loose and devoid of fat.

Skeletal muscle **M** of orbicularis oculi (and levator palpebrae in the upper eyelids) lies immediately superficial to the tarsal plate and is separated from it by a layer of connective tissue **A** which, in the upper lid, represents a forward continuation of the sub-aponeurotic layer of the scalp. The clinical importance of this is that blood or inflammatory exudates collecting above the scalp aponeurosis may track forward into the superficial planes of the eyelid; being extremely lax, this area may become markedly swollen. The connective tissue layer also contains the sensory nerves of the eyelid.

Within the tarsal plate lie some 12–30 *tarsal (Meibomian) glands* **G** oriented vertically and opening at the free margin of the eyelid via minute foramina. These glands are modified sebaceous glands each consisting of a long central duct into which open numerous sebaceous acini. In addition, associated with the eyelashes **E** are sebaceous glands known as the *glands of Zeis* and modified apocrine sweat glands known as the *glands of Moll*. Together, the glands of the eyelid produce an oily layer which is thought to cover the tear layer thereby preventing evaporation of the tears.

The ear

The ear or vestibulo-cochlear apparatus provides for the dual sensory functions of maintenance of equilibrium and hearing (stato-acoustic system).

Structurally the system may be divided into three parts, the *external ear*, the *middle ear* and the *internal ear*. The specific sensory receptors for both movement and sound are situated in a membranous structure located in the internal ear while the external and middle ear are concerned with reception, transmission and amplification of incoming sound waves.

Fig. 21.19 The ear *(illustration opposite)*

The main structural elements of the vestibulo-cochlear apparatus are illustrated in this diagram.

1. External ear: the external ear is responsible for reception of sound waves which are funnelled onto the ear drum (*tympanic membrane*). It consists of the *auricle (pinna)*, a modified horn-shaped structure composed of elastic cartilage covered by skin, which converges onto the *external auditory meatus (canal)*. Elastic cartilage also forms the walls of the outer third of the canal whilst the inner two-thirds of the canal lie in the petrous part of the temporal bone. The canal is lined by hairy skin containing sebaceous glands and modified apocrine sweat glands which secrete a waxy material called *cerumen*.

2. Middle ear: The middle ear, located in a cavity in the petrous temporal bone, is separated from the external auditory meatus by the tympanic membrane. Sound waves impinging on the tympanic membrane are converted into mechanical vibrations which are then amplified by a system of levers made up of three small bones (*ossicles*), the *malleus*, *incus* and *stapes*, and transmitted across the air-filled middle ear to the fluid-filled inner ear cavity. The ossicles articulate with one another via synovial joints and the malleus and incus pivot on tiny ligaments which are attached to the wall of the middle ear cavity. Small slips of muscle, the *tensor tympani* and *stapedius* pass to the mid point of the tympanic membrane and *stapes* bone respectively and damp down excessive vibrations which might otherwise damage the delicate auditory apparatus. The middle ear cavity communicates anteriorly with the nasopharynx via the *auditory (Eustachian) tube* which permits equalisation of pressure changes with the external environment. Posteriorly, the middle ear cavity communicates with numerous interconnected air spaces which lighten the mass of the mastoid part of the bone. The whole of the middle ear and mastoid cavities are lined by simple squamous or cuboidal epithelium.

3. Internal ear: The internal ear consists of an interconnected fluid-filled *membranous labyrinth* lying within a labyrinth of spaces of complementary shape in the temporal bone (the *osseous labyrinth*). The membranous labyrinth is bound down to the walls of the osseous labyrinth in various places but in the main is separated from the bony walls by a fluid-filled space. The fluid within the membranous labyrinth is known as *endolymph* and the fluid in the surrounding peri-membranous space is known as *perilymph*. The peri-membranous space is directly connected with the subarachnoid space and, like the latter, is crossed by delicate fibrous strands and lined by flattened squamous epithelium; the perilymphatic fluid is thus similar in composition to CSF. In contrast, the membranous labyrinth is a closed system but an extension of it, the *endolymphatic duct*, connects with a sac, the *endolymphatic sac*, lying in the subdural space of the underlying brain. The membranous labyrinth is lined by a simple epithelium except in the endolymphatic sac where the cells are columnar with morphological features suggesting that this is the site of endolymph absorption.

The osseous labyrinth may be divided into three main areas:

(a) The vestibule. The central space of the osseous labyrinth is called the *vestibule*; it gives rise to three *semi-circular canals* posteriorly, and the *cochlear* anteriorly. The vestibule contains two components of the membranous labyrinth namely the *utricle* and the *saccule*, which are connected by a short, Y-shaped duct from which arises the endolymphatic duct. The walls of the utricle and saccule each contain a specialised area of sensory receptor cells known as a *macula* (see Fig. 21.27) from which axons pass into the *vestibular nerve* as part of the sensory input for the sense of equilibrium. Laterally, the vestibule is separated from the middle ear cavity by a thin bony plate containing two fenestrations, one oval and the other round in shape. The *oval window* is occluded by the base of the stirrup-shaped stapes bone and its surrounding *annular ligament* whereby vibrations are transmitted to the perilymph from the tympanic membrane via the ossicle chain. The *round window* is closed by a membrane similar to the tympanic membrane and it is thus sometimes described as the *secondary tympanic membrane*. This membrane permits vibrations which have passed to sensory receptors for sound to be dissipated (see later).

(b) The semi-circular canals. Three semicircular canals arise from the posterior aspect of the vestibule, two being disposed in vertical planes at right angles to one another and the other in a near horizontal plane. Within each semicircular canal, is a semicircular membranous duct filled with endolymph and continuous at both ends with the utricle; near one end of each semi-circular membranous duct is a dilated area called the *ampulla*. In each ampulla, there is a ridge called the *crista ampullaris* (see Fig. 21.8) containing sensory receptors with axons converging on the vestibular nerve. Together with the receptors of the maculae of the utricle and saccule, these receptors form the sensory afferents for the function of balance and equilibrium.

(c) The cochlear. The cochlear occupies a conical, spiral-shaped space in the temporal bone extending from the anterior aspect of the vestibule; the space is roughly similar in shape to that inside the shell of a cone-shaped snail or shellfish. The membranous component of the cochlear arises from the saccule and spirals upwards with its blind end attached at the apex of the osseous space. The membranous canal is triangular in cross-section and attached to the bony walls of the cochlear in such a manner as to divide the osseous space into three spiral compartments (see Fig. 21.24). The middle compartment, the *scala media*, contains endolymph and the upper and lower compartments contain perilymph. At the base of the cochlear, the upper perilymph compartment is directly continuous with the perilymph of the vestibule and thus via this space, called the *scala vestibuli*, vibrations pass through the perilymph towards the apex of the cochlear. At the apex, the scala vestibuli becomes continuous with the lower perilymphatic space of the cochlear spiral via a minute hole called the *helicotrema*. This lower space terminates at the secondary tympanic membrane covering the round window and 'spent' vibrations are thus dissipated; the lower perilymphatic space is therefore known as the *scala tympani*. The sensory receptors for sound are located in a spiral-shaped structure known as the *organ of Corti* shown in detail in Figure 21.25.

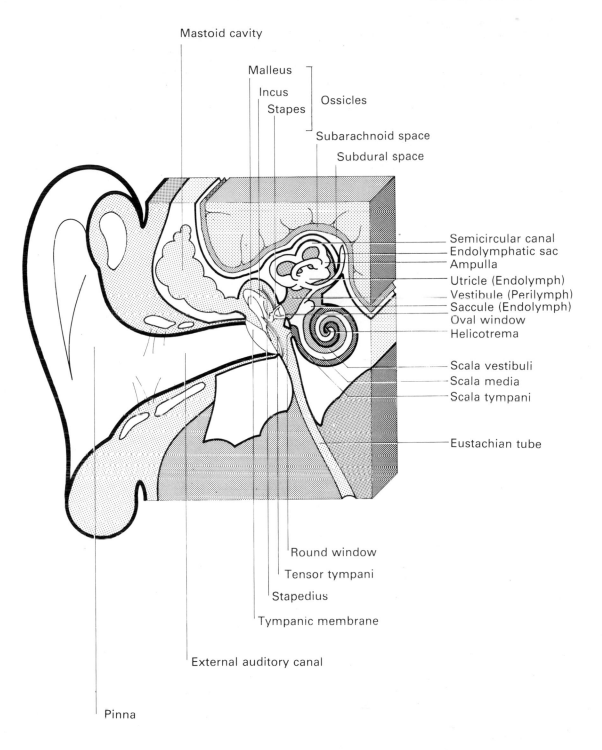

Mastoid cavity

Malleus

Incus

Stapes

Ossicles

Subarachnoid space

Subdural space

Semicircular canal
Endolymphatic sac
Ampulla
Utricle (Endolymph)
Vestibule (Perilymph)
Saccule (Endolymph)
Oval window
Helicotrema

Scala vestibuli
Scala media
Scala tympani

Eustachian tube

Round window

Tensor tympani

Stapedius

Tympanic membrane

External auditory canal

Pinna

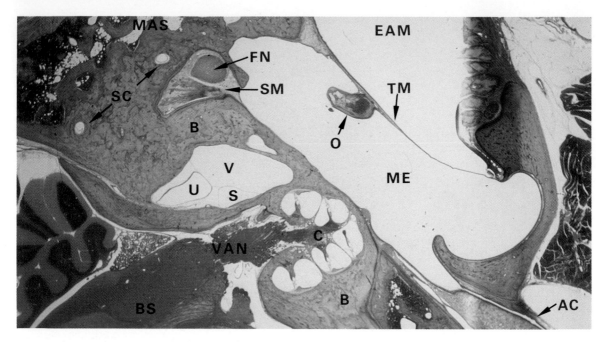

Fig. 21.20 The ear

(H & E × 8)

This micrograph shows a horizontal section through the vestibulo-cochlear apparatus which lies within the temporal bone **B**. The tympanic membrane **TM** can be seen stretched between the tympanic plate of the temporal bone anteriorly and the lateral part of the petrous temporal bone posteriorly, dividing the external auditory meatus **EAM** from the cavity of the middle ear **ME**. Part of one of the ossicles **O**, the handle of the malleus, can be seen attached to the inner aspect of the tympanic membrane. From the anterior aspect of the middle ear chamber, the auditory canal **AC** (Eustachian canal) passes forwards towards the nasopharynx and in the mastoid part of the temporal bone there are numerous irregular mastoid air spaces **MAS**.

Near the centre of the field is the vestibule of the inner ear **V** containing two delicate membranous structures, the utricle **U** and saccule **S** more anteriorly. Two of the semicircular canals **SC** can be identified deep in the posterior part of the petrous temporal bone. Immediately posterior to the middle ear cavity, the facial nerve **FN** is seen in transverse section as it passes inferiorly, and just medial to it lies the stapedius muscle **SM**.

Anterior to the vestibule, the conical spiral of the cochlear **C** has been cut in longitudinal section through its central bony axis. From the base of the cochlear, the vestibulo-auditory nerve **VAN** passes towards the brain stem **BS**, behind which the cerebellum is easily recognisable.

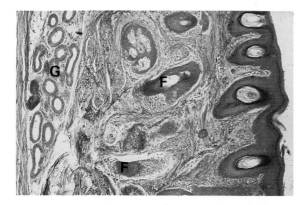

Fig. 21.21 External auditory meatus

(H & E × 100)

The external auditory meatus is the canal leading from the auricle to the tympanic membrane. The wall of the outer third is formed by elastic cartilage whereas the inner two-thirds is formed by the temporal bone. The canal is lined by skin which is devoid of the usual dermal papillae and closely bound down to the underlying cartilage or bone by a dense collagenous dermis. The skin of the outer third (as shown here) has fine hairs and the dermis contains numerous coiled tubular *ceruminous glands* **G** which secrete wax (cerumen) and which represent specialised apocrine sweat glands (see Fig. 9.13). The ceruminous glands open directly onto the surface or into the sebaceous glands associated with hair follicles **F**. The meatal hairs provide protection from foreign bodies whilst the cerumen protects the skin of the external meatus from moisture and infection.

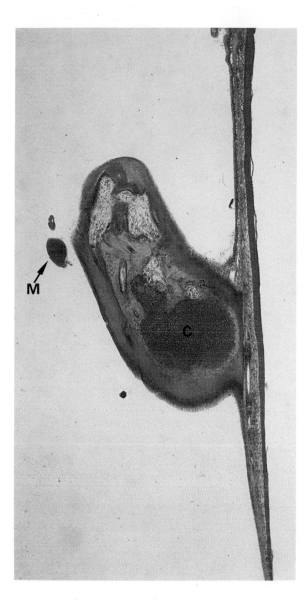

Fig. 21.22 Tympanic membrane and ossicle

(H & E × 20)

The tympanic membrane or ear drum is a thin fibrous membrane separating the external auditory canal from the cavity of the middle ear. With the exception of a small triangular area superiorly, the *pars flaccida*, the membrane is tense (*pars tensa*), being firmly attached to the surrounding bone by a fibrocartilaginous ring. The handle of the malleus is attached to the centre of the membrane, the chain of ossicles pulling the membrane slightly inwards.

The tympanic membrane is made up of three layers, an external *cuticular layer*, an intermediate *fibrous layer* and an inner *mucous layer*. The cuticular layer consists of thin, hairless skin, the epidermis being only about 10 cells thick and the basal layer being flat and devoid of the usual epidermal ridges. The thin dermis contains plump fibroblasts and a fine vascular network.

The intermediate fibrous layer consists of an outer layer of fibres radiating from the centre of the membrane towards the circumference and an inner layer of fibres disposed circumferentially at the periphery. These fibres have long been assumed to be collagen associated with a fine meshwork of elastin; however, recent evidence suggests that the fibres are of a unique composition especially adapted for the function of the membrane.

The inner mucous layer represents a continuation of the modified respiratory-type mucous membrane lining the middle ear cavity but in this situation it is merely a single layer of cuboidal cells devoid of cilia and goblet cells. The underlying lamina propria is thin with a blood supply separate from that of the dermis of the cuticular layer. A similar modified respiratory type mucosa invests the ossicles, small muscles and nerves exposed to the middle ear cavity.

The ossicles consist of compact bone formed by endochondral ossification which accounts for the cartilage **C** seen in this specimen from a kitten. Note also the tensor tympani muscle **M**.

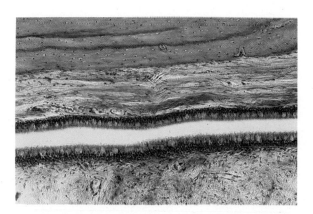

Fig. 21.23 Auditory (Eustachian) canal

(H & E × 320)

The auditory canal connects the cavity of the middle ear with the nasopharynx and allows for equalisation of air pressure between the middle ear and the external environment. From the middle ear, the tube first passes through bone but towards the pharynx; the wall is supported on two sides by cartilage and on the remaining two sides by fibrous tissue.

The tube is lined by typical pseudostratified respiratory epithelium with numerous goblet cells particularly towards the pharyngeal end. The salpingo-pharyngeus and tensor and levator veli palati muscles are connected to the fibrocartilaginous part of the tube causing it to dilate during swallowing.

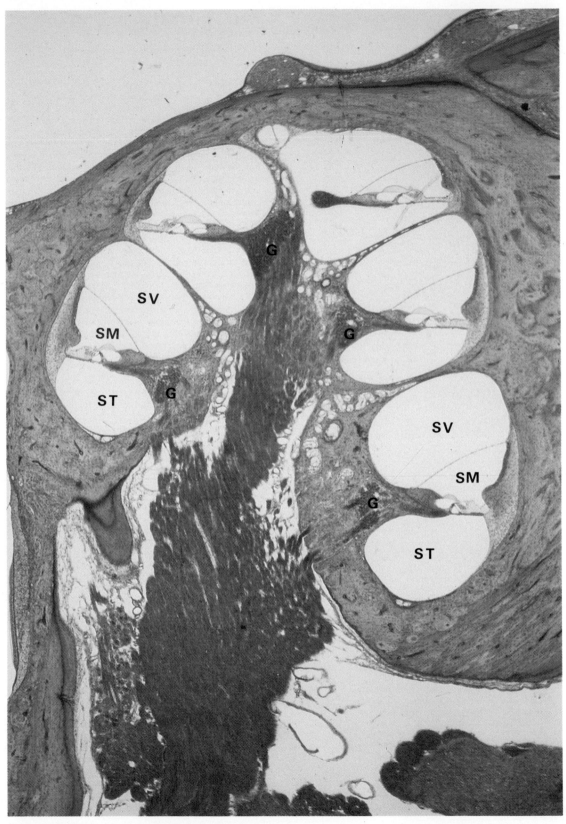

(a)

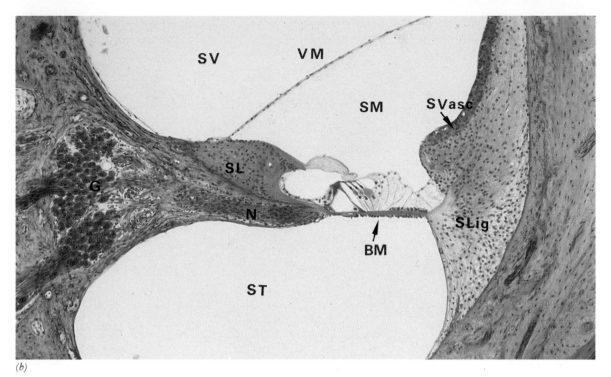

(b)

Fig. 21.24 Cochlear *(illustration (a) opposite)*

(H & E (a) × 20 (b) × 96)

The cochlear is the component of the internal ear which contains the auditory sensory organ. The conical, spiral-shaped form of the cochlear can be visualised in micrograph (a) which shows a cochlear cut in a plane of section which includes its long bony axis. Note that the cavity in the petrous temporal bone is reminiscent of the space inside a conical snail shell. The cochlear has two-and-a-half full turns and in this section therefore, five separate cross sections of the cochlear can be seen, each turn of the spiral being separated from the next by a spicule of bone. A corkscrew-like bony structure, the *modiolus*, forms the central axis of the cochlear.

Each turn of the cochlear canal can be seen to be divided into three compartments as shown in micrograph (b). The central compartment, the scala media **SM**, is roughly triangular in cross section, with the apex attached to a spicule of bone spiralling outwards from the modiolus and known as the *osseous spiral lamina*. Above the free edge of the osseous spiral lamina is a thickened mass of connective tissue known as the *spiral limbus* **SL**. The base of the scala media is thickened and attached to the outer wall of the cochlear. The membrane making up the walls of the scala media represents that part of the membranous labyrinth extending up into the cochlear from the saccule, and the scala media is thus filled with endolymph.

Above the scala media is the scala vestibuli **SV** originating in the vestibule near the oval window and base of stapes; vibrations are conducted towards the apex of the cochlear in the perilymph of the scala vestibuli. Below the scala media is the perilymphatic space which spirals down from the apex to the secondary tympanic membrane, the scala tympani **ST**.

The membrane separating the scala media and the scala tympani known as the *basilar membrane* **BM** supports the organ of Corti, which contains the auditory receptor cells; the organ of Corti is described in detail in Figure 21.25. The cells of the organ of Corti are derived from the simple epithelium lining the membranous labyrinth which embryologically is of ectodermal origin. The basilar membrane is composed of fibrous connective tissue. Axially, it is attached to the osseous spiral lamina and laterally to the *spiral ligament* **SLig** which consists of a marked thickening of the endosteum of the lateral wall of the cochlear canal. The thickened outer wall of the scala media is highly vascular and lined by a stratified epithelium; this area, known as the *stria vascularis* **SVasc** is responsible for maintaining the correct ionic composition of endolymph.

The membrane between the scala media and scala vestibuli, the *vestibular (or Reissner's) membrane* **VM**, is composed of extremely delicate fibrous tissue lined by simple squamous epithelium on both sides. The scala vestibuli and scala tympani are lined by a simple unspecialised squamous epithelium of mesodermal origin.

In micrograph (b) bundles of afferent nerve fibres **N** can be seen arising from the base of the organ of Corti and converging towards the *spiral ganglion* **G** in the modiolus at the base of the spiral lamina. These ganglion cells represent the cell bodies of bipolar sensory neurones, and their proximal axons form the auditory component of the 8th cranial nerve (see Fig. 21.26).

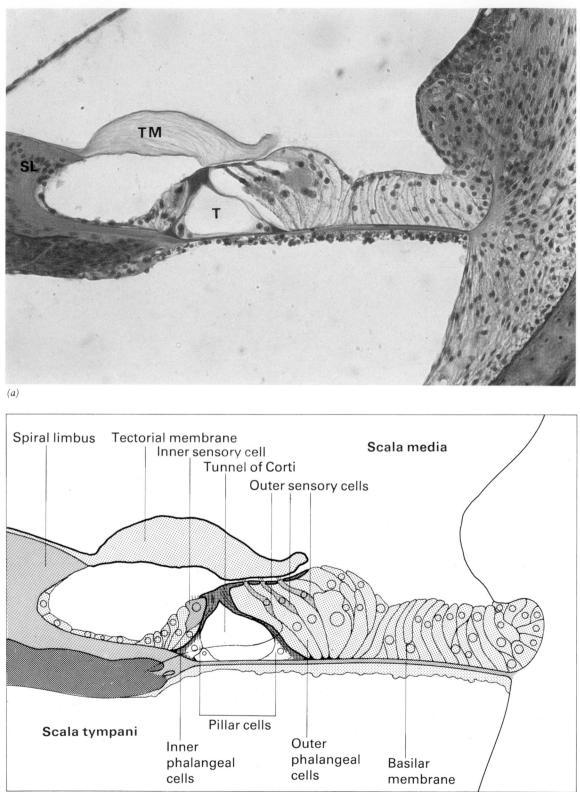

(a)

(b)

Fig. 21.25 Organ of Corti *(illustrations opposite)*

(a) H & E × 480 (b) Schematic diagram

The organ of Corti is a highly specialised epithelial structure containing receptor cells which convert (transduce) mechanical energy in the form of vibrations into electrochemical energy resulting in excitation of auditory sensory receptors.

The organ of Corti lies in the scala media supported on the basilar membrane. The basilar membrane consists of a thin sheet of fibrous connective tissue stretched between the osseous spiral lamina of the modiolus and the spiral ligament laterally; its under surface, exposed to the scala tympani, is lined by a simple epithelium. The basilar membrane is thinnest at the base of the cochlear and becomes progressively thicker as it spirals towards the apex.

The organ of Corti consists of two basic types of cells, *sensory (hair) cells* and *support cells* of several different types. At the centre of the organ is a triangular-shaped canal, the *inner tunnel* or *tunnel of Corti* **T** bounded on each side by a single row of tall columnar cells called *pillar cells*. Each pillar cell contains a dense bundle (pillar) of microtubules and the pillars on either side of the tunnel of Corti converge at the surface and then curve laterally to form a thin, hood-like structure containing small fenestrations. The cell bodies of the pillar cells lie in the acute angles formed by the pillars and the basilar membrane at the floor of the tunnel.

On the inner aspect of the inner row of pillar cells is a single row of flask-shaped cells called *inner phalangeal cells* which support a single row of *inner sensory (hair) cells*. The phalangeal cells contain microtubules, some of which

support the base of the hair cells while others extend to the free surface around the hair cells. Beyond the outer row of pillar cells there are three to five rows of *outer phalangeal cells* which support the same number of rows of *outer sensory (hair) cells*. Cytoplasmic extensions of the phalangeal cells extend to the surface between and around the hair cells and their microtubules support the fenestrated hood-like structure formed by the pillar cells. Through the fenestrations project the free ends of the sensory cells. A variety of other specialised epithelial cells provide the remaining support for the organ of Corti.

The sensory cells are known as hair cells because numerous stereocilia i.e. very long microvilli (see Fig. 5.23) project from their free ends. As previously described, the spiral ganglion of the cochlear contains bipolar cell bodies of first order sensory neurones. From here, fibres pass towards the base of the rows of hair cells, those going to the outer hair cells traversing the tunnel of Corti. The end of each fibre ramifies into a number of dendrites which make synaptic contact with several hair cells; each sensory cell may synapse with dendrites of several different sensory neurones. In addition, inhibitory neurones arising in the brain stem send fibres which also synapse with the sensory cells and exert a suppressive effect.

From the layer of *border cells* which cover the spiral limbus **SL**, there extends a flap-like mass of glycosaminoglycans called the *tectorial membrane* **TM** which overlies the sensory cells and into which the tips of the stereocilia of the sensory cells are embedded.

Function of the organ of Corti

Details of the exact physiological processes for the sense of hearing remain to be discovered. However, in brief, the mechanism is as follows. Sound waves are funnelled into the external auditory meatus and impinge on the tympanic membrane which vibrates at the appropriate frequency. These vibrations are transmitted to the stapes bone via the malleus and incus and, in the process, their amplitude is enhanced about tenfold. The base of the stapes, which lies in the oval window, conducts the vibrations into the perilymph of the vestibule of the inner ear and pressure waves pass from here into the scala vestibuli of the cochlear. These pressure waves are probably conducted directly to the endolymph of the scala media across the delicate vestibular membrane from which vibrations are induced in the basilar membrane upon which rests the organ of Corti. From here, 'spent' vibrations are transmitted into the perilymph of the secondary tympanic membrane over the round window.

The basilar membrane is thinnest at the base of the cochlear and thickest at the apex, and it appears that at

every point on the spiral, the membrane is 'tuned' to vibrate to a particular frequency of sound waves reaching the ear; the overall range of frequencies encompassed is of the order of 11 octaves with the highest frequencies (pitch) being sensed towards the base of the cochlear and progressively lower frequencies being sensed along the spiral towards the apex. For any given sound frequency, only one specific point of the basilar membrane and organ of Corti is thought to vibrate and thereby activate the receptor cells to initiate afferent sensory impulses which then pass to the auditory cortex of the brain. The process of transduction of mechanical energy into electro-chemical energy probably results from deformation of the stereocilia of the sensory cells.

The sensory input from the cochlear is integrated in the brain stem and auditory cortex from which efferent suppressor pathways can modulate receptor activity to enhance auditory acuity.

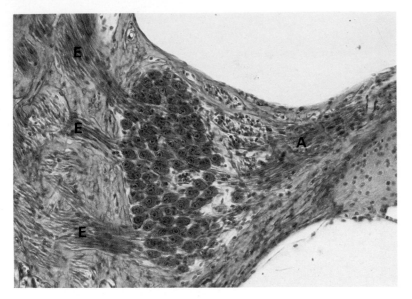

Fig. 21.26 Spiral ganglion

(H & E × 320)

The spiral ganglion is a spiral-shaped mass of nerve cell bodies lying in a canal at the extremity of the osseous spiral lamina of the modiolus.

As seen in this micrograph, the ganglion cells have the typical appearance of somatic ganglion cells (see Fig. 7.19) and represent the cell bodies of bipolar sensory neurones relaying information from the receptors of the organ of Corti to the brain.

Note the afferent fibres **A** entering the ganglion from the organ of Corti and numerous bundles of efferent fibres **E** which pass to the centre of the modiolus to form the *cochlear nerve*, the auditory component of the eighth cranial nerve; the cochlear nerve is readily seen in Figure 21.24 (a).

Fig. 21.27 Receptor organs of the saccule and utricle

(H & E (a) × 480 (b) × 600 (c) Scanning EM × 5000 (d) Schematic diagram)

The saccule and utricle are two dilated regions of the membranous labyrinth lying within the vestibule of the inner ear and filled with endolymph. The walls of each are composed of a fibrous, connective tissue membrane which is bound down in places to the periosteum of the vestibule and in other areas attached to the periosteum by fibrous strands, the intervening space being filled with perilymph. Internally, the saccule and utricle are lined by simple cuboidal epithelium but in each there is a region of highly specialised epithelium called the macula, shown in micrographs (a) and (b), containing receptor cells which contribute part of the sensory input to that part of the brain responsible for maintaining balance and equilibrium. The macula of the utricle is oriented at right angles to that of the saccule.

The maculae are made up of two basic cell types, *sensory cells* and *support cells*. The support cells are tall and columnar with basally-located nuclei and microvilli at their free surface. The receptor cells lie between the support cells with their nuclei placed more centrally. Each receptor cell has a single, eccentrically-located cilium of typical conformation (see Fig. 5.21) and many stereocilia (long microvilli) projecting from its surface giving rise to the name *hair cells*. The 'hairs' are embedded in a thick, gelatinous plaque of glycoprotein probably secreted by the supporting cells; this is lost during histological preparation. At the surface of the glycoprotein layer is a mass of crystals mainly composed of calcium carbonate and known as *otoliths*; these are shown in micrograph (c).

There are two different forms of sensory cells. The first type is bulbous in shape, stains poorly, and the nuclei tend to lie at a lower level than those of the second type which are more slender in shape. The bulbous receptor cells are invested by a meshwork of dendritic processes of afferent sensory neurones, whereas the others have only small dendritic processes at their bases. The receptor cells also have synaptic connections with modulatory (inhibitory) neurones from the CNS.

Function of the maculae

The function of the maculae is believed to relate mainly to the maintenance of balance by providing sensory information about the static position of the head in space. This is of particular importance when the eyes are closed, or in the dark or under water, and the maculae are consequently more developed in animals other than humans.

When the head is moved from a position of equilibrium, the otolithic membrane tends to move with respect to the receptor cells thus bending their stereocilia. When the stereocilia are bent in the direction of the cilium, the receptor cell undergoes excitation and when the relative movement is in the opposite direction, excitation is inhibited.

The neuronal pathways of the balance and equilibrium mechanism are extremely complex and the sensory input from the maculae is integrated with that of proprioceptors, muscle spindles etc. to elicit reflex responses directed towards the maintenance of postural equilibrium.

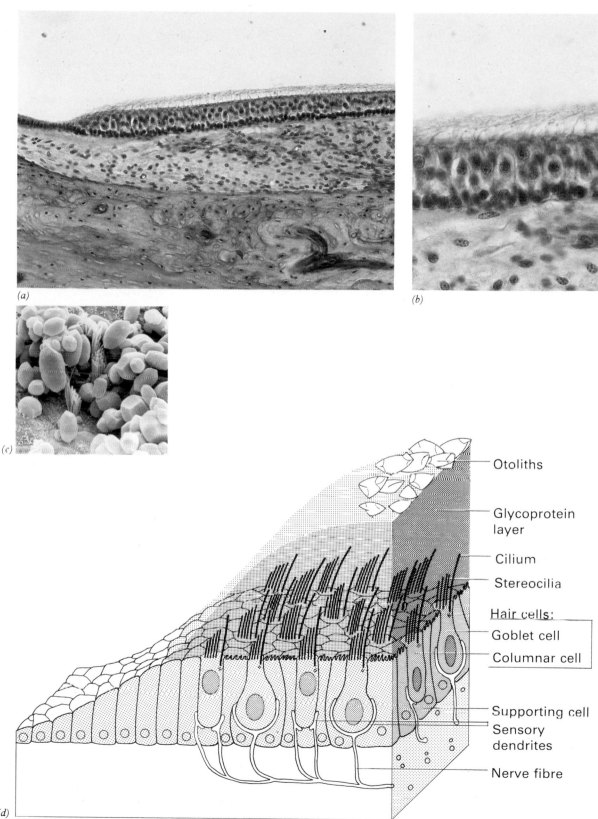

(a)

(b)

(c)

(d)

Otoliths

Glycoprotein layer

Cilium

Stereocilia

Hair cells:

Goblet cell

Columnar cell

Supporting cell

Sensory dendrites

Nerve fibre

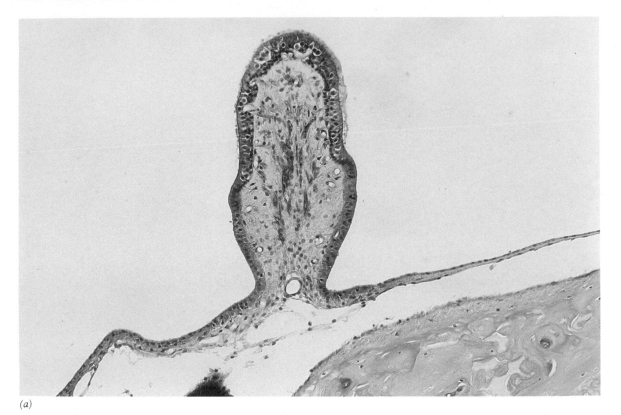

(a)

Fig. 21.28 Receptor organs of the semi-circular canals

(a) Masson's trichrome × 200 (b) Schematic diagram (opposite)

Three semicircular canals arise from the vestibule of the inner ear each containing a membranous semicircular duct which opens at both ends into the utricle. At one end of each duct is a dilated portion, the ampulla, which contains a receptor organ called the crista.ampullaris.

Each crista ampullaris is an elongated epithelial structure situated on a ridge of connective tissue arising from the membranous wall of the ampulla and oriented at right angles to the direction of flow of the endolymph in the semicircular canal. Structurally, the cristae ampullares bear many similarities to the maculae of the utricle and saccule (see Fig. 21.27). The receptor cells are of two morphological forms, one globular and the other more slender, the former being invested by a basket of sensory dendrites, and the latter having small dendritic endings at its base only. The receptor cells are supported by a single layer of columnar cells which is continuous with the simple cuboidal epithelium lining the rest of the membranous labyrinth.

Like those of the maculae, the receptor cells of the cristae each have numerous stereocilia and a single cilium, the cilium being situated at the margin of the cell nearest to the utricle. The stereocilia and cilia of the sensory receptors are embedded in a ridge of gelatinous glycoprotein which is tall and cone-shaped in cross section giving rise to the term

cupula. In contrast to the macula, the cupula does not contain otolithic crystals.

Function of the crista ampullaris

When the head is moved in the plane of a particular semicircular canal, the inertia of the endolymph acts so as to deflect the cupula in the opposite direction. The stereocilia of the sensory cells are then deflected towards or away from the cilia resulting in excitation or inhibition respectively.

In each ear there are three semicircular canals, two in vertical planes and one in a near-horizontal plane. Each is paired with a semicircular canal in the other ear, the members of each pair being oriented in parallel. The sensory input from the cristae ampullares mainly concerns changes in the direction and rate of movement of the head. Afferent impulses pass via bipolar sensory neurones with cell bodies in the vestibular ganglion which lies at the base of the internal auditory meatus. Afferent fibres pass via the vestibular part of the eighth cranial nerve to the brain stem, cerebellum and cerebral cortex where sensory information from various other sources is integrated for the maintenance of balance, position sense and equilibrium.

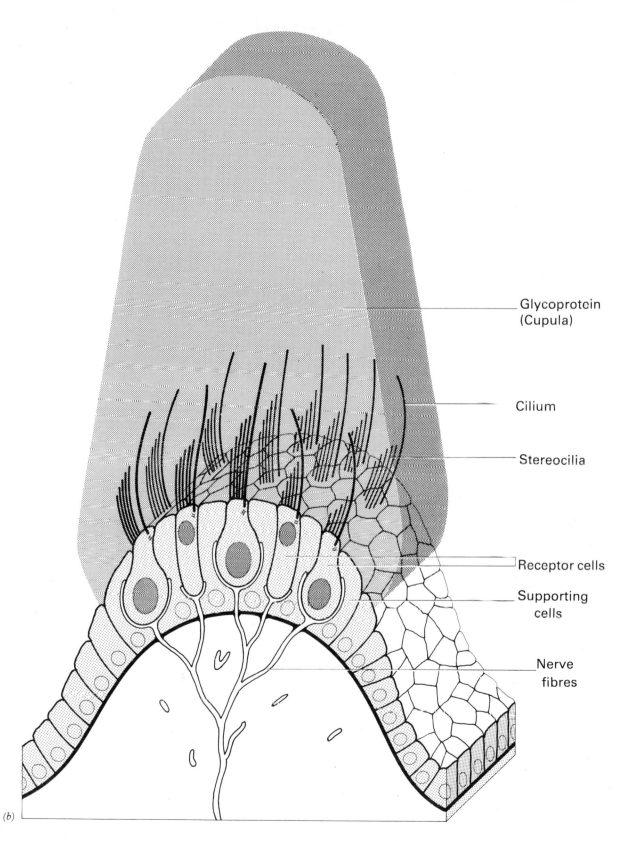

Glycoprotein
(Cupula)

Cilium

Stereocilia

Receptor cells

Supporting
cells

Nerve
fibres

(b)

Notes on staining techniques

1. Haematoxylin and eosin (H & E)

This is the most commonly used technique in animal histology and routine pathology. The basic dye haematoxylin stains acidic structures a purplish blue. Nuclei and rough endoplasmic reticulum, for example, both have a strong affinity for this dye owing to their high content of DNA and RNA respectively. In contrast, eosin is an acidic dye which stains basic structures red or pink. Most cytoplasmic proteins are basic and hence cytoplasm generally stains pink or pinkish red. In general, when the H & E staining technique is applied to animal cells, nuclei stain blue and cytoplasm stains pink or red.

2. Periodic acid-Schiff reaction (PAS)

Staining techniques which specifically stain components of cells and tissues are called histochemical staining techniques. Such techniques are invaluable for the understanding of cell and tissue structure and function, and for making a diagnosis on diseased tissues. The PAS reaction stains glycogen a deep red colour, traditionally described as magenta. The mucin produced by goblet cells of the gastro-intestinal and respiratory tracts stains magenta with this technique (and is therefore termed PAS positive). Basement membranes and the brush borders of kidney tubules and the small and large intestines are also PAS positive, as is cartilage and to some extent collagen.

3. Masson's trichrome

This technique is a so-called connective tissue technique since it is used to demonstrate connective tissue elements, principally collagen. As its name implies, the staining technique produces three colours; nuclei and other basophilic structures are stained blue, collagen is stained green or blue depending on which variant of the technique is used, and cytoplasm, muscle, erythrocytes and keratin are stained bright red.

4. Alcian blue

Alcian blue is a mucin stain which may be used in conjunction with other staining methods such as H & E or van Gieson (see below). Certain types of mucin, but not all, are stained blue by the Alcian blue method, as is cartilage. When the technique is combined with van Gieson, the Alcian blue colour becomes green.

5. Van Gieson

This is another connective tissue method in which collagen is stained red, nuclei blue and red cells and cytoplasm yellow. When used in combination with an elastic stain, elastin is stained blue/black in addition to the results described above. This staining technique is particularly useful for blood vessels and skin.

6. Reticulin stain

This method demonstrates the reticulin fibres of connective tissue which are stained blue/black by this technique. Nuclei may be counterstained blue with haematoxylin or red with the dye, neutral red.

7. Azan

This technique is traditionally classed as a connective tissue method but is excellent for demonstrating fine cytological detail, especially in epithelium. Nuclei are stained bright red; collagen, basement membrane and mucin are stained blue; muscle and red blood cells are stained orange to red.

8. Giemsa

This technique is a standard method for staining blood cells and other smears of cells e.g. bone marrow. Nuclei are stained dark blue to violet, background cytoplasm pale blue and erythrocytes pale pink.

9. Toluidine blue

This is a basic stain which stains acidic components various shades of blue. It is commonly employed on very thin, resin embedded specimens. Some tissue components are able to turn the blue dye red, a phenomenon known as metachromasia.

10. Silver and gold methods

These methods were extremely popular at the end of the nineteenth century and are occasionally used today to demonstrate such fine structures as cell processes, e.g. in neurones, motor end-plates and intercellular junctions. Depending on the method used, the end product is either black, brown or golden.

11. Chrome alum/haematoxylin

This method is rarely used and is similar to the H & E method in principle, in that nuclei are stained blue and cytoplasm is stained red. Empirically this method demonstrates the alpha cells of the pancreas as pink cells and the beta cells as blue.

12. Isamine blue/eosin

This method is also similar to the H & E method but the blue component is rather more intense.

13. Nissl and methylene blue methods

These techniques use a basic dye to stain the rough endoplasmic reticulum found in neurones: when this is seen as clumps it is called Nissl substance.

14. Sudan black and osmium

These dyes stain lipid-containing structures, such as myelin, a brownish-black colour.

Index

Acetyl choline, 103, 104
Acetylcholinesterase, 104, 105
Acidophilia, 23
Acid phosphatase, 8
Acinus, 76
Acrosomal head cap, 282
Acrosomal vesicle, 281, 282
Actin, 20, 85
Adipocytes, 52, 58
  brown, 58–60
  white, 58, 59
Adrenal gland, 267–271
Adrenaline, 267, 271
Adrenocorticotrophic hormone,
  258–260, 269
Adventitia
  of gastro-intestinal tract, 204
  of respiratory tract, 179
  of urinary bladder, 256, 257
  tunica adventitia—see Tunica
    adventitia
Agranulocyte, 38
Aldosterone, 239, 250, 255, 269
Alkaline phosphatase, 39, 220
Alpha
  particles, 19
  granules, 46
  cells, 272, 273
Alveolar ducts
  of breast, 305, 306
  of lung, 178, 186
Alveolar sacs, 178, 186
Alveoli
  of breast, 305–307
  of lungs, 178, 187–190
Alveolus of tooth, 192
  alveolar ridge, 192
Amacrine cells, 321, 323
Ameloblast, 195
Anaphase, 30, 31
Angiotensin, 255
Anulus fibrosus, 160
Antibodies, 161, 163
Antidiuretic hormone, 239, 250, 252,
  258, 259, 262
Antigen, 161, 163
Anal canal, 224
Apocrine secretion, 75
Appendix, 203, 224
APUD cells, 275, 276
Aqueous humor, 318, 325
Arachnoid mater, 112, 113
Arachnoid villi, 112
Areola, of breast, 305
Argentaffin cells, 274
Argyrophil cells, 274
Arrector pili, 134, 135, 138
Arteries
  arterial system, 118, 121, 122
  arterio-venous shunts, 123
  coronary, 118, 119

elastic, 121
  muscular, 122
  pulmonary, 179, 185
Arterioles, 121, 122
Astrocytes, 110, 111
ATP-ase, 87, 229
Atretic follicles, of ovary, 290, 295
Auerbach's (myenteric) plexus, 204,
  206
Autophagy, 7
Autoregulation, 123
Axon, 96
Axoneme, 72
  of cilia, 72
  of flagella, 283

Band form of granulocyte—see Stab
  cell
Barr body, 10, 39
Basal body, 20, 34, 72
Basal lamina, 71
Basement membrane, 64, 71
  collagen type in, 53
Basophil, 38, 42
Basophilia, 23, 24
Bellini, ducts of, 238–240, 252, 256
Beta
  cells, 272
  particles, 19
Betz cells, 315
Bile, 217, 225, 232
  biliary system, 225–227, 229–231
  canaliculi, 226, 229–231
  duct, 226, 227, 232
Bilroth, cords of, 176, 177
Bladder
  gall,—see Gall bladder
  urinary, 236, 257
Blood, 36–51
  blood-brain barrier, 113
  blood vascular system, 118–128
Bombesin, 274
Bone, 142, 144–157
  bone marrow, 47, 151, 152
  bony end plate, 159
  cartilage bones, 152
  development, 152–157
  histological preparation of, 145
  lamellar bone, 145
    compact, 145, 148
    cortical, 146, 148
    cancellous, 145, 151
  membrane bones, 152
  repair, 157
  woven bone, 145
Bowman's capsule, 238, 239, 241–247
Bowman's glands, 317
Bowman's membrane, 328
Bowman's space, 238, 239, 241–247
Breast, 289, 304–307
Bronchus, 178–180, 184

Bronchiole, 178–180, 185
  respiratory, 186
  terminal, 186
Brown
  adipocyte—see Adipocyte, brown
  adipose tissue—see Tissue, adipose,
    brown
Bruch's membrane, 320, 322
Brunner's glands, 214
Brush border, 66, 73
  of intestinal lining cells, 219–221
  of proximal convoluted tubule, 248,
    249
Bulbo-urethral glands—see Cowper,
  bulbo-urethral glands of

Caecum, 203, 222
Cajal, horizontal cells of, 315
Calcitonin, 264–266
Calcium hydroxyapatite
  in bone, 144, 150
  in dentine, 193
  in enamel, 195
Calcium homeostasis, 147, 150, 263,
  266
Callus, 157
Calyx, renal, 237, 256
Canaliculi
  of biliary system,—see Bile,
    canaliculi
  of bone, 146, 147
Capacitation, of spermatozoa, 288
Capillaries, 118, 123–126
Cardia, of stomach, 208
Cartilage, 142–144
  articular, 158, 159
  cartilaginous joints, 158
  elastic, 142, 144
  fibro-cartilage, 142, 144, 160
  growth, 142
  hyaline, 142, 143
Caveoli, 90
Cell, 2–34
  cell cycle, 28
  cell membrane—see Plasma
    membrane
  replication, 28–34
Cementocytes, 197
Cementum, 192, 193, 197
Centrioles, 20, 34
Centromere, 29
Centrosome, 20, 34
Cerebellum, 312
Cerebral cortex, 314, 315
Cerebro-spinal fluid (CSF), 110, 112
Cerumen, 330, 332
Ceruminous glands, 332
Cervix, uterine, 289, 303
Chiasma formation, 32, 33
Cholecystokinin-pancreozymin (CCK),
  214, 232, 233, 274

Chondroblast, 142, 143
Chondrocyte, 142–144
Choroid, of eye, 318–320
Choroid plexus, 112
Chromaffin cells, 271
Chromatid, 29, 30, 32
Chromatin, 10
Chromophil cells, 260
Chromophobe cells, 260
Chromosomes, 29–33
Chylomicrons, 217, 220, 221
Chymotrypsin, 214, 233
Cilia, 67, 71, 72, 183
Ciliary body, 318–320, 325
   ciliary processes, 325
Circulatory system, 118–129
Clara cells, 186, 188
Clear (C) cells—see Parafollicular cells
Cochlear, 330–332, 334–337
Collagen, 52–56
Collecting duct, of kidney, 238, 239,
   250, 252
Collecting tubule, of kidney, 238, 239,
   250, 252, 253
Colon, 203, 204, 222, 223
Colostrum, 306
Complement, 163
Cone cells, of retina, 318, 321–324
Conjunctiva, 328
Constrictor pupillae, 326
Cornea, 318, 320, 328
   corneo-scleral layer, of eye, 318
Corona radiata, 293
Corpora amylacea, 287
Corpus albicans, 290, 294, 295
Corpus cavernosum, 287
Corpus luteum, 290, 294
   of pregnancy, 295
Corpus spongiosum—see Corpus
   cavernosum
Corti, organ of, 330, 334–337
Cortisol, 269
Cowper, bulbo-urethral glands of, 277,
   288
Crista ampullaris, 330, 340, 341
Crista, mitochondrial, 17–19
Cumulus oophorus, 293
Cupula, 340
Cystic duct, 232
Cytokinesis, 29–31
Cytoplasm, 2
Cytoskeleton, 2, 20, 21
Cytosol, 2

Delta cells, 272
Demilune, secretory, 77, 201
Dendrites, 96
Dental pulp—see Pulp, of tooth
Dentine, 192–196
Dermis, 130
Descemet's membrane, 328
Desmosome, 74
Diapedesis, 124
Diaphysis, 145, 155
Diarthrosis, 158
Differentiation, cellular, 28
Dilator pupillae, 326
Diploid number of chromosomes, 29,
   32, 33

Diplosome, 34
Disse, space of, 230–231
Distal convoluted tubule, 238, 239,
   250, 251
   and juxtaglomerular apparatus, 255,
   256
Division, cellular—see Mitosis
Drumstick chromosome, 39
Ductuli efferentes, 277, 284
Ductus deferens, 277, 285
Duodenum, 203, 204, 214
Dura mater, 112, 113
Dynein, 72

Ear, 329–341
Ejaculatory duct, 277, 286
Elastin, 53, 57
   in elastic arteries, 121
   in lungs, 190
   internal elastic lamina, 122
   external elastic lamina, 122
Electron microscopy, transmission, 2
   scanning—see Scanning electron
   microscopy
Enamel, 192–195
   organ, 195
Endocardium, 118, 119
Endocrine glands, 78, 258–276
Endocytosis, 6, 7
Endometrium, 298–302
Endomysium, 80
Endoneurium, 106, 107
Endoplasmic reticulum, 2
   rough, 12
   smooth, 13
Endosteum, 145
Endothelium, 64, 118, 123–126
Energy production and storage 17–19
Enterochromaffin cells, 274
Enterocytes, 218–221
Enteroglucagon, 274
Enterokinase, 214, 233
Eosinophil, 38, 40, 41
   appearance in section, 62
Eosinophilia, 23
Ependymal cells, 110, 111
Epicardium, 118, 119
Epidermis, 130–132
   epidermal appendages, 130, 134
Epididymis, 277, 278, 285
Epimysium, 80
Epinephrine—see Adrenaline
Epineurium, 106
Epiphysis, 145, 155
   epiphyseal plate, 155–157
Epithelium, 64
   epithelial tissues, 64–78
Erythroblasts, 48–50
Erythrocytes, 36, 37
   appearance in section, 62
Erythropoiesis, 48–50
Erythropoietin, 47, 49, 236
Euchromatin, 10
Eustachian tube, 178, 333
Exfoliative cytology, 303
Exocytosis, 6, 16
Exteroceptors, 114
Extracellular material, 52, 53

Eye, 318–329
Eyelid, 329

Fabricius, bursa of, 163
Fallopian tube—see Oviduct
Female reproductive system, 289–307
Fenestrated capillaries—see Capillaries
Fibroblast, 52, 54, 55
Fibrocyte, 54
Fibronectin, 53
Fixation, for histology, 22, 23
Flagellum, 282, 283
Fluorescence microscopy, 24, 104
Follicle stimulating hormone, 258–260,
   292, 296, 302
Follicular cells, of ovary, 292
Formalin induced fluorescence—see
   Fluorescence microscopy
Fovea, of eye, 318, 319, 324
Freeze-etching, 11
Frozen section, 23, 213
Fuzzy coat, 5

Gall bladder, 232
Gamete, 32
Gametogenesis, 32
   in females, 257, 261
   in males, 279
Ganglion, 96
   parasympathetic, 109
   spinal, 109
   sympathetic, 109
Gap junction, 74
Gastric inhibitory polypeptide (GIP),
   274
Gastric mucosa, 184, 185
Gastrin, 208, 211, 213, 233, 274, 276
Gastrin (G) cells, 213
Gastro-intestinal endocrine system,
   203, 211, 213, 274–276
Gastro-intestinal tract, 203–224
   general structure, 204
Germinal centres
   of lymph nodes, 166–169
   of spleen, 175
Germinal epithelium, of ovary, 292
Gingiva, 192, 197
Glands, 64
   exocrine, 64, 75–77
   endocrine, 64, 78
Glisson's capsule, 229
Glial cells—see Neuroglia
Glomerulus, 238–247
Glomus body, 141
Glucagon, 272, 273
Glucocorticoids, 267–269
Glycocalyx, 5
Glycogen, 18, 19, 26, 228
   rosettes, 18, 19
Glycoproteins, structural, 53
Glycosaminoglycan, 52
Goblet cell, 70
Golgi apparatus (body, complex), 2,
   14, 15, 24
Gonadotrophic hormones, 258–260
Graafian follicle, 293
Granulocyte, 38
   formation (granulopoiesis), 48–50

Grey matter, 110, 308
Ground section, 145
Ground substance, 52
Growth hormone, 258–260
Growth plate—*see* Epiphysis,
    epiphyseal plate
Gustatory cells, 316
Gut-associated lymphoid tissue
    (GALT), 172, 173

Haematoxylin and Eosin (H&E)—*see*
    Staining methods
Haemoglobin, 36, 38
Haemopoiesis, 36, 47–50
Hairs, 134–137
Haploid number of chromosomes, 32,
    33
Hassal's corpuscles, 164, 165
Haversian canal, 146–148
Haversian systems, 146–148
Heart
    conducting system, 120
    muscle—*see* Muscle, cardiac
    structure of wall, 118, 119
Hemi-desmosome, 74, 132
Henle, loop of, 238–240, 250, 253
Helicine arteries, 288, 290
Heparin, 42, 61
Hepatocytes, 225–231
Hertwig's sheath, 195
Heterochromatin, 10
Histaminase, 41
Histamine, 42, 61
Histiocytes, 44, 60
Histological techniques, 22, 23
    for bone, 145
    for the nervous system, 308
    histochemistry, 2, 22
    histochemical method for electron
        microscopy, 8
    histochemical methods for light
        microscopy, 25, 39, 87, 104, 220,
        228, 229, 276
    staining methods—*see* Staining
        methods
Histones, 10
Holocrine secretion, 75
Howell-Jolly bodies, 50
Howship's lacunae, 150
Human chorionic gonadotrophin, 294
Human placental lactogen, 306
Hyaloid canal, 318
Hyaluronic acid, 52
Hyaluronidase, 52, 283
Hypodermis, 130
Hypophysis—*see* Pituitary gland

Ileum, 203
    ileo-caecal junction, 222
Immune system, 161–177
Immunohistochemistry, 2
    examples of, 25, 273
Inflammation, 161
Insulin, 272
Intercalated disc, 91–94
Intercalated ducts, 201
Interferon, 161
Interoceptors, 114
Interphase, 28

Interstitial cells of the testis—*see*
    Leydig cells
Interstitial cell stimulating hormone
    (ICSH), 284
Interstitial systems of bone, 146, 148
Intervertebral disc, 158, 160
Intrinsic factor, 212
Iris, 318–320, 326

Jejunum—*see* Small intestine
Joints, 158–160
    intervertebral, 160
    synovial, 158, 159
Junctional complex, 74
Juxtaglomerular apparatus, 254, 255

Keratin, 69, 131
    keratinisation, 69, 132
Keratohyaline granules, 132
Kerckring, valves of—*see* Plica
    circulares
Kidney, 236–256
Killer cells, 163
Kinetochore, 30, 34
Kupffer cells, 228

Lacis cells, 254, 255
Lacrimal gland, 328
Lactation, 306, 307
Lacteal, 217, 219, 220
Lactiferous duct, 305
Lactiferous sinus, 305
Lamina propria
    definition, 178
Laminin, 53
Langerhans cell, 132
Langerhans, islet of, 233, 272, 273
Large intestine, 203, 204, 222, 223
Larynx, 178, 179
Lens, 318–320, 327
Leptomeninges, 112
Leucocytes, 36, 38
    defence function, 60
    in connective tissue, 62
    mononuclear—*see* Agranulocytes
Leydig cells, 279, 284
Lieberkuhn, crypts of, 217, 218
Ligaments, 142, 159
    periodontal—*see* Periodontal
        membrane
Light microscopy, 2, 22
Lip, 191, 192
Lipase, 220
Lipid, 19, 26
    biosynthesis, 13
    droplets, 19
    in brown adipocytes, 26, 59
    in white adipocytes, 58, 60
Lipofuscin granules, 7, 27, 109
Liver, 225–231
Luteinising hormone, 258–260, 294,
    298, 302
Lymph nodes, 161, 166–171
    lymphatic vessels, 129
    lymphoid follicles, 166–169
Lymphoblast, 48, 49, 163, 170
Lymphocyte, 38, 43
    appearance in section, 62
    in immune system, 161–175

Lymphokines, 63, 163
Lymphopoiesis, 48, 49
Lysosomes, 6, 7, 8
    histochemical markers for, 8, 39
Lysozyme, 39, 328

Macrophages, 38, 62, 63
    tissue fixed macrophages, 44, 60
    dendritic, 168
    alveolar, 187
    macrophage-monocyte system, 44,
        62
    of liver, 228
    of CNS, 110
    in immune mechanisms, 161, 163
Macula densa, 254, 255
Macula lutea, 318, 324
Maculae, of saccule and utricle, 330,
    338, 339
Malassez, epithelial rests of, 197
Male reproductive system, 277–288
Malpighian layer of epidermis—*see*
    Stratum, skin, germinativum
Mammary glands—*see* Breast
Martinotti, cells of, 315
Mast cells, 60, 61
Medulla, of brain stem, 310
Megakaryoblast, 48, 49
Megakaryocyte, 45–49
Meibomian glands, 329
Meiosis, 31, 32
Meissner's corpuscle, 115
Meissner's plexus, 204, 206
Melanin, 27, 133
    synthesis, 133
Melanocytes
    of choroid, 320
    of hair, 137
    of iris, 326
    of skin, 133
Melanocyte stimulating hormone, 133,
    258–260, 262
Melatonin, 273, 274
Membrane
    plasma—*see* Plasma membrane
    structure, 5
    transport mechanisms, 5, 6
Meninges, 110, 112, 113
    of spinal cord, 309
Menstrual cycle, 289, 298
    integration with ovarian cycle, 302
Menstruation, 289, 298, 301, 302
Merkel cells, 114, 132
Merocrine secretion, 75
Mesangium, 241
    mesangial cells, 242, 243, 247
    mesangial substance, 243, 247
Mesaxon, 100, 101
Mesenchyme, 52, 54
Mesothelium, 64
Metachromasia, 61
Metamyelocyte, 48–50
Metaphase, 30, 31
    metaphase plate, 30
Metaphysis, 156, 157
Metarterioles, 123
Microbodies—*see* Peroxisomes
Microcirculation, 123
Microfilaments, 20, 21

Microglia, 110, 111
Microphages, 38
Microtubules, 20–22, 27
Microvilli, 66, 71, 73
Mineralocorticoids, 267–269
Mitochondrion, 2, 17, 25
Mitosis, 28–31, 33, 34
Modiolus, 335
Moll, glands of, 329
Monoblast, 48, 49
Monocyte, 38, 44
    formation (monopoiesis), 48, 49
Monophyletic theory, 47
Morgagni, columns of, 222
Motilin, 274
Motor end plate, 103–105
Motor unit, 79, 104
Movement, cellular, 19, 20
Mucoprotein—see Proteoglycan
Mucous membrane (mucosa)
    definition, 178
    of gastro-intestinal tract, 204, 205
    of upper respiratory tract, 181
    oral, 191, 192
Mucigen, 70
Mucopolysaccharide—see
    Glycosaminoglycan
Mucus, 70
Muller cells, 321
Multivesicular body, 8
Muscle, 79–94
    cardiac, 79, 91–94
    skeletal (striated, voluntary), 79–87
        fibre types, 87
        bony insertion, 149
        tendinous insertion, 159
    visceral (smooth, involuntary), 79,
        88–90
Muscularis mucosae, 204, 206
Muscularis, of gastrointestinal tract,
    204, 206
Myelin, 99
    in peripheral nerves, 107
    sheath, 99, 101, 102
Myeloblast, 48–50
Myelocyte, 48–50
Myeloid tissue—see Bone, marrow
Myeloperoxidase, 39
Myenteric plexus—see Auerbach's
    plexus
Myoblast, 82
Myotube, 82
Myocardium, 118, 119
    cardiac muscle—see Muscle, cardiac
Myoepithelial cells, 75, 202
Myofibrils, 83, 84
Myofilaments, 84, 85
Myoglobin, 87
Myometrium, 298, 301
Myosin, 20, 85

Nails, 140
Nephron, 236, 238, 239
Nervous tissues, 95–116
    central nervous system, 308–315
        cellular constituents of, 110–113
    peripheral nerves, 106–109
Neuroendocrine system, 275
Neuroglia, 110, 111

Neuromuscular junction, 103–105
Neuromuscular spindle, 116
Neurones, 95–99
Neurosecretion, 259–262
Neurotransmitter, 95, 103
Neurovascular bundle, 108, 128
Neutrophils, 38–40
    appearance in section, 62
Nexus—see Gap junction
Nipple, 305
Nissl substance, 97–99
Noradrenaline (norepinephrine), 103,
    104, 267, 270
Normoblast, 48–50
Nose, 178, 181
Nuclear envelope, 2, 10, 11
Nuclear pores, 11
Nucleoli, 10
Nucleoplasm, 2
Nucleoprotein, 20
Nucleus, 2, 9–11, 23, 24
Nucleus pulposus, 160

Odontoblasts, 195, 196
Oesophagus, 203, 204, 207, 208
Oestrogen, 289, 292–294, 298, 302
Oestrus cycle, 289
Olfactory receptors, 317
Oligodendrocytes, 99, 110, 111
Oocyte, 292, 293
Oogenesis, 32, 289–293
Oogonia, 32, 292
Opsonins, 63, 163
Optic nerve, 318–320, 323, 324
Optic papilla (disc), 318, 319, 324
Oral tissues, 191–202
Ora serrata, 318
Organelles, 2
Ossicles of ear, 330–333
Ossification
    endochondral, 152, 154–157
    intramembranous, 152, 153
Osteoblasts, 145, 149, 150, 157
Osteoclasts, 145, 150, 157
Osteocytes, 145–148
Osteoid, 145, 150
Osteoprogenitor cells, 145
Otoliths, 338, 339
Ovary, 289–291
Oviduct, 289, 297
Ovum, 289–293
Oxyntic cells, of stomach—see Parietal
    cells, of stomach
Oxyphil cells, 267
Oxytocin, 258, 259, 262, 306

Pacinian corpuscles, 115, 130
Palate, 192
Pancreas, 233–235
    endocrine component of, 272, 273
Pancreatic polypeptide, 274
Paneth cells, 218
Papillae, of tongue, 198
Paracortex, of lymph node, 169, 170
Parafollicular cells, 264, 265
Paraluteal cells—see Theca luteal cells
Paraneurone, 275
Parathyroid gland, 266, 267
Parathyroid hormone, 266, 267

Paraurethral glands
    of prostate, 286
    of urethra, 287
Parietal cells, of stomach, 209, 210,
    212
Pelvis, renal, 237, 256
Penis, 277, 287, 288
Pepsin, 209, 211
Pepsinogen, 211
Peptic cells, 209, 211
Perfusion methods, 81, 189, 220, 227,
    243, 273
Peri-arteriolar lymphoid sheaths, of
    spleen, 174, 175
Pericardium, 118, 119
Perichondrium, 142, 143
Pericytes, 124
Perikaryon, 96
Perimysium, 80
Perineurium, 106, 107
Periodontal membrane (ligament), 192,
    197
Periodontium, 192
Periosteum, 145, 148–150
Peristalsis, 80, 203, 206
Peroxisomes, 9
Peyer's patch, 172, 173, 216, 217
Phagocytins, 39
Phagocytosis, 6, 7
Phagosome—see Endocytosis
Physaliphorous cells, 160
Pia mater, 112, 113
    pia-arachnoid, 112
Pigmentation—see Skin, pigmentation
Pineal gland, 273, 274
Pinealocytes, 274
Pinocytosis, 6
Pituicytes, 262
Pituitary gland, 258–262
Plasma, 36
    proteins, 36
Plasmablast, 163, 169,
Plasma cell, 62, 163, 169, 171
Plasmalemma—see Plasma membrane
Plasma membrane, 2
    specialisations, 71–74
Platelets, 36, 45, 46, 48, 49
Pleura, 190
Plica circulares, 217
Pneumocytes, 187
    Type I, 187–189
    Type II (surfactant cells), 187–189
Podocytes, 239, 241–247
Poietins, 47
Polar bodies, 32
Polymorphonuclear leucocytes
    (polymorphs), 38
Polyribosomes (polysomes), 9
Pons, 311
Portal lobule, 226
Portal tract, 225–227
Portal triad, 227
Precapillary sphincter, 123
Proerythroblasts, 48–50
Progesterone, 294, 295, 298, 302
Prolactin, 258–260, 306
Prolymphocytes, 48, 49
Promyelocytes, 48, 49
Prophase, 30, 31

Proplasmacyte, 169
Proprioceptors, 114
Prostate gland, 277, 286, 287
Protein synthesis, 9
Proteoglycan, 52
Proximal convoluted tubule, 239, 248, 249
Pulp, of tooth, 192, 196
   pulp cavity, 192, 193
Pupil, of the eye, 318, 326
Purkinje
   cells of the cerebellum, 312
   fibres of the heart, 91, 120
Pus, 40
Pylorus (pyloric antrum), 203, 213
   pyloric sphincter, 214

Ranvier, node of, 102
Rathke's pouch, 259, 262
Receptors—see Sensory receptors
Rectum, 203, 204, 224
   recto-anal junction, 224
Red
   blood cells—see Erythrocytes
   blood cell formation—see
     Erythropoiesis
   marrow—see Bone, marrow
   pulp of spleen, 174, 176
Reinke, crystals of, 284
Reissner's membrane, 335
Releasing hormones, 259
Renal corpuscle, 238-242
Renal papilla, 237, 240, 256
Renal tubule, 238, 239
Renin, 255
   renin-angiotensin-aldosterone
     mechanism, 236, 255
Residual body, 7
Respiration, cellular, 17
Respiratory system, 178-190
   respiratory epithelium, 67, 181-183
Rete testis, 278, 284
Reticulin, 53, 57
Reticulocytes, 38
Reticulo-endothelial system, 60, 61
Reticulum cells, 61
Retina, 318-324
Rhodopsin, 322
Ribosomes, 9
   and rough endoplasmic reticulum, 12
   mitochondrial, 17
Rod cells, of retina, 318, 321-324

Saccule, 330-332, 338, 339
Salivary glands, 200-202
Sarcolemma, 79
Sarcomere, 84, 85
Sarcoplasm, 79
Sarcoplasmic reticulum, 79, 86
Sarcosomes, 79
Satellite cells, 109
Scanning electron microscopy
   of erythrocytes, 37
   of glomerulus, 244, 245
   of intestinal villi, 217
   of otoliths, 338
   of respiratory epithelium, 183

Schlemm, canal of, 318, 319, 325, 326
Schwann cells, 99
   and myelinated axons, 101, 102
   and non-myelinated axons, 100
   in peripheral nerves, 106-108
Sclera, 318-320
Sebaceous glands, 134, 138
Sebum, 134
Secretin, 214, 233, 274
Secretion, 14, 16
   apocrine, 75, 140
   holocrine, 75, 138
   merocrine (eccrine), 75, 139
   secretory granules, 14, 24
   secretory vacuoles, 2
   secretory vesicles, 14, 16
Sectioning, principles of, 23
Semen, 277, 288
Semicircular canals, 330-332, 340, 341
Seminal fluid, 277, 286
Seminal vesicle, 277, 286
Seminiferous tubule, 278-280
Sensory receptors, 114-116
   special sense organs, 318-341
Serosa
   definition, 204
Serotonin, 45, 274
Sertoli cell, 279, 281
Sharpey's fibres
   of bone, 148, 149
   of periodontal membrane, 197
Sinusoids, 123, 126
   lining cells of liver, 228, 230, 231
   of liver, 227, 230, 231
Skeletal tissues, 142-160
Skin, 130-141
Slit pores, 244-247
Slow reacting substance of anaphylaxis
   (SRS-A), 42
Small intestine, 203, 204, 216-222
   digestive processes, 217
Somatostatin, 272, 274, 276
Spermatid, 280-282
Spermatocyte, 280, 181
Spermatogenesis, 32, 279-281
Spermatogonia, 32, 279-282
Spermatozoa, 277-283, 288
Spermiogenesis, 279-282
Spinal cord, 309
Spleen, 161, 173-177
Stab cell, 48-50
Staining methods, 23-27, 342
   histochemical—see Histochemistry
   histological preparation methods—
     see Histological methods
   immunological—see
     Immunohistochemistry
   particular methods,
     Alcian blue, 130, 144, 155-158,
      181, 182, 184, 185, 223
     Aldehyde fucsin, 213
     Azan, 23, 56, 66, 67, 241, 242,
      248, 250, 252, 254, 256, 260, 268,
      269, 290, 292, 293, 297
     Bielchowsky, 312
     Cajal, 110
     Chrome salt fixation, 271
     Cresyl blue, 38
     Cresyl violet, 24

Elastin methods, 57, 120-122,
   128, 144, 184, 186, 190
Giemsa, 24, 29, 31, 36, 39, 40,
   42-45, 47, 50
Gold impregnation, 99, 104
Goldner's trichrome, 150
Golgi-Cox, 99, 312, 315
Gomori's chrome alum
   haematoxylin/phloxine, 77, 272
Ground sections, unstained, 146,
   147, 193, 196, 197
Haematoxylin and Eosin (H&E),
   23, 26, 32 (plus numerous
   examples throughout the book)
Heidenhain's haematoxylin, 84
Iron haematoxylin, 24, 25, 83
Isamine blue, with eosin, 78, 262
Masson's trichrome, 56, 58, 77,
   80, 81, 88, 89, 108, 115, 116, 118,
   119, 127, 130, 135, 137, 148, 207,
   256, 257, 304, 324, 340
Methylene blue, 315
Methyl green/pyronin, 171
Neutral red, 170, 174, 176, 312
Nissl, 99, 315
Orange G, 210, 219
Osmium fixation, 26, 107
Papanicolou, 68, 303
Perfusion methods—see Perfusion
   methods
Periodic acid Schiff (PAS), 26, 70,
   71, 200, 210, 219, 248, 251
Perl's Prussian blue, 228
Phloxine-tartrazine, 218
Phosphotungstic acid, 149
Reticulin methods, 57, 168, 170,
   174, 176, 229
Silver impregnation methods, 27,
   65, 71, 114, 115, 240
Sudan black, 102, 220
Supravital methods—see
   Supravital staining
Toluidine blue, 61, 72, 92, 132,
   133, 143, 170, 183, 187, 219, 223,
   243
van Gieson, 106, 107, 120, 324,
   328
Weigart-Pal, 309
Steroid hormones, 267-270
Stereocilia, 71, 73, 285
Stomach, 203, 204, 208-214
Stratum, skin
   corneum, 131, 132
   germinativum (basale), 131, 132
   granulosum, 131, 132
   lucidum, 131, 132
   spinosum, 131, 132
Stratum, uterine
   basilis, 298-301
   compactum, 298-301
   functionalis, 298-301
   spongiosum, 298-301
Striated border—see Brush border
Striated ducts, 201, 202
Subarachnoid space, 112, 113
Subcutaneous layer of skin—see
   Hypodermis
Subdural space, 112
Submucosa

Submucosa (cont'd.)
  definition, 178
Substance P, 274
Substantia nigra, 313
Succinate dehydrogenase, 87
Supravital staining, 38
Surfactant, 187–189
  cells—see Pneumocytes, Type II
Suspensory ligament of the eye, 318,
  319, 325
Sweat glands, 130, 134, 139
  apocrine, 140
  merocrine, 139
Symphysis, 158
Synapse, 95, 103–105
Synchondrosis, 158
Syncytium, 91
Syndesmosis, 158
Synostosis, 158
Synovium, 158, 159
  synovial fluid, 158, 159

Taeniae coli, 222
Taste bud, 199, 316
Tectorial membrane, 336, 337
Telophase, 30, 31
Tendon, 142, 159
Terminal bouton, 96, 99, 103, 104
Testis, 277–281
Testosterone, 284
Thalamus, 313
Theca, of ovarian follicle, 292–294
Theca luteal cells, 294
Thermoregulation
  by brown adipose tissue, 58–60
  by skin, 130, 134, 139, 141
Thrombocytes—see Platelets
Thrombosthenin, 46
Thymosine, 164
Thymus, 161–165
Thyroglobulin, 264, 265
Thyroid gland, 263–265
Thyroid hormone, 263–265
Thyroid stimulating hormone, 258–260

Tissue
  adipose, 52, 58–60
    brown, 58–60
    white, 58–59
  areolar, 56
  connective, 52–63
  elastic, 57
  epithelial—see Epithelium
  mucous, 54
  reticular, 57
Tongue, 198, 199
Tonofibrils, 20, 132
Tonsil,
  lingual, 199
  palatine, 172
Tooth, 192–197
  development, 194, 195
Trachea, 178, 179, 182, 183
Tropocollagen, 53, 54
Tropoelastin, 53, 57
Trypsin, 214, 233
Tubulin, 20
Tunica albuginea
  of ovary, 290
  of testis, 278
Tunica, of blood vessels
  adventitia, 118
  intima, 118
  media, 118
Tunica vaginalis, 278
Tympanic membrane, 330–333

Ureter, 236, 237, 256
Urethra, 236, 277, 286–288
Urinary system, 236–257
  urinary epithelium, 69, 257
Uterine tube—see Oviduct
Uterus, 289, 290, 298–303
Utricle, 330–332, 338, 339
Uvea (uveal tract), 318–320

Vagina, 289, 290, 304
Valves
  in heart, 120

  in lymphatic vessels, 129
  in veins, 127
Vasa recta, 239, 240, 250, 253
Vasa vasorum, 118, 121, 128
Vas deferens—see Ductus deferens
Vasoactive intestinal peptide (VIP),
  274
Vater, ampulla of, 232
Veins, 127, 128
Vena cava, 128
Venules, 123, 126, 127
Vestibulo-cochlear apparatus—see Ear
Villi, intestinal, 216–220
Vitamin D, 130
Vitreous body, 318
Vitreous humor, 318
Vocal cords, 178
Volkmann's canals, 146, 147
Von Ebner's glands, 199, 316
Vulva, 289

Weil, cell free zone of, 196
White
  adipose tissue—see Tissue, adipose,
    white
  blood cells—see Leucocytes
  pulp of spleen, 174, 175
  matter, 110, 308

Yellow
  marrow—see Bone, marrow

Zeis, glands of, 329
Zona, of adrenal cortex
  fasciculata, 268, 269
  glomerulosa, 268, 269
  reticularis, 268, 269
Zona granulosa, 292, 293
Zona pellucida, 292
Zygote, 32
Zymogen, 234
  zymogenic cells of stomach—see
    Peptic cells